The Public Health Response to 2009 H1N1

The Public Health Response to 2009 H1N1

A Systems Perspective

Edited by

MICHAEL A. STOTO

MELISSA A. HIGDON

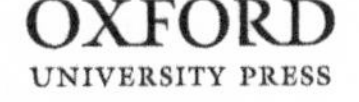

OXFORD
UNIVERSITY PRESS

Oxford University Press is a department of the University of Oxford. It furthers the University's objective of excellence in research, scholarship, and education by publishing worldwide.

Oxford New York
Auckland Cape Town Dar es Salaam Hong Kong Karachi
Kuala Lumpur Madrid Melbourne Mexico City Nairobi
New Delhi Shanghai Taipei Toronto

With offices in
Argentina Austria Brazil Chile Czech Republic France Greece
Guatemala Hungary Italy Japan Poland Portugal Singapore
South Korea Switzerland Thailand Turkey Ukraine Vietnam

Oxford is a registered trademark of Oxford University Press in the UK and certain other countries.

Published in the United States of America by
Oxford University Press
198 Madison Avenue, New York, NY 10016

Library of Congress Cataloging-in-Publication Data
The public health response to 2009 H1N1 : a systems perspective / edited by Michael A. Stoto, Melissa A. Higdon.
p. ; cm.
Includes bibliographical references.
ISBN 978-0-19-020924-7 (alk. paper)
I. Stoto, Michael A., editor. II. Higdon, Melissa A., editor.
[DNLM: 1. Influenza A Virus, H1N1 Subtype. 2. Influenza, Human—prevention & control. 3. Civil Defense—organization & administration. 4. Communicable Disease Control—organization & administration. 5. Influenza, Human—epidemiology.
6. Public Health Surveillance. WC 515]
RA644.I6
614.5'18—dc23
2014035162

9 8 7 6 5 4 3 2 1
Printed in the United States of America
on acid-free paper

CONTENTS

CONTRIBUTORS

Tomás J. Aragón, MD, DrPH
City and County of San Francisco
Population Health Division
San Francisco Department of Public Health
University of California, Berkeley School of Public Health
Berkeley, CA

Allison T. Chamberlain, MS
Emory Preparedness and Emergency Response Research Center
Department of Epidemiology
Emory University
Atlanta, GA

Edward W. Chan, PhD
Engineering and Applied Sciences Department
RAND Corporation
Santa Monica, CA

Maria Pia Fantini, MD
Department of Biomedical and Neuromotor Sciences
University of Bologna
Bologna, Italy

Andrew S. Hackbarth, MPhil
RAND Corporation
Santa Monica, CA

Sam F. Halabi, JD
University of Tulsa College of Law
O'Neill Institute for National and Global Health Law
Georgetown University
Washington, DC

Melissa A. Higdon, MPH
Harvard School of Public Health
Boston, MA

Jennifer C. Hunter, DrPH, MPH
School of Public Health
University of California
Berkeley, CA

Tamar Klaiman, PhD, MPH
University of the Sciences
Philadelphia, PA

John D. Kraemer, JD, MPH
Department of Health Systems Administration
Georgetown University
Washington, DC

Matthew W. Lewis, PhD
Behavioral and Policy Sciences Department
RAND Corporation
Santa Monica, CA

Leesa Lin, MS
Harvard School of Public Health
Boston, MA

Pierluigi Macini, MD
Society of Hygiene, Preventive Medicine and Public Health

Christopher Nelson, PhD
RAND Corporation
Santa Monica, CA

Katherine O'Connell, RN
Progressive Care Unit
Cooper University Hospital
Camden, NJ

Brit K. Oiulfstad, DVM, MPH
Acute Communicable Disease Control Program
Department of Public Health
Los Angeles County
Los Angeles, CA

Alonzo Plough, PhD, MPH
Department of Public Health
Los Angeles County
Los Angeles, CA

Daniela C. Rodriguez, DrPH
Department of International Health
Johns Hopkins University
Baltimore, MD

Elena Savoia, MD, MPH
Harvard School of Public Health
Boston, MA

Katherine Seib, MSPH
Department of Medicine, Division of Infectious Diseases
Emory University
Atlanta, GA

Michael A. Stoto, PhD
Department of Health Systems Administration
Georgetown University
Washington, DC

Christine A. Vaughan, PhD
Behavioral and Policy Sciences Department
RAND Corporation
Santa Monica, CA

Kasisomayajula Viswanath, PhD
Department of Social and Behavioral Sciences
Harvard School of Public Health
Boston, MA

Ellen A. S. Whitney, MPH
Emory Preparedness and Emergency Response Research Center
Department of Epidemiology
Emory University
Atlanta, GA

Ying Zhang, PhD
Department of Health Systems Administration
Georgetown University
Washington, DC

CHAPTER 1 | Introduction

MICHAEL A. STOTO

Introduction

The 2009 H1N1 pandemic required a concerted response effort from—and tested—the entire public health emergency preparedness (PHEP) system in the United States and other countries. The pandemic was quickly identified and characterized by laboratories in the United States and Mexico, triggering pandemic influenza plans around the globe. However, public health surveillance systems were arguably less effective in tracking the pandemic over time and identifying groups accurately at higher risk of experiencing its consequences. Some school systems moved quickly to close to protect children and limit the spread of pH1N1 (the pandemic virus) in the community, but the epidemiologic impact of this strategy might not have justified the costs. In less than a year, a new vaccine was developed and produced, and—despite production delays in and widespread concerns about its safety—more than 80 million people were eventually immunized, including 34% of the population groups targeted initially. However, approximately half of the 162 million 2009 H1N1 vaccine doses produced went unused. Globally, 78 million doses were sent to 77 countries, but most arrived long after they would have done the most good (Fineberg, 2014).

The National Health Security Strategy (NHSS) identifies quality improvement as a strategic objective and calls for the development, refinement, and widespread implementation of quality improvement tools. The draft of the first NHSS Biennial Implementation Plan (released for public comment in 2010) further calls for efforts to "collect data on performance measures from real incidents . . . analyze performance data to identify gaps, [and] recommend and apply programs to mitigate those gaps" (CDC, 2010a, 2010b). In the spirit of the NHSS's directive, this publication, *The Public Health Response to 2009 H1N1: A Systems Perspective* focuses on learning from the public health system's response to pH1N1. The objectives are (1) to learn from the United States' and the global H1N1 experience about PHEP capabilities,

(2) to identify the implications for measuring the level of preparedness in current public health systems, and (3) to illustrate a variety of rigorous research methods that can be used to learn from exceptional events such as public health emergencies.

The analysis takes a systems perspective in which "public health systems" are understood to include not only government health agencies but also healthcare providers, community organizations such as schools and the media, and many others. The Institute of Medicine has defined the public health system as the "complex network of individuals and organizations that have the potential to play critical roles in creating the conditions for health" (Institute of Medicine, 2003, p. 28). For PHEP, this system includes not only federal, state, and local health departments, but also hospitals and health care providers, fire departments, schools, the media, and many other public and private organizations (Institute of Medicine, 2008; Klaiman, 2012).

The remainder of this chapter provides an outline of the major events of the pandemic to set the stage for the analyses that follow and a discussion of the qualitative research methods used in the analysis. The body of the book is organized according to the Institute of Medicine's core public health functions: assessment, policy development, and assurance. These functions are reflected in the primary public health response capabilities in the Linking Assessment and Measurement to Performance (LAMPS) public health emergency preparedness logic model (Figure 1-1) developed by Stoto and colleagues (2012). As a point of reference, the corresponding public health preparedness capabilities prepared by the Centers for Disease Control and Prevention (CDC) Division of State and Local Readiness (Centers for Disease Control and Prevention, 2011) are noted.

Chapters 2 and 3 address assessment—specifically, outbreak detection and characterization—and surveillance, respectively, to provide situational awareness. Both are covered by the CDC biosurveillance capabilities 12 (public health laboratory testing) and 13 (public health surveillance and epidemiological investigation). These chapters are drawn from the work of Zhang, Stoto, and colleagues investigating the impact of advances in global surveillance and notification systems on the 2009 H1N1 pandemic (Stoto, 2012; Zhang, 2013), and the effectiveness of public health surveillance systems in the United States—and specifically at Georgetown University—for providing situational awareness throughout the pandemic.

The next group of chapters (Chapters 4 and 5) explores policy development and implementation during the pandemic. In Chapter 4, Klaiman and colleagues explore the excess variability in U.S. school closure decisions in response to the pandemic as a window to the interface between policies developed at the national level before the pandemic and its implementation at the state and local levels during the actual event. School closures are an example of the nonpharmaceutical interventions addressed by CDC capability 11 (Klaiman, 2011). In Chapter 5, Lewis and colleagues address the challenges

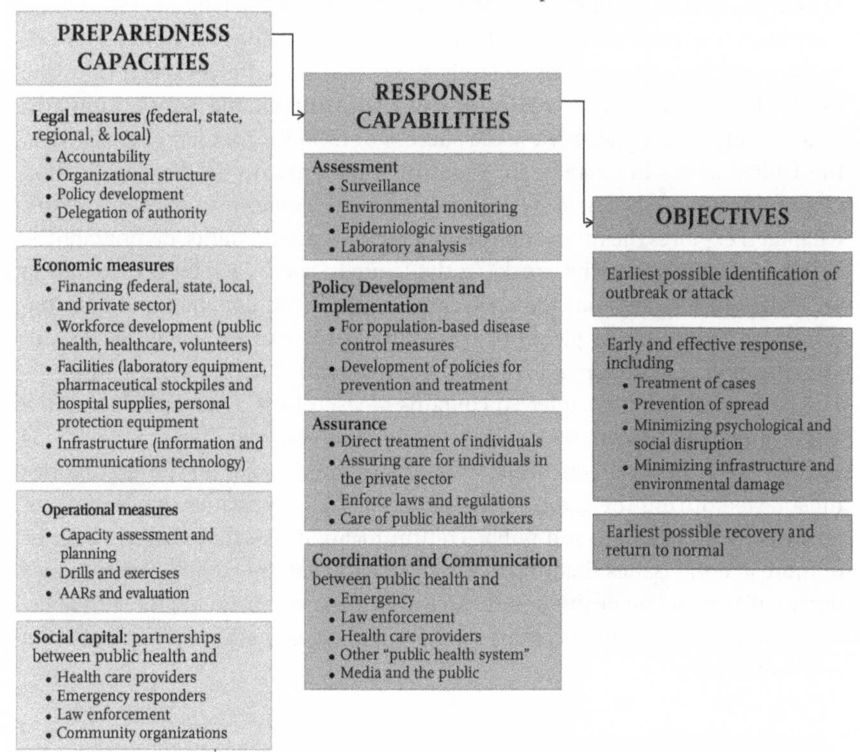

FIGURE 1-1 Public health emergency preparedness logic model (Stoto, M.A., Nelson, C.D., and the LAMPS investigators. (2012b). Measuring and assessing public health emergency preparedness: a methodological primer. Accessed on March 3, 2013 at http://lamps.sph.harvard.edu/images/stories/MeasurementWhitePaper.pdf).

of managing long-duration, moderate-acuity public health incidents based on the experience of the Los Angeles County Department of Public Health (LACDPH). Both of these chapters address CDC capabilities 3 (emergency operations coordination) and 6 (information sharing).

The third set of chapters (Chapters 6–12) focuses on the public health "assurance" function that, in the context of emergency preparedness, primarily means dispensing medical countermeasures. These functions are covered by the CDC countermeasures and mitigation capabilities, especially 8 (medical countermeasure dispensing) and 9 (medical materiel management and distribution). Set in the spring wave, before the pH1N1 vaccine was available, in Chapter 6 Hunter and colleagues explore the management of antiviral drugs by local health departments (LHDs) in California. The remaining chapters in this group explore, from a number of perspectives, what became the largest mass vaccination campaign in U.S. history. In Chapter 7, Chamberlain and colleagues use a national survey to explore the perspectives of 64 city, state, and territorial immunization program managers. Higdon and Stoto use a Massachusetts case study in Chapter 8 to explore how the national vaccination campaign was implemented at the local level. In Chapter 9, Savoia and colleagues use similar methods to study the response in Italy—specifically, the Emilia Romagna region—and compare it with the United States. Similarly, Klaiman and colleagues review the success of local vaccination campaigns in the United States in Chapter 10. Based on a national survey developed using communications theory, a systematic literature review, and focus groups, Chapter 11 explores the interaction among socioeconomic status, demographics, beliefs, and pH1N1 vaccine uptake in the United States. Chapter 12, expanding on Halabi (2014), assesses the obstacles to vaccination donation and distribution faced by the major global pharmaceutical companies, the World Health Organization, and donor and recipient governments during the pandemic.

The final chapter (Chapter 13) contains crosscutting conclusions about the implications of the analysis for PHEP policy and practice. These suppositions include some general conclusions about the three major PHEP capabilities most tested during the 2009 H1N1 pandemic: biosurveillance, medical countermeasure dispensing, and public communication. We then discuss a series of more general issues that must be addressed to ensure an effective response during future public health emergencies. We conclude this chapter with a discussion of the implications of our analyses for ongoing efforts to measure and improve PHEP.

History

In spring 2009, a novel strain of influenza virus, now denoted pH1N1, emerged in North America and spread to the rest of the world in less than two months (World Health Organization, 2009). Because of the potentially severe health consequences of a pandemic influenza, the detection of cases in California and Mexico set off a coordinated wave of activity across the public health system to minimize public health consequences. A timeline of these events is presented in Table 1-1.

The 2009 H1N1 influenza outbreak did not conform to anticipated pandemic influenza scenarios in that it originated in North America, rather than Southeast Asia. Adding to the sense of urgency, previous pandemic response planning efforts had focused primarily on a different influenza virus: subtype (A)H5N1. So, the first public health challenge was to track the spread of the new virus and characterize its epidemiologic properties to guide and monitor the effects of response efforts. Existing public health surveillance and laboratory systems rapidly developed a case definition and new testing procedures, but public health laboratories soon became overloaded with samples to be tested, and surveillance definitions and procedures were changed as necessary to handle the load.

TABLE 1-1 Summary Timeline of 2009 H1N1 Events

DATE	DESCRIPTION
February–March	First pH1N1 cases emerge in Mexico and the United States
April 21–30	CDC and Mexico issue alerts; United States declares public health emergency (April 26); CDC, state, and local HDs activate emergency operations centers; WHO declares PHEIC (April 25) and raises pandemic threat to level 4 (April 27)
May	Cases spread throughout the United States and world, vaccine production begins and CDC announces the first doses will be delivered in late September or early October
June 11	WHO raises pandemic threat to level 6; spring wave of cases diminishes
July 29	ACIP issues priority groups for pH1N1 vaccine
August	CDC and state HDs encourage local HDs to activate plans to administer vaccine in late September
Late August	Fall wave cases peak in the South
Late October	Vaccine begins to ship (23 million doses by October 30)
November	Fall wave cases peak in the Northeast; vaccine widely available and clinics held
December	Vaccine priorities relaxed; demand for vaccine declines

Advisory Committee on Immunization Practice (ACIP); Centers for Disease Control and Prevention (CDC); Health Department (HD); Public Health Emergencies of International Concern (PHEIC); World Health Organization (WHO).

On April 26, 2009, the United States declared a public health emergency in response to the threat posed by the new influenza virus. With no vaccine immediately available, this declaration led the CDC to ship large quantities of medical provisions from the Strategic National Stockpile to state health departments around the nation in an effort to mitigate and control outbreaks of the novel virus.

By June 11, 2009, the virus had spread so extensively around the world that the World Health Organization declared a global pandemic was underway (World Health Organization, 2009). This declaration reflected the fact that the virus had spread throughout multiple parts of the world, but was not indicative of the severity of the illness in those infected. Most people in the United States who became ill from 2009 H1N1 influenza recovered without hospitalization, and in many cases without medical treatment. However, the pattern of those who did become seriously ill and required hospitalization was different from seasonal influenza, which usually has the greatest impact on older adults. Data from the initial wave of influenza in the spring showed the highest rate of hospitalization was in children younger than five years, followed by young people age 5 to 24 years. Data also showed that pregnant women, along with people with underlying chronic medical conditions, were at particularly high risk for hospitalization and death (Centers for Disease Control and Prevention, 2009a, 2009b).

As concern about pandemic influenza in the United States grew in recent years, school closings were seen increasingly as a means of "social distancing," capable of slowing the spread of disease through the population (Ferguson et al., 2006). Thus, when novel influenza H1N1 emerged suddenly in 2009, it was not surprising that more than 726 K–12 schools in the United States closed, affecting 368,282 students (Cauchemez et al., 2009; Stein and Wilgorn, 2009). School closures during the pandemic's first wave occurred in several rough phases. Initially, schools were closed on a somewhat ad hoc basis. After the CDC issued preliminary guidance on April 26, schools with confirmed or suspected pH1N1 cases generally closed for at least seven days. On May 1, the CDC changed its guidance to suggest 14 days of closure, and most schools with cases closed with the intent to remain shuttered for 14 days. After CDC guidance changed again on May 5 to say that closure was, in general, not necessary, most schools did not close after a case was identified.

One of the major aspects of the public health response to the 2009 H1N1 pandemic was a national influenza vaccination campaign. Efforts to produce a vaccine for the 2009 H1N1 virus began within days of detection of the first cases in the United States. The CDC began immediately to develop a high-yield vaccine virus that would be effective against the new virus. After it was developed, it was sent to vaccine manufacturers to begin production, although at that point the U.S. government had not yet determined whether the vaccination campaign would be implemented. Throughout the summer, the National Institutes of Health conducted clinical trials on pilot lots of the vaccine, and the Food and Drug Administration developed a plan for licensing the vaccine.

The CDC Advisory Committee on Immunization Practices (ACIP) met on July 29 to develop the guidance for the mass vaccination campaign, and ultimately recommended a target group that included an estimated 159 million Americans, of which 62 million were designated to be the highest priority should vaccine supplies be inadequate. Recommendations were based on available clinical and epidemiologic data, and input from the general public. ACIP assumed that approximately 120 million doses of vaccine would be available by mid October, and that individuals would require two doses of the vaccine to be fully immunized (Schnirring, 2009). As data from clinical trials became available in the fall, the CDC ultimately recommended that a single dose would be sufficient to protect people 10 years and older. Children younger than 10 years would require two doses. ACIP recommended that vaccination efforts focus on five initial target groups:

1. Pregnant women
2. People who lived with or cared for infants younger than six months
3. Healthcare and emergency medical services personnel
4. Infants age six months and older through young adults aged 24 years
5. Adults age 25 through 64 years who were at a greater risk for complications because of chronic health disorders or compromised immune systems (Centers for Disease Control and Prevention Advisory Committee on Immunization Practices, 2009)

Although the purchase and distribution of vaccine was a federal responsibility, organizing and implementing population-wide immunization campaigns was delegated primarily to state and local health departments, which required state-level immunization programs to activate plans to expand their vaccine management and distribution capabilities (Rambhia et al., 2010). Thus, working in parallel with the process of developing, licensing, and producing the vaccine, federal, state, tribal, territorial, and local public health officials started to plan an ambitious vaccination program.

The prototype of the national vaccine distribution strategy was the federal Vaccines for Children program, through which healthcare providers work routinely with their state and local health departments to provide recommended pediatric vaccines to eligible children. In preparation for the vaccination campaign, the CDC expanded its contract with McKesson Corporation for the Vaccines for Children program to enable centralized distribution of the 2009 H1N1 vaccine. Funded by the federal government, the vaccine was allocated to states in proportion to their populations. State health departments, in turn, worked with LHDs and other partners to develop plans to distribute and administer the vaccine within the state. Because of the scope and short time frame of the campaign, unprecedented efforts were made to strengthen existing vaccine distribution partnerships and to integrate new partners into the distribution and administration system, particularly for vaccination of pregnant women, other high-risk adults, and children. These partners included healthcare providers, health systems, pharmacies, community organizations, health insurers, and large companies with occupational health clinics, among others.

In September 2009, the National Institutes of Health announced that results of the clinical trials indicated the vaccine was safe and effective. The Food and Drug Administration approved four of the 2009 H1N1 influenza vaccines (a fifth was later approved in November), and the CDC had organized a centralized distribution system for shipping the vaccine to public and private provider vaccination sites based on orders placed by the states. With these pieces in place, the national vaccination campaign was launched at the beginning of October.

Initially, health departments were informed they could expect to receive shipments of vaccine in advance of the fall "wave," but various technical issues delayed vaccine manufacture (McKesson Corp, 2009). However, decisions regarding how to implement the vaccine programs were left to be made by authorities at the state and local levels. Vaccine began to arrive in local communities in mid October, just as the influenza epidemic was reaching its peak. Mass vaccination pursued in anticipation of additional waves of disease continuing throughout the winter influenza season, however, according to guidance from ACIP. Because ACIP guidance was nonbinding, health departments were free to adapt the guidance to local conditions. The mass vaccination campaign started in October 2009 (Schnirring, 2009), with most localities focusing on limited vulnerable populations. Given that only 23.2 million doses had been shipped by October 30, 2009, communities had to make decisions quickly on how to break down priority groups further and how to communicate these decisions to vaccinators and to the public. Vaccinators were challenged with determining whether to turn away individuals who sought vaccine but did not fall into priority or "subpriority" groups.

Determining how to disseminate the H1N1 influenza vaccine rapidly to thousands of new and existing vaccine providers and the public was a major challenge for state and local health departments because of the changing estimates of when the vaccine would be available, uncertainties in distribution, and prioritization strategies. Because LHDs held primary responsibility for implementing public and school-based clinics, practices varied widely. Public clinics were often modeled after existing mass dispensing plans, whereas many school-based clinics had to be designed and implemented during the response. Because the national campaign was unique in its initial urgency, limited supply of vaccine, and high public demand, LHDs could not depend on previous experience or established "best practices" to decide how to administer vaccines to the public most efficiently. Many state-level immunization programs worked closely and in unique ways with their state-level emergency preparedness offices to use incident command structures and emergency operations centers to help manage response activities and personnel efficiently and consistently. The high demand for vaccine during a time of uncertainty regarding vaccine delivery timing and quantity made this especially challenging. As a result, there were extensive local differences in vaccination processes (Institute of Medicine, 2010), which suggests there is room for improvement in the quality of the response across locations (Association of State and Territorial Health Officials, 2010).

Eventually, the 2009 H1N1 vaccination campaign was the largest such effort in U.S. history. In less than a year, for instance, a new 2009 H1N1 vaccine was developed, produced, and delivered to 81 million people. From another perspective, however, the response had its limitations. For instance, less than half the population was vaccinated and nearly half of the 162 million 2009 H1N1 vaccine doses produced went unused (Association of State and Territorial Health Officials, 2010; Institute of Medicine, 2010; National Association of County and City Health Officials, 2010).

Methods

As mentioned earlier, the U.S. NHSS calls for efforts to "collect data on performance measures from real incidents . . . analyze performance data to identify gaps, [and] recommend and apply programs to mitigate those gaps" (CDC, 2010b). To address this goal, public health professionals have been using after-action reports/improvement plans (AARs/IPs) as instruments and opportunities for learning from experience, but their utility and effectiveness has varied. This was demonstrated by an analysis of a series of AARs/IPs describing the response to the 2009 H1N1 pandemic and hurricanes Katrina, Gustav, and Ike. The reports varied widely in terms of their intended uses and users, scope, timing, and format. The analysis in many AARs lacked a description of the public health system or the agency's performance on the capabilities being examined. The lack of probing analyses reflected in AARs/IPs may be a result of concerns about revealing weaknesses that could jeopardize funding, lack of skilled staff to perform the analysis, lack of time (especially given the extended nature of the event), or lack of objectivity in assessing performance (Savoia et al., 2012).

Learning about public health systems' emergency response capabilities is challenging because actual events are unique, and both the epidemiologic facts and the context varies from one community to another. In other words, there is no replication, a centerpiece of the scientific method. In addition, public health emergencies are often characterized by uncertainty and require flexibility in the use of a combination of basic PHEP system capacities. As a result, assessing the response is more complex than checking whether a plan has been followed. When the focus is on improvement rather than accountability, and on complex PHEP *systems* rather than their components or individuals, qualitative assessment of the system capabilities of PHEP systems can be more useful than quantitative metrics.

Ensuring that after-action assessments of actual experience with the PHEP system are rigorous can be challenging, but a well-established body of social science methods provides a useful approach (Stoto et al., 2013). For example, based on discussions at an international symposium on Health Policy and Systems Research, Gilson (2011) summarizes a series of concrete processes for ensuring rigor in case study and qualitative data collection and analysis (Box 1-1). Because the focus is on public health systems rather than individuals, Yin's (2009) classic book on case study methods, now in its fourth edition, is also relevant. March and colleagues (1991) and Weick and Sutcliffe (2001) offer more specific suggestions relevant to PHEP. The realist evaluation perspective (Pawson and Tilley, 1997) also has much to offer.

Because one of the goals of this book is to illustrate a variety of rigorous research methods that can be used to learn from exceptional events such as public health emergencies, we conclude the introduction with a detailed discussion of the qualitative methods used, organized according to Gilson's (2011) framework.

Use Theory

Gilson (2011) recommends the use of theory to guide sample selection, data collection and analysis, and to influence interpretive analysis. "Theory" in this context is meant broadly, ranging from basic social science theories about risk communication to preparedness doctrine as embodied in the National Incident Management Strategy or the NHSS.

Box 1-1 PROCESSES FOR ENSURING RIGOR IN CASE STUDY AND QUALITATIVE DATA COLLECTION AND ANALYSIS*

- *Prolonged engagement with the subject of inquiry.* Although ethnographers may spend years in the field, health policy and systems research tends to draw on lengthy and perhaps repeated interviews with respondents, and/or days and weeks of engagement within a case study site
- *Use of theory.* To guide sample selection, data collection and analysis, and draw into interpretive analysis
- *Case selection.* Purposive selection to allow prior theory and initial assumptions to be tested or to examine "average" or unusual experience
- *Sampling.* Of people, places, times, etc., initially, to include as many as possible of the factors that might influence the behavior of those people central to the topic of focus (subsequently extend in the light of early findings) Gather views from wide range of perspectives and respondents rather than letting one viewpoint dominate
- *Multiple methods.* For each case study site: Two sets of formal interviews with all sampled staff, Researcher observation & informal discussion, Interviews with patients, Interviews with facility supervisors and area managers
- *Triangulation.* Looking for patterns of convergence and divergence by comparing results across multiple sources of evidence (e.g., across interviewees, and between interview and other data), between researchers, across methodological approaches, with theory
- *Negative case analysis.* Looking for evidence that contradicts your explanations and theory, and refining them in response to this evidence
- *Peer debriefing and support.* Review of findings and reports by other researchers
- *Respondent validation (member checking).* Review of findings and reports by respondents
- *Clear report of methods of data collection and analysis (audit trail).* Keeping a full record of activities that can be opened to others and presenting a full account of how methods evolved to the research audience

*Reproduced with permission from: Gilson, L. (2011). Building the field of health policy and systems research: social science matters. *PLoS Medicine, 8*, e1001079.

In this book, the use of theory begins with the use of the LAMPS PHEP logic model (Figure 1-1) and the CDC public health preparedness capabilities (Centers for Disease Control and Prevention, 2011) as an overall organizing principle. Chapters 5, 6, and 7, for example, all examine how emergency response doctrine, as represented in the National Incident Management System, fared in the 2009 pandemic.

More specifically, in Chapter 11, Savoia and colleagues demonstrate the value of a formal, theory-based approach to survey development that includes a thorough literature review, the development of a structural influence model, focus groups in multiple languages, and the use of Web-based survey methods. In Chapter 4, Klaiman and colleagues examine how the "theory" of social distancing, based on epidemiologic models and historical analysis, met the reality of 2009 school closure decisions.

Alternatively, case studies can be used to develop and test new theories. In Chapter 5, for instance, Lewis and colleagues illustrate the use of a systematic methodology in the tradition of grounded theory to analyze the LACDPH response to the 2009 H1N1 pandemic. This approach included (1) a large-sample survey to elicit major themes from a broad group of stakeholders; (2) focus groups with key organizations involved in the response to address challenges identified by the survey, and groups that used diagramming to elicit root causes and potential corrective actions; (3) individual leadership interviews that focused on priorities identified earlier; and (4) a "change conference" to present the findings to the LACDPH executive leadership.

In Chapter 8, Stoto and Higdon adopt a "realist evaluation" approach to identify "what works for whom in what circumstances and in what respects" (Pawson and Tilley, 1997, p. 2). From a methodological perspective, the challenge is to identify how program mechanisms (M) interact with contextual factors (C) to result in positive, negative, or neutral outcomes (O). In this perspective, C + M = O stories, (or mini theories from case studies) are tested in other circumstances. The C + M = O stories identified in this analysis are summarized in Table 1-2.

Select Cases

Gilson (2011) recommended a purposive—rather than a random—approach to selecting cases to allow prior theory and initial assumptions to be tested, or to examine both "average" and unusual experiences. For instance, Klaiman and colleagues (Chapter 10) first used a "positive deviance" approach to identify

TABLE 1-2 Sample C + M = O Stories

OUTCOME: SUCCESSFUL ADMINISTRATION OF PH1N1 VACCINE	
CONTEXT	MECHANISM
Typical health department with a good relationship with schools	Use school-based clinics to administer vaccine
Small health departments in a rural setting	Pool resources to conduct regional clinics
Large group practice with an emergency medical response system	Use emergency medical response to set appointments automatically for patients for whom vaccine is appropriate
Network of community health centers with strong relationships to populations served	Use community health centers to administer vaccine

high-performing LHDs and, second, to study them to ascertain model immunization practices—what seems to work in what circumstances.

It can also be useful to conduct a series of parallel case studies in which cases are chosen intentionally to reflect a variety of settings, such as health department types, geographic areas, and populations served, and to test theories about the determinants of effective PHEP systems (Yin, 2009). Chapters 8 and 9 illustrate this with parallel case studies, using similar methods, in Massachusetts and the Emilia Romagna region in Italy.

Gilson (2011) also recommends negative case analysis (i.e., looking specifically for evidence that contradicts current explanations and theory, and refining them in response to this evidence). For example, the analysis of influenza surveillance systems in Chapters 2 and 3 offer a number of surprises relative to pandemic planning assumptions. In terms of the epidemiology, it was assumed that a pandemic viral strain would emerge in Asia and would be virulent in addition to its ease of transmittal; it was not assumed that children would be at a higher risk for infection or severe consequences. As a result, school closing policies based on the premise that children were efficient vectors for community transmission lost their rationale when it appeared that children were the ones who needed protection (Chapter 4).

Experience More Interpretations

Particularly when dealing with single, unique cases, March and colleagues (1991) stress the need for multiple observers to increase the number of interpretations, which creates a mosaic of conflicting lessons. In particular, Weick and Sutcliffe (2001) recommend that researchers resist the temptation to "normalize" unexpected events. In the face of system failure, they argue, it is natural to look for evidence that confirms expectations, that postpones the realization that something unexpected is developing. Rather, experience that calls into question planning assumptions is more important than experience that confirms them (Weick and Sutcliffe, 2001).

In Chapter 6, Hunter and colleagues illustrate the use of a rigorous mixed-methods approach to describe the range of methods used by LHDs in California to manage antiviral activities and to gain a better understanding of the related challenges experienced. First, a multidisciplinary focus group of pandemic influenza planners from key stakeholder groups in California was convened to generate ideas and to identify critical themes related to the local implementation of antiviral activities during the H1N1 influenza response. These qualitative data informed the development of a Web-based survey that was distributed to all 61 LHDs in California for the purpose of assessing the experiences of a representative sample of local health agencies in a large region. Similarly, in Chapter 7, Chamberlain and colleagues use an Internet-based survey to identify the perspectives of 64 city, state, and territorial immunization program managers. The 35-question survey asked immunization program managers about their health department's management structure during the H1N1 vaccination campaign, including whether the department had used an incident command system, the role of their incident commander, and whether they opened an emergency operations center. The survey also gathered perceptions of the helpfulness of existing pandemic influenza plans. The extent of collaboration with state-level emergency preparedness programs was assessed through questions regarding the degree of collaboration with those programs before the pandemic, and the delineation of tasks between the two programs during the H1N1 vaccination campaign.

The "facilitated look-backs" (Aledort et al., 2006) used in preparing the Massachusetts and Emilia Romagna region case studies (Chapters 8 and 9) provided an opportunity to review events that occurred during the pandemic from the point of view of state and local health departments, healthcare providers, school systems, and others to explore different interpretations of events and perceptions of what happened.

Experience More Preferences

As mentioned, to learn as much from single, unique cases, March and colleagues (1991) recommend gathering as much information as possible on the preferences and values organizations use distinguish successes from failures. This approach can be seen in Chapter 5, in which Lewis and colleagues use a grounded theory case study approach with formal surveys of a broad group of stakeholders and focus groups with key organizations involved in the response to identify insights about managing long-duration, moderate-acuity public health incidents. The in-depth case studies of Massachusetts and the Emilia Romagna region (Chapters 8 and 9) are other examples of this approach.

Use Multiple Methods

Gilson (2011) recommends the use of multiple research methods within case studies. At one level, this is the approach adopted by Lewis and colleagues in Chapter 5, when they describe their use of a large-sample survey, focus groups with key organizations, individual leadership interviews, and a "change conference" to analyze the LACDPH's response to the 2009 H1N1 pandemic. Similarly, Stoto and Higdon (Chapter 8) and Savoia and colleagues (Chapter 9) used facilitated look-backs and group and individual interviews to prepare their case studies.

More generally, because these three chapters and the analyses of Chamberlain and colleagues (Chapter 7) and Klaiman and colleagues (Chapter 10) all focused on dispensing pH1N1 vaccinations, they can be viewed as parallel analyses of the same general "case" using different research methods.

Use Triangulation

Gilson (2011) and Yin (2009) both suggest looking for patterns of convergence and divergence by comparing results across multiple sources of evidence (e.g., across interviewees, and between interview and other data), among researchers, across methodological approaches, with theory. In Chapter 3, for instance, Stoto and Zhang, compare multiple data sources to identify a consistent pattern of biases in 2009 H1N1 surveillance data (Stoto, 2012; Zhang, 2011). This approach helps to address the lack of a gold standard to describe the actual trends in the rate of pH1N1 infection and its consequences over time.

Prolong Engagement with the Subject of Inquiry, Respondent Validation, and Peer Debriefing

As described by Gilson (2001), health policy and systems research tends to draw on lengthy and perhaps repeated interviews with respondents, and/or days and weeks of engagement in a case study site. Pawson and Tilley (1997) and Greenhalgh (2009) make a similar point about evaluations in the realist perspective. Rather than maintaining an arms-length relationship with research subjects, this approach to assessment incorporates reviews of preliminary findings and reports by the PHEP practitioners whose systems are being evaluated. Review of findings and reports by other researchers is also critical. As described earlier, the case studies of Los Angeles (Chapter 5), Massachusetts (Chapter 8), and the Emilia Romagna region (Chapter 9) were all prepared using this approach.

Prolonged engagement with the subject can also take place after the data have been gathered. In Chapter 6, for instance, Hunter and colleagues describe a process of careful note-taking and analysis of focus group data, followed by participant validation of summaries and themes. Chamberlain and colleagues (Chapter 7) describe a process they used to code free text responses to qualitative survey questions and analyze the results for themes. Although their methods were less formal, Klaiman and colleagues (Chapters 4 and 10) also spent a substantial amount of time reviewing data to identify themes and results.

Similarly, in their analysis of advances in global surveillance and notification systems (Chapter 2), Zhang and Stoto describe a "critical events" approach for analyzing the policy implications of data from real incidents on public health system emergency response capabilities. This approach involves three critical steps, each of which requires professional judgment and knowledge of public health systems. First, the analyst must prepare a timeline that describes key events in both the epidemiology and the public health response. This task can be a challenge because early events are not, in and of themselves, seen as noteworthy and, typically, are not recorded as they occur. Second, based on this timeline, the analyst must identify the critical events, which are events of more complexity than the recognition of a cluster of cases, but less complex than the emergence of a new pathogen. Critical events represent opportunities when the response might have occurred sooner or later than it did, depending on the public health system's capabilities. Last, the analyst must identify the factors that allowed the events to occur when they did, rather than earlier or later. In a standard root-cause analysis, these are the "root causes." This task requires knowledge of how public health systems are supposed to perform and the factors that can degrade this performance. It is also useful to consider what might have happened had the critical events turned out differently, an approach that March and colleagues (1991) describe as a "simulating experience."

Report Methods of Data Collection and Analysis Clearly (Audit Trail)

Gilson (2011) notes the importance of keeping a full record of activities that can be opened to others, and presenting to the research audience a full account of how methods evolved. This task can be difficult when studying actual events, which can be drawn out, when the focus is, naturally, on dealing with the public health emergency. Debriefing participants "within the hour," as Weick and Sutcliffe (2001) advocate, can be difficult during public health emergencies, but the principle of recording the "facts" in real time and saving the analysis for later is important. For example, although not a CDC requirement, the expectation that state and local health department AARs and IPs were required to be completed within 60 days of the 2009 H1N1 outbreak made it difficult to conduct a thorough analysis of the public health system response (Stoto et al. 2013).

To address this problem, the National Transportation Safety Board requires a preliminary report within five days of an airplane crash, focusing only on the basic facts, and a factual report with additional information concerning the occurrence within a few months. A final report, which includes a statement of the probable cause, may not be completed for months or until after the investigation has been completed (National Transportation Safety Board, no date).

Acknowledgments and Disclosures

This research was conducted with funding support awarded to the Harvard School of Public Health under cooperative agreements with the U.S. CDC (grant no. 5P01TP000307-01). The authors are grateful for comments from John Brownstein, Melissa Higdon, Tamar Klaiman, John Kraemer, Larissa May, Christopher Nelson, Hilary Placzek, Ellen Whitney, Ying Zhang, the staff of the CDC Public Health Surveillance Program Office, and others who commented on presentations.

References

Aledort, J. E., Lurie, N., Ricci, K. (2006). Facilitated look-backs: a new quality improvement tool for management of routine annual and pandemic influenza.

RAND TR-320. Accessed March 3, 2013, at http://www.rand.org/pubs/technical_reports/TR320.html.

Cauchemez, S., Ferguson, N. M., Wachtel, C., Tegnell, A., Saour, G., Duncan, B., Nicoll, A. (2009). Closure of schools during an influenza pandemic. *The Lancet Infectious Diseases, 9*, 473–481.

Centers for Disease Control and Prevention. (2009a). Deaths related to 2009 pandemic influenza A(H1N1) among American Indian/Alaska Natives: 12 states, 2009. *Morbidity and Mortality Weekly Report, 58*(48), 1341–1344.

Centers for Disease Control and Prevention. (2009b). Novel influenza A(H5N1) virus infections in three pregnant women: United States, April–May 2009. *Morbidity and Mortality Weekly Report, 58*(18), 497–500.

Centers for Disease Control and Prevention. (2010a). The 2009 H1N1 pandemic: summary highlights, April 2009–April 2010. Accessed March 3, 2013, at http://www.cdc.gov/h1n1flu/cdcresponse.htm.

Centers for Disease Control and Prevention. (2011). Public health preparedness capabilities: national standards for state and local planning. Accessed March 3, 2013, at http://www.cdc.gov/phpr/capabilities.

Centers for Disease Control and Prevention. (2010b). Implementation Plan for the National Health Security Strategy of the United States of America. Accessed on October 2, 2014 at http://www.phe.gov/Preparedness/planning/authority/nhss/ip/Documents/nhss-ip.pdf.

Centers for Disease Control and Prevention Advisory Committee on Immunization Practices. (2009). Use of influenza A (2009) monovalent vaccine: recommendations of the Advisory Committee on Immunization Practices. *Morbidity and Mortality Weekly Report, 58*(RR10), 1–8.

Ferguson, N. M., Cummings, D. A. T., Fraser, C., Cajka, J. C., Cooley, P. C., Burke, D. S. (2006). Strategies for mitigating an influenza pandemic. *Nature, 442*, 448–452.

Fineberg, H. V. (2014). Pandemic preparedness and response: lessons from the H1N1 influenza of 2009. *The New England Journal of Medicine, 370*, 1335–1342.

Gilson, L. (2011). Building the field of health policy and systems research: social science matters. *PLoS Medicine, 8*, e1001079.

Greenhalgh, T. (2009). How do you modernize a health service? A realist evaluation of whole-scale transformation in London. *Milbank Quarterly, 87*, 391–416.

Halabi, S. F. (2014). The uncertain future of vaccine development and deployment for influenza pandemic. Briefing paper no. 8. Accessed March 19, 2014, at http://www.law.georgetown.edu/oneillinstitute/resources/documents/Briefing8 Halabi.pdf.

Institute of Medicine. (2003). The future of the public's health in the 21st century. Accessed March 3, 2013, at http://www.nap.edu/catalog.php?record_id=10548.

Institute of Medicine. (2008). Research priorities in emergency preparedness and response for public health systems: a letter report. Accessed March 3, 2013, at http://www.iom.edu/Activities/Research/PreparednessEMS.aspx.

Institute of Medicine. (2010). The 2009 H1N1 influenza vaccination campaign: summary of a workshop series. Accessed March 3, 2013, at http://iom.edu/Reports/2010/The-2009-H1N1-Influenza-Vaccination-Campaign.aspx.

Klaiman, T., Kraemer, J. D., Stoto, M. A. (2011). Variability in school closure decisions in response to 2009 H1N1. *BMC Public Health, 11*, 73–82.

Klaiman, T., O'Connell, K., Stoto, M. A. (2012). Local health department public vaccination clinic success during 2009 pH1N1. *Journal of Public Health Management and Practice, 11*, 17–24.

March, J. G., Sproull, L. S., Tamuz, M. (1991). A model of adaptive organizational search. *Organization Science, 2*, 1–13.

McKesson Corp. (2009). CDC expands existing vaccine distribution partnership with McKesson to include H1N1 flu vaccine. Accessed March 3, 2013, at http://www.mckesson.com/en_us/McKesson.com/Our%2BBusinesses/McKesson%2BSpecialty%2BHealth/Newsroom/CDC%2BExpands%2BExisting%2BVaccine%2BDistribution%2BPartnership%2Bwith%2BMcKesson%2Bto%2BInclude%2BH1N1%2BFlu%2BVaccine.html.

National Association of County and City Health Officials. (2010). NACCHO H1N1 policy workshop report. Accessed March 3, 2013, at http://www.naccho.org/topics/H1N1/upload/NACCHO-WORKSHOP-REPORT-IN-TEMPLATE-with-chart.pdf.

National Transportation Safety Board. (no date). Aviation Accident/Incident Database. Accessed March 3, 2013, at http://www.asias.faa.gov/portal/page/portal/ASIAS_PAGES/LEARN_ABOUTS/ntsb_la.html

Pawson, R., Tilley, N. (1997). *Realist evaluation*. New York: Sage.

Rambhia, K. J., Watson, M., Sell, T. K., Waldhorn, R., Toner, E. (2010). Mass vaccination for the 2009 H1N1 pandemic: approaches, challenges, and recommendations. *Biosecurity Bioterrorism, 8*(4), 321–330.

Savoia, E., Agboola, A., Biddinger, P. (2012). Use of after action reports (AARs) to promote organizational and systems learning in emergency preparedness. *International Journal of Environmental Research and Public Health, 9*, 2949–2963.

Schnirring, L. (2009). U.S. H1N1 vaccine delayed as cases and deaths rise. *CIDRAP News*. Accessed March 3, 2013, at http://www.cidrap.umn.edu/cidrap/content/influenza/swineflu/news/oct1609vaccine.html.

Stein, R., Wilgorn, D. (2009). Fort Worth shutters all schools: WHO warns of a likely pandemic. *Washington Post*. Health Section, May 1, 2009. Accessed October 2, 2014 at http://www.washingtonpost.com/wp-dyn/content/article/2009/04/30/AR2009043001133.html.

Stoto, M. A. (2012). The effectiveness of U.S. public health surveillance systems for situational awareness during the 2009 H1N1 pandemic: a retrospective analysis. *PLoS One, 7*, e40984.

Stoto, M. A., Nelson, C. D., Klaiman, T. (2013). Getting from what to why: using qualitative methods in public health systems research. Academy Health issue brief. Accessed November 1, 2013, at http://www.academyhealth.org/files/publications/QMforPH.pdf.

Stoto, M. A., Nelson, C. D., LAMPS investigators. (2012). Measuring and assessing public health emergency preparedness: a methodological primer. Accessed March 3, 2013, at http://lamps.sph.harvard.edu/images/stories/MeasurementWhitePaper.pdf.

Weick, K., Sutcliffe, K. (2001). *Managing the unexpected: assuring high performance in an age of complexity.* New York: Jossey-Bass.
World Health Organization. (2009). World now at the start of 2009 influenza pandemic: statement by Dr. Margaret Chan, Director-General of the World Health Organization. Accessed March 3, 2013, at http://www.who.int/mediacentre/news/statements/2009/h1n1_pandemic_phase6_20090611/en/index.html.
Yin, R. (2009). *Case study research: design and methods.* New York: Sage.
Zhang, Y., May, L., Stoto, M. A. (2011). Evaluating syndromic surveillance systems at institutions of higher education (IHEs) during the 2009 H1N1 influenza pandemic. *BMC Public Health, 11,* 591–600.

CHAPTER 2

Did Advances in Global Surveillance and Notification Systems Make a Difference in the 2009 H1N1 Pandemic?

MICHAEL A. STOTO AND YING ZHANG

Introduction

In the past decade, many new advanced systems for disease surveillance and notification have been developed and implemented throughout the world (Hitchcock et al., 2007). These systems generally fall into two categories: indicator-based surveillance and notification. *Indicator-based surveillance systems* gather and analyze original data, especially those indicative of emerging health problems in the population (Paquet et al., 2006). More recent advances include enhancements of traditional case reporting and laboratory capabilities, and the development and implementation of "syndromic surveillance" systems that collect and analyze statistical data on health trends, such as symptoms reported by people seeking care in emergency departments or other healthcare settings, or even sales of prescription or over-the-counter flu medicines or Web searches (Stoto, 2007). *Notification systems*, on the other hand, provide a means for communicating about the evidence that emerges from indicator-based surveillance systems to understand more completely the implications of local results and to enable a global response if warranted. Notification systems in a large part stem from the adoption and implementation of international health regulations (IHR) and include efforts such as the Global Public Health Intelligence Network (GPHIN), ProMED Mail, HealthMap, Argus, and Veratect (described later), which search the Internet and other sources to identify disease outbreaks that might not have been apparent to health officials. These systems, also known as *event-based surveillance systems* (Paquet, 2006), have the potential to detect outbreaks based on indirect evidence of illness not reported to local health officials.

The outbreak of a novel strain of A(H1N1) influenza virus, A/California/7/2009, now referred to as pH1N1, provided an opportunity to see how well these systems functioned in practice as an integrated public health surveillance system. The epidemiology of pH1N1 has been well described elsewhere (Jhung et al., 2011; Chowell et al., 2011; Swerdlow et al., 2011), and adding to this understanding is not the goal of this chapter. Rather, taking advantage of this opportunity, the primary objective is to identify the strengths and weaknesses of current global disease surveillance and notification systems to improve their performance in the future. Specifically, we ask whether and how advances in global surveillance and notification systems put in place during the past decade made a difference in the public health response to the 2009 H1N1 pandemic. We also identify the policy implications of the findings for future enhancements to global surveillance and notification systems and for how preparedness should be assessed.

As a secondary objective, this analysis illustrates the use of "critical event analysis," part of the toolkit for systematic quality improvement (QI), a perspective called for in the U.S. National Health Security Strategy (NHSS) (U.S. Department of Health and Human Services, 2009a). Emphasizing processes (chains of events that produce specific outcomes) and systems of people and information, the QI approach refers to a range of specific practices including procedures and system changes based on their effects on measurable outcomes, the reduction of unnecessary variability in outcomes while preserving system differences critical to the specific environment, continuous improvement rather than one-time initiatives, and critical event/failure mode analysis. The NHSS implementation guide also calls for the development, refinement, and wide-spread implementation of QI tools. In particular, this includes "efforts to collect data on performance measures from real incidents . . . analyze performance data to identify gaps, [and] recommend and apply programs to mitigate those gaps" (U.S. Department of Health and Human Services, 2009b).

Methods

This analysis is an in-depth case study that draws on information from a systematic review of the scientific literature, official documents, websites, and news reports. In particular, we constructed a timeline (Figure 2-1) in which three kinds of events are represented and distinguished by a color code (explained in the Results section): (1) the emergence and spread of the pH1N1 virus itself, (2) local health officials' awareness and understanding of the emerging outbreak, and (3) notifications about and global health officials' awareness of the events and their implications. The primary sources for this analysis were a timeline published by *Science* Insider, an online publication associated with *Science* magazine (Cohen, 2009a), other scientific and lay publications as indicated in the text, and two of the authors' contemporaneous notes. In a number of cases the sources differed, so we used our judgment to determine which fit best with the other time points. This uncertainty is represented in the text with phrases such as "In early April . . . ."

With the events classified in this way, we then conducted a critical event analysis focused on the surveillance process rather than the epidemiologic facts. Specifically, we first identified critical events, incidents that advanced the recognition of what we now know as a global pandemic. These events are points in time when the public health system might have responded sooner or later than it did, depending on the system's capabilities. We then tried to identify the factors that allowed the events to occur when they did, rather than earlier or later, consistent with root-cause analysis. In particular, we asked (1) when health officials in Mexico, the United States, and at the global level became aware of the epidemiologic facts of the unfolding pandemic; (2) whether an earlier recognition could have been possible; (3) whether advances in surveillance notification systems seem likely to have hastened the detection of the outbreak; and (4) whether there are improvements that might be possible through enhanced practices, procedures, or new systems. We sought to analyze decisions based on the information that was available, or could have been available, to the decision-makers at the time. Because illustrating the strengths and weaknesses of this approach is one of our objectives, we discuss the challenges, limitations, and opportunities presented by this approach in detail in the Conclusions.

Results

The Mexican Outbreak

The exact location of the first human cases of pH1N1 infection is not known; however, retrospective analyses have identified cases dating back to February and March 2009 in at least three locations throughout Mexico, as indicated in Figure 2-1. The earliest confirmed cases occurred on February 24 in the state of San Luis Potosí in central Mexico (Cohen, 2009b) and the first confirmed case in Mexico City had its onset on March 11 (Centers for Disease Control and Prevention, 2009a). There was also an outbreak of influenzalike illness in preschool children in the state of Tlaxcala in central Mexico starting March 5 (Lopez-Gatell, 2009a). Starting March 15, a major respiratory disease outbreak occurred in La Gloria in the state of Veracruz. This outbreak was originally attributed to a large pig farm on the outskirts of town, but when three children became seriously ill in late March and early April, health authorities in Veracruz began to suspect an atypical influenza (Cohen, 2009a; Weaver and Tuckman, 2009). Consistent with Pan American Health Organization (PAHO)/World Health Organization (WHO) recommendations at the time, surveillance was conducted using use immunofluorescence, which has low sensitivity in practice. In addition, Mexico's Instituto de Diagnóstico y Referencia Epidemiológicos

Sunday	Monday	Tuesday	Wednesday	Thursday	Friday	Saturday
22-Feb	23	24	25	26	27	28
		Earliest confirmed case in San Luis Potosi				
1-Mar	2	3	4	5	6	7
				Onset of influenza-like respiratory illness in preschool		
8	9	10	11	12	13	14
			First confirmed case in Mexico City		National alert issued regarding Tlaxcala outbreak	
15	16	17	18	19	20	21
La Gloria outbreak begins						
22	23	24	25	26	27	28
					Onset in Oaxaca diabetic	Onset in California Patient B
29	30	31	1-Apr	2	3	4
	Onset in California Patient B		NHRC finds untypable flu virus in Patient A			
	Children seriously ill in La Gloria		HealthMap reports about La Gloria			
5	6	7	8	9	10	11
	Veratect issues alert about Mexican outbreak Local news story about La Gloria	InDRE identifies unsubtypable influenza A strain in sample from La Gloria		PAHO accesses Veratect alert about Mexican outbreak	GPHIN notifies WHO of acute respiratory illness in Marshfield Clinic unable to subtype Patient A	PAHO asks Mexican IHR focal point to verify La Gloria
12 (Easter)	13	14	15	16 (Obama visit)	17	18
Mexico notifies PAHO of cluster of respiratory illness in La Gloria	Wisconsin state lab unable to subtype Patient A, sends to CDC Oaxaca diabetic dies Mexico notifies US and Canada of cluster of unexplained respiratory illness in La Gloria	CDC identifies H1N1 of swine origin in Patient A SINAVE aware of severe pneumonia and excess number of influenza cases and outbreaks throughout Mexico	Veracruz briefs the Mexican Directorate General of Epidemiology regarding La Gloria outbreak investigation	Veratect alerts CDC & WHO re Oaxaca Mexico, US, Canada teleconference to discuss unusual epidemiology of influenza in the three countries	CDC identifies H1N1 of swine origin in Patient B US alerts PAHO about the two isolates of a novel swine-origin H1N1 Mexican press conference regarding atypical influenza and excess morbidity and mortality Mexico notifies PAHO of Oaxaca case	InDRE/NML teleconference to discuss novel agent
New York City students travel to Cancun, Mexico						
19	20	21	22	23	24	25
Active surveillance finds excess demand for health services and high case fatality rate in pneumonia cases in Mexico City hospitals	Veratect alerts CDC re Mexico Onset in New York City students	Mexico reports atypical influenza in different cities, sends samples to NML and CDC CDC issues alert re novel virus in California	Mexico alerts PAHO of atypical influenza and pneumonia, noting possible relation to novel H1N1 in the US	CDC and NML confirm novel H1N1 in Mexican samples NYC DHMH notified of more than 100 cases at New York City school	Schools closed in Mexico City First ProMed reports published NYC DHMH suspects outbreak is H1N1 and begins investigation	WHO declares a Public Health Emergency of International Concern Canada reports cases
4107 respiratory specimens sent to U.S. WHO and NREVSS collaborating laboratories, of which 6.7% were influenza-positive						
26	27	28	29	30	1-May	2
CDC declares a public health emergency New Zealand, France, Israel, Brazil and Spain report suspect cases	CDC issues Mexican travel recommendation WHO raises pandemic threat level from phase 3 to phase 4 European countries report suspect cases	Schools closed throughout Mexico Suspect cases reported in Middle East and Asia-Pacific region	CDC confirms pH1N1 in New York City cases	300 US schools closed	Mexico suspends non-essential government and private business services	
35,381 respiratory specimens sent to U.S. WHO and NREVSS collaborating laboratories, of which 12.1% were influenza-positive						
3	4	5 (Cinco de Mayo)	6	7	8-Jan	9
33,653 respiratory specimens sent to U.S. WHO and NREVSS collaborating laboratories, of which 14.62% were influenza-positive						

Key	Mexico		United States		World-wide awareness
	Epidemiology	Official awareness	Epidemiology	Official awareness	

(InDRE) used real-time polymerase chain reaction (rt-PCR) for molecular diagnosis, but of course probes for the pandemic strain were not available until afterward, so the pandemic was not recognized at this time.

In addition, a 39-year-old woman with new-onset diabetes mellitus in Oaxaca developed severe respiratory illness on March 27 and eventually died of this illness on April 13 (Cordova-Villalobos et al., 2009). In addition, an excessive amount of influenzalike illness was experienced in the Distrito Federal (Mexico City) in mid-March (Cohen, 2009a).

By mid-April, Mexican national health authorities were aware of these and other respiratory illness outbreaks throughout the country through the National Surveillance System SINAVE (Sistema Nacional de Vigilancia Epidemiologica). This system receives weekly reports on 117 notifiable conditions from nearly all of the more than 19,000 hospitals, clinics, and doctors' offices in Mexico, and also monitors 520 sentinel influenza surveillance units covering all 32 states (Ministry of Health Mexico, 2012). On March 13, the Mexican Directorate General of Epidemiology issued an alert about the outbreak of influenzalike illness in preschool children the previous week in Tlaxcala (Lopez-Gatell, 2009a) (the Mexican public health system's awareness of the outbreak and response is represented by text with a solid dark background in Figure 2-1). On April 6, a local news story reported that 60% of La Gloria residents were infected, and there were three deaths (Weaver and Tuckman, 2009). The following day, InDRE identified an influenza A viral strain that could not be subtyped (i.e., a different strain than those known to be circulating at that time) in a sample from La Gloria. In DRE had previously identified "unsubtypable" samples from Mexico City, San Luis Potosí, and Baja, California. By April 14, SINAVE was aware there had been an increase in the number of cases and outbreaks of seasonal influenza observed since February (Frenk, 2009; Lopez-Gatell, 2009a). SINAVE was also notified through both official and unofficial channels of cases of severe laboratory-confirmed pneumonia, with high fatality, in young previously healthy adults between the ages of 20 and 40 years in Mexico City and the states of México,

---

FIGURE 2-1 Timeline of H1N1 events. Epidemiologic events are indicated in light shades (solid for Mexico and striped for the United States), local awareness and understanding of these events in dark shades, and global notifications and awareness of these events are not shaded. CDC, Centers for Disease Control and Prevention; DHMH, Department of Health and Mental Hygiene; GPHIN, Global Public Health Intelligence Network; IHR, international health regulations; InDRE, Instituto de Diagnóstico y Referencia Epidemiológicos; NML, National Microbiology Laboratory; NREVSS, National Respiratory and Enteric Virus Surveillance System; NHRC, Naval Health Research Center; NYC, New York City; PAHO, Pan American Health Organization; SINAVE, Sistema Nacional de Vigilancia Epidemiologica; U.S., United States; WHO, World Health Organization.

Veracruz, and San Luis Potosí (Chowell et al., 2009; Cohen, 2009a; Lezana, 2009). Active surveillance of Mexico City hospitals starting on April 17 triggered by these reports found excess demand for health services and a high case fatality rate in pneumonia cases (Lopez-Gatell, 2009a).

The clinical and epidemiologic characteristics of the cases that had come to light by mid-April varied, and respiratory illness during the winter could easily have been regarded as seasonal influenza. Many of the cases were determined to have influenza B, a trend that was also being observed in the United States (Cohen, 2009c). But, a severe respiratory infection that, unlike seasonal influenza, affected children and young adults together with prompts from the WHO(as discussed later) led the Directorate General of Epidemiology to "connect the dots" between the outbreaks across the country by mid-April.

On April 15, Veracruz officials briefed the Directorate General of Epidemiology regarding the La Gloria outbreak investigation, with PAHO officers in attendance. Two days later, authorities conducted a press conference to warn about the atypical influenza season with an increasing morbidity trend and excess mortality. After notification about the emergence of novel H1N1 in the United States and interactions with Canadian health officials and the U.S. Centers for Disease Control and Prevention (CDC; as described later), Mexico notified PAHO (the WHO regional office for the Americas) of a potential atypical pneumonia outbreak on April 22, closed schools in Mexico City on April 24 and throughout Mexico on April 28, and did not open high schools and universities until May 7. On May 1, nonessential government and private-sector business services were suspended. The number of confirmed cases peaked shortly afterward but rebounded for a second peak in June and July, by which time the entire country was affected (Ministry of Health Mexico, 2010).

The United States Outbreak

In late March, a nine-year-old girl and a 10-year old boy in southern California became ill with influenza (U.S. epidemiologic dates are represented by text with a striped light background in Figure 2-1) (Centers for Disease Control and Prevention, 2009b). An experimental diagnostic device was being tested by the Naval Health Research Center (NHRC) in San Diego requiring that respiratory samples be collected and analyzed. On April 1, the NHRC found an unsubtypable influenza A virus in one of these samples (the U.S. public health system's awareness of the outbreak and response is represented by text with a striped dark background in Figure 2-1). By protocol, respiratory samples were sent to the designated reference laboratory, the Marshfield Clinic in Wisconsin, which on April 10 confirmed that the pathogen was influenza A virus, but could not identify the strain any further. Also according to protocol, a part of the sample was sent to the Wisconsin State Laboratory of Hygiene, which confirmed the finding on April 13 and forwarded the sample to the CDC for additional analysis. On April 14, the CDC identified the subtype as pH1N1 of swine origin, and on April 17 found pH1N1 in another specimen from the

NHRC in San Diego. Following a call with California health officials on April 19, the CDC issued an alert and notified the WHO on April 21 (Cohen, 2009a).

Between April 10 and 19, 14 students from a high school in Queens, New York, traveled to Mexico (all but one to Cancun) during their spring recess and developed flu symptoms the week of April 19. On April 23, two days after the CDC alert, the school nurse notified the New York City Department of Health and Mental Hygiene (DHMH) that approximately 100 students were being sent home with flu symptoms. The DHMH notified the CDC that afternoon and began an investigation April 24. The following day, the DHMH reported that most laboratory specimens from these students tested positive by rt-PCR for influenza A with no human H1 or H3 subtypes detected, indicating the virus was probably pH1N1. On April 29, the CDC confirmed by rt-PCR that most specimens were positive for pH1N1 (Centers for Disease Control and Prevention, 2009b).

On April 26, aware of the New York outbreak, as well as 20 cases from California and Texas, the U.S. Department of Health and Human Services (2009c) declared a public health emergency in the United States. The following day, the CDC issued "a travel health warning recommending that United States travelers postpone all non-essential travel to Mexico" (Centers for Disease Control and Prevention, 2009c). About 300 schools in the United States were closed by April 30, when the accumulated pH1N1 cases numbered more than 100 nationwide. An immediate consequence was an increase in the number of U.S. respiratory specimens sent for testing by the WHO and the National Respiratory and Enteric Virus Surveillance System (NREVSS) collaborating laboratories from 4,219, of which 7.7% were influenza-positive, in the week ending April 25 (week 16) to 14,330, of which 13.2% were influenza-positive, in the week ending May 2 (week 17). The number of specimens, along with the percent influenza-positive, peaked at 7,844 (41.9%) in the week ending June 20 (week 24). By the end of the summer, the first wave had waned, but pH1N1 cases had been confirmed in every U.S. continental state (Centers for Disease Control and Prevention, 2009d, 2009e, 2009f).

International Awareness and Global Spread

Health officials outside of Mexico were potentially aware of what was eventually determined to be the 2009 H1N1 pandemic as early as April 1, when HealthMap first disseminated local media reports about a "mysterious" influenzalike illness in La Gloria (global epidemiology and response are represented by text with no shading in Figure 2-1). The HealthMap system combines automated, around-the-clock data collection and processing with expert review and analysis to aggregate reports according to type of disease and geographic location. HealthMap sifts through large volumes of information on events, obtained from a broad range of online sources in multiple languages, to provide a comprehensive view of ongoing global disease activity through a publicly available website (Brownstein et al., 2010). Throughout the month of April, HealthMap also identified informal local Spanish-language sources reporting the spread of the epidemic throughout Mexico.

On April 6, Veratect, a private firm based in Kirkland, Washington, that conducts disease surveillance, issued an alert based on information from La Gloria and other sources of a "strange" outbreak of acute respiratory infection that led to bronchial pneumonia in some pediatric cases. This alert was available to the CDC, WHO, PAHO, and several U.S. city and state public health officials that subscribe to Veratect's service, and records indicate that the PAHO accessed it on April 9 and 10 (Wilson, pers. comm., December 3, 2009).

On April 10, the GPHIN notified the WHO of acute respiratory illness in La Gloria (Brownstein et al., 2010), and on the following day the PAHO IHR focal point (the point of contact with the WHO under the IHR) requested verification. On Sunday, April 12, Mexico's Director General of Epidemiology, Hugo López-Gatell, who served as the Mexican IHR focal point, confirmed the existence of acute respiratory infections, but said the initial epidemiologic investigation produced no evidence of a link to fecal contamination from pig farms (Cohen, 2009a). Dr. López-Gatell considered this outbreak to be a potential "public health emergency of international concern" (PHEIC) because it met IHR criteria (severe public health impact and an unusual event) and provided a detailed report to the PAHO. On April 13, based on a trilateral collaboration agreement, this communication was shared with the IHR focal points in the United States and Canada, and was discussed in a teleconference on April 16. Concerned that this pattern was similar to severe acute respiratory syndrome (SARS),the WHO requested verification (Harris, 2009), and Mexican authorities quickly responded that lab tests had failed to find any connection to a SARS-like or even a flu virus. On April 17, Dr. López-Gatell sought information from local officials about a cluster of cases of acute respiratory illness in a hospital in Oaxaca and was told there was no cluster, but rather a single patient with diabetes with a severe case of acute respiratory illness, presumably of viral origin (Cohen, 2009c). The same day, Mexico notified the PAHO of this case, noting the possibility that it could be related to the cases of pH1N1 in the United States.

On April 17, InDRE Director Celia Alpuche contacted the Canadian National Microbiology Laboratory (NML), part of the Public Health Agency of Canada, for help in dealing with the situation that was developing. Dr. Alpuche knew the NML's director, Frank Plummer, through the Global Health Security Action Group and other international collaborations, and valued his expertise dealing with SARS and other unknown pathogens. In a teleconference the following day, InDRE and NML officials concluded the outbreak was likely to be a novel agent, unrelated to influenza. After a conference call between Mexico, Canada, the United States, and the PAHO, Mexican samples were sent to the NML and the CDC; on April 23, both labs identified the viral subtype aspH1N1. This collaboration was possible because of the Security and Prosperity Partnership of North America, a trilateral agreement between the United States, Canada, and Mexico launched in March 2005. The CDC Morbidity and Mortality Weekly Report on two California children confirmed with swine influenza A was posted on the ProMED website on April 21, which was the first report regarding pH1N1 (ProMED, 2009). On April 24, ProMED also reported severe respiratory illness clusters in Mexico and connected them with the U.S. cases (ProMED, 2009).

Aware of the developments in Mexico and Canada, Veratect attempted to contact the CDC, and California and Texas officials on April 16 and 17. On April 20, Veratect attempted urgently to contact the CDC. James Wilson, Veratect Medical Director, said in December 2009 that he had been more concerned about this situation than any other in many years of surveillance work (Wilson, pers. comm., December 3. 2009). However, Dr. Wilson was quoted in the *Washington Post* on May 3, 2009, as having said "I suspect this is probably a false alarm."

On April 22, Mexico's IHR focal point alerted the PAHO about an unusual outbreak of atypical pneumonia in young adults and indicated a probable relation of these events to the outbreak in La Gloria (Lopez-Gatell, 2009b). On April 25, the Mexican epidemiologic evidence, together with the laboratory results confirming the pH1N1 subtype in both Mexican and U.S. cases, led the WHO to declare a "Public Health Emergency of International Concern" (Chan, 2009). During the next few days, Canada, plus a number of countries in Europe, the Middle East, and Asian-Pacific regions, reported suspected cases. Reflecting the rapid spread of the virus, the WHO raised the global pandemic threat level from phase 3 to phase 4 on April 27. By May 6, the WHO had reported 1,893 confirmed cases in 23 countries. Because cases were identified in these countries so shortly after reagents were available for testing, it is likely the virus was actually circulating days to weeks earlier.

Implications for Policy and Practice

A/California/7/2009, now known as pH1N1, was circulating in Mexico and the United States in March 2009 and perhaps earlier. That it was a novel pathogen came to the world's attention in April because of three critical events: the identification of novel pH1N1 in two California children and its subsequent connection to the Mexican cases, the recognition that multiple and apparently disparate disease outbreaks throughout Mexico were connected, and the recognition that an outbreak in New York City was connected to the Mexican and California cases.

The first critical event was the identification of pH1N1 in two California children through the NHRC's surveillance research program. Because the epidemiologic information suggested human-to-human transmission, this triggered a series of events involving three laboratories (the Marshfield Clinic, the Wisconsin State Laboratory of Hygiene, and eventually the CDC, which identified the pathogen). Although the first child became ill on March 28, the

CDC did not identify pH1N1, a potential public health emergency of international importance under the IHR, until the second child was also determined to have pH1N1 on April 17, three weeks later and five days after Mexico had notified of a potential PHEIC regarding the La Gloria outbreak. In retrospect, one might ask whether this identification could have occurred earlier. A review of the timing of the events suggests that it could have, but only if health officials in California, Wisconsin, and the CDC knew it was a novel pathogen, which of course they did not know. To find two children with unsubtypable influenza at the end of the flu season is not remarkable, and indeed it is only because of the research being conducted at the NHRC that these cases came to light at all.

The second critical event (which actually started earlier than the first) was the recognition that a number of disease outbreaks throughout Mexico with apparently different epidemiologic characteristics represented a single phenomenon and thus were a potential PHEIC. Health authorities in Veracruz and Tlaxcala were aware of outbreaks with an unusual high frequency of severe pneumonia in otherwise healthy young people in March, and in the week of April 5, national authorities came to realize the outbreaks were related, resulting in the first international alert on Sunday, April 12. However it was not recognized that the responsible pathogen was pH1N1 until April 23, two days after the CDC identified the new virus strain and published its alert about pH1N1 in the children from California. Two labs in Canada and the United States were able to test samples from Mexico and determine quickly—in only two days—that pH1N1 was the pathogen.

Although the samples were sent earlier than the established protocol in response to Mexican authorities' growing concerns, one might ask whether samples could or should have been sent for testing earlier. As indicated in Figure 2-1, during the week of April 12, which happened to begin on Easter Sunday and which coincidentally included a visit of President Obama to Mexico City, the CDC was identifying pH1N1 in the first two cases and Mexican authorities were conferring with the PAHO and their North American counterparts about the situation. Although GPHIN, HealthMap, and Veratect had been issuing alerts about events in Mexico for more than a week, no one seems to have connected the outbreaks in Mexico and the United States until early in the week of April 19. Had that connection been made earlier, it is possible that the WHO could have declared a PHEIC before Saturday, April 25. Mexican, U.S., and Canadian officials held a trilateral teleconference on April 16, but U.S. participants did not mention the isolation of novel pH1N1, about which they alerted the PAHO one day later. Given the uncertainties and the concern that both Mexican and American health officials must have had about the situation in their own countries during the week of April 12, it is understandable they did not make the connection. Only in retrospect did it become clear that each had the key to the other's epidemiologic puzzle.

The final critical event was the recognition, on April 24, of an outbreak of pH1N1 in New York City high school students who had traveled to Cancun, Mexico, during their Easter recess the previous week. This recognition, only days after the first student became ill, was possible because a school nurse and New York City health officials were aware of pH1N1 and the Mexican situation through alerts and the news media earlier in the week of April 19. Although the New York Department of Health and Mental Hygiene would have definitely investigated an event of this magnitude, knowledge of the CDC and Mexican alerts a few days earlier added urgency to the situation (Fine, pers. comm., Feb. 5, 2011). This in turn contributed to understanding the outbreak's epidemiology and presumably helped trigger the declaration of a health emergency in the United States on April 26, as well as the WHO's alert the previous day. Because the report was filed immediately after the students became ill, and was acted on immediately, it seems unlikely that this could have happened any earlier.

In retrospect, considering the chain of critical events, if the California samples had been tested with more urgency during the week of April 5 rather than that of April 12, and if the results had been reported to Mexican authorities earlier, it seems possible that global alerts about pH1N1 could have been advanced by about one week, to April 18. By this time, however, the virus had spread throughout Mexico and the United States, especially because of Easter travel. So even with the earliest possible recognition of the emerging pandemic, it seems unlikely that the worldwide spread could have been contained. And of course what now seems clear in retrospect was far from clear in April 2009. Indeed, coming at the end of the normal flu season, no single Mexican or American surveillance finding was exceptional, so without the international communication that occurred in 2009, the pandemic could have taken longer to detect and to characterize than it did.

Although it is impossible to quantify the effect, it could have taken much longer for the world to become aware that a new pandemic subtype had emerged. One must only consider the years of effort it took to identify and characterize the human immunodeficiency virus three decades ago, and the resulting confusion (Altman, 2011). Global recognition of the emergence of SARS in 2003, five years earlier, was delayed for weeks despite some awareness of its effect in China (Zhong and Zeng, 2006). In their analysis of 281 WHO–verified nonendemic human infectious disease outbreaks that occurred between 1996 and 2009, Chan and colleagues (2010) found the median time from outbreak start to outbreak discovery decreased from 29.5 days in 1996 to 13.5 days in 2009, and the median time from outbreak start to public communication about the outbreak decreased from 40 days in 1996 to 19 days in 2009. Both the Mexican and the U.S. responses compare favorably with these statistics, and our analysis of the impact of notification systems is consistent the hypothesis of Chan and colleagues (2010) that the improvement was largely a result of the proliferation of Internet–based notification systems. The analysis of Chan and colleagues (2010), however, only addressed the recognition of single outbreaks. Recognizing that the same pathogen was responsible for outbreaks at various locations throughout Mexico and in southern California and New York City, and moreover that the pathogen was a newly emerged viral subtype, is more challenging. It is rare for subtypes to be identified so quickly (Morens, pers. comm., February 5, 2011), but modifications in the protocol to assess the importance of nonsubtypable strains before its definitive confirmation may provide opportunities for more timely responses.

Analysis of these critical events shows how global investments in disease surveillance and notification, coupled with a heightened awareness of pandemic influenza, contributed to an enhanced public health response to pH1N1. First, enhanced laboratory capacity in the United States and Canada led to earlier identification and characterization of pH1N1. Among other things, this recognition triggered national and global pandemic plans, PCR-based tests were developed quickly to aid in surveillance and clinical decision-making, and a vaccine seed strain was developed quickly that led to the development of the pandemic vaccine in time to be used during the second pandemic wave in fall 2009 (although not before that wave began), in which the CDC took a leading role. In particular, the early detection was the result primarily of the existence of an experimental influenza surveillance system developed and operated by the U.S. Navy's NHRC in southern California, which identified the first two cases. Laboratory response networks initiated or enhanced in recent years were also critical because they enabled the involvement of the CDC and Canada's NML, which had the capacity to recognize pH1N1 as novel. This includes the collaboration among Mexico's InDRE, the NML, and the CDC that was possible because of the Security and Prosperity Partnership of North America agreement as well as protocols and relationships that facilitated collaboration among the NHRC, the Marshfield Clinic, the Wisconsin State Laboratory of Hygiene, the New York City Department of Health and Mental Hygiene, and the CDC.

Second, enhanced global notification systems led to earlier detection and characterization of the outbreak by helping to "connect the dots" between cases in California, Mexico, and New York City. Through SINAVE and other sources, Mexican officials were aware, for instance, of a serious problem the week of April 12, but it was not until the CDC's publication regarding pH1N1 in California the following week that they sent samples and realized the two outbreaks were the same. After the pandemic, and with the support of the United States and Canada, Mexico has also developed its own capabilities for rt-PCR testing throughout the country, facilitating much faster diagnosis. Similarly, without the awareness that the same virus that was making children ill in California and circulating widely—and seriously affecting young people—in Mexico, during the week of April 19, the school nurse in Queens and New York City health officials might not have taken the outbreak as seriously as they did in students who had traveled to Mexico the previous week. The notification systems that contributed to these results include the IHR, voluntary reporting systems such as ProMED, and active searching activities by GPHIN, HealthMap, Argus, and Veratect. In addition, some have speculated that countries' awareness that outbreaks within their borders will soon come to light through these channels increases the likelihood they will report these outbreaks themselves (Katz, 2009).

The early events in the 2009 H1N1 pandemic thus illustrate the important contribution of the 2005 IHR and the paradigm shift that accompanied it. This includes the definition of a PHEIC as a comprehensive and flexible representation of health hazards, the algorithm for risk assessment (Annex 2 of the IHR), and the existence of national focal points that can (and are mandated to) communicate directly with the WHO rather than go through diplomatic channels. In this experience, the IHR system was also instrumental in speeding two-way communications between Mexico and the PAHO and between the United States and the PAHO. Similarly, the North American Plan for Avian and Pandemic Influenza (NAPAPI) facilitated communication among Mexican, U.S., and Canadian health authorities (U.S. Department of State, 2007). On the other hand, Mexico, Canada, and the United States currently have no official protocols for sharing information from event-based surveillance sources such as GPHIN, HealthMap and Veratect. The second edition of the NAPAPI, published in April 2012, seeks to develop a more effective international sharing mechanism based on the lessons learned from the 2009 pandemic (U.S. Department of State, 2012).

Syndromic surveillance systems played an important role in detecting the pH1N1 outbreak, but a different one than is commonly used to justify them—that such systems can detect outbreaks before conventional surveillance systems and enable a rapid public health response (Stoto, 2007). Because pH1N1 emerged during the normal flu season, there were too few cases to have been detected by standard alerting algorithms. In the United States, for instance, the earliest appearance of the pandemic did not trigger a quantitative alert in any syndromic surveillance system, although four of the earliest cases presented at providers who were members of the CDC's U.S. Outpatient Influenza-like Illness Surveillance Network (ILINet), and were tested and flagged for attention (Lipsitch et al., 2011). In Mexico, however, general acute respiratory illness with no laboratory diagnosis is a notifiable condition. A sharp increase in such reports to SINAVE in early April, along with an analysis indicating an atypical age distribution (Chowell et al., 2009), helped Mexican officials realize the problem they were seeing was widespread, and led authorities to conduct active surveillance for severe pneumonia starting April 17, influenzalike illness in patients visiting primary healthcare units and hospitals, and influenza-related deaths (Chowell et al., 2011).

Conclusions

An analysis of this sort is clearly limited in two important respects. First, because public health experts in the midst of deciphering the facts of a disease outbreak rarely take notes—it is often not clear until days or weeks into an outbreak that there is anything worth recording—any retrospective analysis is subject to recall bias colored by the epidemiologic data and explanations that eventually emerged (Weick and Sutcliffe, 2011). For instance, facts and events that might not have seemed important in isolation at the time take on added significance after the fact if they fit the epidemiologic story that was eventually constructed. Second, it is impossible to know what would have occurred in counterfactual circumstances—if, for example, a certain surveillance system had not existed. For instance, the fact that by 2009 the world was four to five years into a period of enhanced concern about pandemic influenza means that even in the absence of any concrete surveillance and notification enhancements, it is likely that the public health response was better than what might have been expected before the avian influenza outbreak that started in Hong Kong in 1997 and the SARS outbreak in 2003.

Despite these limitations, a systematic analysis of three critical events that occurred during March and April 2009—identification of pH1N1 in samples from two children from California, the recognition that multiple and apparently disparate disease outbreaks throughout Mexico represented a single phenomenon related to the California cases, and the recognition that an outbreak of influenza in New York City high school students were part of the same picture—shows that enhanced laboratory-based surveillance coupled with improved global notification systems did seem to have improved the global public health response to pH1N1. The surveillance enhancements that made this possible include an experimental influenza surveillance system operated by the NHRC in southern California and laboratory response networks linking Mexico's InDRE, Canada's NML, and the CDC, as well as private and public health laboratories in the United States. The global notification systems that contributed to these results include formal and informal channels as well as activities such as GPHIN, HealthMap, ProMED Mail, Argus, and Veratect, which actively search the Internet for evidence of disease outbreaks. At the national level, starting in May 2008, Mexican authorities held a weekly meeting, named "Epidemiologic Pulse," to scan and assess epidemiologic events in Mexico and the world. This session played a key role in integrating the information from formal and informal sources that emerged nearly a year later. PAHO officials attended the April 15 session at which the La Gloria situation was discussed. The trilateral teleconference the following day was enabled by NAPAPI, a nonlegally-binding agreement prepared under the Security and Prosperity Partnership of North America treaty (U.S. Department of State, 2007). Because most of these resources did not exist a decade earlier, it seems likely the investments in building these systems, together with a heightened awareness of pandemic influenza, enabled a more rapid and effective global public health response to H1N1.

Considering the chain of critical events, it is possible that global alerts about pH1N1 could have been advanced by about one week to April 18. However, because the virus had already spread throughout Mexico, the United States, and elsewhere by that time, it seems unlikely an earlier global alert would have made a difference in containing the worldwide spread of the virus. Rather, recognizing there are many false positives in epidemiology, and what now seems clear in retrospect was far from clear in April 2009, the picture that emerges from this analysis is a global public health system, and particularly public health agencies in Mexico, Canada, and the United States, that worked together effectively to solve a challenging epidemiologic puzzle in a reasonably timely fashion.

This analysis also illustrates the challenges of early detection and characterization in public health emergencies. First, although in retrospect the events described in this analysis clearly add up to tell the story of the emergence of a new pandemic viral subtype, many of the events—even large numbers of respiratory illness cases at the end of the winter flu season—taken in isolation were not sufficient to cause alarm. Given the number of such "signals" that truly are isolated events, it is not useful or appropriate for local, national, or international public health agencies to react with alarm on every such occasion. Second, as with most novel pathogens, the emergence of pH1N1 was characterized by uncertainty that took weeks to months to resolve. Many emergency preparedness professionals, however, still think in terms of single cases triggering a response in hours or at most days, and this thinking is reflected in such key public health preparedness documents as the CDC's 2011 *Public Health Preparedness Capabilities: National Standards for State and Local Planning* (Division of State and Local Readiness in the Office of Public Health Preparedness and Response, Centers for Disease Control and Prevention, 2011).

Epidemiologists familiar with the emergence of novel pathogens rightly compare the rapidly evolving facts and scientific knowledge with the "fog of war" (Stoto et al., 2005), and the United Kingdom's Pandemic Influenza Preparedness Programme has shown how it should be factored into public health preparedness planning (Pandemic Influenza Preparedness Team, 2011). Similarly, recognition that it may take time to understand and characterize an emerging threat has important implications for implementation of the IHR, which define a PHEIC through a flow chart (Gostin, 2004; Katz, 2009) that implicitly presumes a bright line between a PHEIC and other outbreaks.

More broadly, this recognition means it is important to expect and plan for uncertainty in preparing for the emergence of a new pathogen. This task requires attention to response *capabilities* in addition to preparedness *capacities*. For instance, the CDC's and the Trust for America's Health's most recent state-by-state assessments of public health preparedness focus on ensuring that state and local public health laboratories can respond rapidly, can identify or rule out particular known biological agents, and have the workforce and surge capacity to process large numbers of samples during an emergency (Office of Public Health Preparedness and Response, 2010; Trust for America's Health, 2010). Similarly, the Global Health Security Agenda announced in February 2014 that it seeks to build capacity by developing and strengthening diagnostic and laboratory systems, and global networks for sharing biosurveillance information and training, and by deploying a workforce to ensure the effective functioning of these systems (U.S. Department of Health and Human Services, 2014). Although such capabilities seem necessary for some events, they are not sufficient, and none of these measures would have ensured the public health system could have identified the emergence of and characterized pH1N1 as well and as efficiently as it was done in Mexico and the United States in April 2009. Rather, the surveillance system capabilities that were most essential were the availability of laboratory networks capable of identifying a novel pathogen, notification systems that made health officials aware of the epidemiologic facts emerging from numerous locations in at least two countries, and the intelligence necessary to connect the dots and understand their implications.

Last, this analysis illustrates the potential of the critical events approach for collecting, analyzing, and understanding the policy implications of data from real incidents on public health system' emergency response capabilities. There are three critical components of this approach; each requires professional judgment and knowledge of public health systems.

First, the analyst must prepare a timeline that describes key events in both the epidemiology and the public health response, such as the one in Figure 2-1. This task can be a challenge because, as noted previously, early events are not, in and of themselves, seen as noteworthy and are typically not recorded as they occur. Situation reports that are now prepared routinely by emergency response organizations can be helpful, but are typically not started until there is an indication of a problem. For instance, the CDC did not activate its Emergency Operations Center for pH1N1 until April 22, 2009, which was more than a month after the outbreak began in Mexico. Alternatively, it would be useful to record retrospectively the officials' knowledge and understanding of events as soon as possible after it becomes clear a public health emergency is underway.

Second, based on this timeline, one must identify the critical events. These are events of more complexity than the recognition of a cluster of cases, but less than the emergence of a new pathogen. They represent opportunities when the response might have occurred sooner or later than it did, depending on the public health system's capabilities. This is comparable, in a standard root-cause analysis, with the choke points in the process map when errors occur. For this analysis, for instance, we choose incidents that advanced the recognition of, and enabled a response to, the global pandemic. Identifying these events was challenging, but the careful creation of a timeline was an essential first step.

Last, the analyst must identify the factors that allowed the events to occur when they did, rather than earlier or later. In a standard root-cause analysis, these are the root causes. This task requires knowledge of how public health systems are supposed to perform and the factors that can degrade this performance. It is also useful to consider what might have happened had the critical events turned out differently, an approach that March and colleagues describe as "simulating experience" (March et al., 1991).

Learning about public health systems' emergency response capabilities is challenging because actual events are unique, and both the epidemiologic facts and the context varies from one community to another. In other words, there is no replication—a centerpiece of the scientific method. In this context, our analysis of the global public health system's ability to detect the pH1N1 pandemic gains rigor not by statistical analysis of repeated events, but rather by a detailed analysis of the timing of events in Mexico, the United States, and the rest of the world. The kind of analysis described here is far more extensive and probing than is commonly seen in the after-action reports prepared by health departments after exercises or actual events (Stoto et al., 2013) and illustrates the potential of the critical events approach for learning about public health system' emergency response capabilities from real incidents that the NHSS implementation guide calls for (U.S. Department of Health and Human Services, 2009b; Stoto, 2014).

Acknowledgments and Disclosures

This research was conducted with funding support awarded to the Harvard School of Public Health under cooperative agreements with the U.S. CDC (grant no. 5P01TP000307). The authors are grateful for comments from John Brownstein, Melissa Higdon, Tamar Klaiman, John Kraemer, Larissa May, Christopher Nelson, Hilary Placzek, Ellen Whitney, Ying Zhang, the staff of the CDC Public Health Surveillance Program Office, and others who commented on presentations. The data and conclusions have been previously published in:

- Zhang, Y., Lopez-Gatell, H., Alpuche-Aranda, C., Stoto, M.A. (2013). Did advances in global surveillance and notification systems make a difference in the 2009 H1N1 pandemic?–A retrospective analysis. *PLoS ONE 8*, e59893.

References

Altman, L.K. (2011). 30 Years in, we are still learning*from AIDS. The New York Times*, D1. Accessed May 11, 2011, at http://www.nytimes.com/2011/05/31/health/31aids.html.

Brownstein, J.S., Freifeld, C.C., Chan, E.H., Keller, M., Sonricker, A.L. (2010).Information technology and global surveillance of cases of 2009 H1N1 influenza. *The New England Journal of Medicine, 362*(18), 1731–1735.

Centers for Disease Control and Prevention. (2009a). CDC—seasonal influenza (flu)—weekly report: influenza summary update 2008–2009 influenza season week 33 ending August 22, 2009. Accessed January 18, 2011, at http://www.cdc.gov/flu/weekly/weeklyarchives2008-2009/weekly33.htm.

Centers for Disease Control and Prevention. (2009b). CDC—seasonal influenza (flu)—weekly report: influenza summary update 2008–2009 influenza season week 34 ending august 29, 2009. Accessed January 18, 2011, at http://www.cdc.gov/flu/weekly/weeklyarchives2008-2009/weekly34.htm.

Centers for Disease Control and Prevention. (2009c). CDC—seasonal influenza (flu)—weekly report: influenza summary update 2008–2009 influenza season week 35 ending September 5, 2009. Accessed January 18, 2011, at http://www.cdc.gov/flu/weekly/weeklyarchives2008-2009/weekly35.htm.

Centers for Disease Control and Prevention. (2009d). Swine influenza A (H1N1) infection in two children: southern California, March–April 2009. *MMWR Morbidity and Mortality Weekly Report, 58*(15), 400–402.

Centers for Disease Control and Prevention. (2009e). Swine-origin influenza A (H1N1) virus infections in a school: New York City, April 2009. *MMWR Morbidity and Mortality Weekly Report, 58*(17), 470–472.

Centers for Disease Control and Prevention. (2009f). Update: novel influenza A (H1N1) virus infections—worldwide, May 6, 2009. *MMWR Morbidity and Mortality Weekly Report, 58*(17), 453–458.

Chan, M. (2009). Swine influenza: statement by WHO Director-General, Dr. Margaret Chan. Accessed February 25, 2011, at http://www.who.int/mediacentre/news/statements/2009/h1n1_20090425/en/index.html.

Chan, E.H., Brewer, T.F., Madoff, L.C., Pollack, M.P., Sonricker, A.L. (2010). Global capacity for emerging infectious disease detection. *Proceedings of the National Academy of Sciences of the United States of America, 107*(50), 21701–21706.

Chowell, G., Bertozzi, S.M., Colchero, M.A., Lopez-Gatell, H., Alpuche-Aranda, C. (2009). Severe respiratory disease concurrent with the circulation of H1N1 influenza. *The New England Journal of Medicine, 361*(7), 674–679.

Chowell, G., Echevarrã-Zuno, S., Viboud, C., Simonsen, L., Tamerius, J. (2011). Characterizing the epidemiology of the 2009 influenza A/H1N1 pandemic in Mexico. *PLoS Medicine, 8*(5), e1000436.

Cohen, J. (2009a). Exclusive: interview with head of Mexico's top swine flu lab. Accessed January 18, 2011, at http://news.sciencemag.org/scienceinsider/2009/05/exclusive-inter.html.

Cohen, J. (2009b). Swine flu outbreak, day by day. Accessed June 1, 2011, at http://news.sciencemag.org/scienceinsider/special/swine-flu-timeline.html.

Cohen, J. (2009c). Yet another new patient zero in swine flu pandemic. Accessed February 25, 2011, at http://news.sciencemag.org/scienceinsider/2009/07/yet-another-new.html.

Cordova-Villalobos, J.A., Sarti, E., Arzoz-Padres, J., Manuell-Lee, G., Mendez, J.R. (2009). The influenza A (H1N1) epidemic in Mexico: lessons learned. *Health Research Policy and Systems*, 7,21.

Division of State and Local Readiness in the Office of Public Health Preparedness and Response, Centers for Disease Control and Prevention. (2011). Public health preparedness capabilities: national standards for state and local planning. Accessed May 31, 2011, at http://www.cdc.gov/phpr/capabilities/.

Frenk, J. (2009). Mexico's fast diagnosis. *The New York Times*, A23. Accessed January 18, 2011, at http://www.nytimes.com/2009/05/01/opinion/01frenk.html.

Gostin, L.O. (2004). International infectious disease law: revision of the world health organization's international health regulations. *Journal of the American Medical Association, 291*(21), 2623–2627.
Harris G. (2009). Questions linger over the value of a global illness surveillance system. *The New York Times*, A7. Accessed January 18, 2011, at http://www.nytimes.com/2009/05/02/health/02global.html.
Hitchcock, P., Chamberlain, A., Van Wagoner, M., Inglesby, T.V., O'Toole, T. (2007). Challenges to global surveillance and response to infectious disease outbreaks of international importance. *Biosecurity and Bioterrorism, 5*(3), 206–227.
Jhung, M.A., Swerdlow, D., Olsen, S.J., Jernigan, D., Biggerstaff, M. (2011). Epidemiology of 2009 pandemic influenza A(H1N1) in the United States. *Clinical Infectious Diseases*, 52(Suppl 1), S13–S26.
Katz, R. (2009). Use of revised international health regulations during influenza A (H1N1) epidemic, 2009. *Emerging Infectious Diseases, 15*(8), 1165–1170.
Lezana, M. (2009). Mitigating the spread of A/H1N1: lessons learned from past outbreaks. Accessed June 25, 2009, at http://mcmsc.asu.edu/conferences/files/Miguel%20%C3%80ongel%20Lezana%20Fern%CE%ACndez%20-%20H%201N1%E2%80%A8%20Epidemic%20in%20Mexico,%E2%80%A8Lessons%20Learned.pdf.
Lipsitch, M., Finelli, L., Heffernan, R.T., Leung, G.M., Redd, S.C. (2011). Improving the evidence base for decision making during a pandemic: the example of 2009 influenza A/H1N1. *Biosecurity and Bioterrorism, 9*(2), 89–115.
Lopez-Gatell, H. (2009a). Emergency notification of potential public health importance (PHEIC): outbreak of acute respiratory disease at La Gloria, Perote, Veracruz, Mexico, April 12th, 2009.
Lopez-Gatell, H. (2009b). Keynote lecture: influenza A (H1N1): a pandemic expected? Presented at the 30th National Congress of the Mexican Association of Infectious Disease and Clinical Microbiology. Guadalajara, Jalisco, Mexico.
March, J.G., Sproull, L.S., Tamuz, M. (1991). Learning from samples of one or fewer. *Organization Science, 2*(1), 1–13.
Ministry of Health Mexico. (2010). Influenza estadísticas: situación actual de la epidemia (31 de Mayo de 2010). Accessed February 25, 2011, at http://portal.salud.gob.mx/opencms/opencms/sites/salud/descargas/pdf/influenza/situacion_actual_epidemia_310510.pdf.
Ministry of Health Mexico. (2012). Centro nacional de vigilancia epidemiologica y control de enfermedades [National Center of Epidemiological Surveillance and Diseases Control]. Accessed July 11, 2012, at http://www.dgepi.salud.gob.mx/.
Office of Public Health Preparedness and Response. (2010). 2010 Report: public health preparedness: strengthening the nation's emergency response state by state. Accessed February 21, 2011, at http://www.bt.cdc.gov/publications/2010phprep/pdf/complete_PHPREP_report.pdf.
Pandemic Influenza Preparedness Team. (2011). UK influenza pandemic preparedness strategy 2011: strategy for consultation. Accessed May 30, 2011, at http://www.dh.gov.uk/en/Consultations/Liveconsultations/DH_125316.
Paquet, C., Coulombier, D., Kaiser, R., Ciotti, M. (2006) Epidemic intelligence: a new framework for strengthening disease surveillance in Europe. *Eurosurveillance, 11*(12), 212–214.

ProMED. (2009). Influenza A (H1N1) virus, swine, human. Accessed December 20, 2012, at http://www.promedmail.org/direct.php?id=20090422.1516.

Stoto, M.A. (2007). Syndromic surveillance in public health practice. In: Institute of Medicine, editor. *Global infectious disease surveillance and detection: assessing the challenges—finding solutions, workshop summary*. Washington, DC: National Academy Press.

Stoto, M.A. (2014). Biosurveillance capability requirements for the Global Health Security Agenda: lessons from the 2009 H1N1 pandemic. *Biosecurity and Bioterrorism, 12*, 225–230.

Stoto, M.A., Dausey, D.J., Davis, L.M., Leuschner, K., Lurie, N. (2005). Learning from experience: the public health response to WestNile virus, SARS, monkeypox, and hepatitis A outbreaks in the United States. RAND Health, TR-285-DHHS. Accessed May 31, 2011, at http://www.rand.org/pubs/technical_reports/TR285.html.

Stoto, M.A., Nelson, C., Higdon, M.A., Kraemer, J.D., Singleton, C.M. (2013). Learning about after action reporting from the 2009 H1N1 pandemic: a workshop summary. *Journal of Public Health Management and Practice, 19*, 420–427.

Swerdlow, D.L., Finelli, L., Bridges, C.B. (2011). 2009 H1N1 influenza pandemic: field and epidemiologic investigations in the United States at the start of the first pandemic of the 21st century. *Clinical Infectious Diseases, 52*(Suppl 1), S1–S3.

Trust for America's Health. (2010). Ready or not 2010: protecting the public's health from disease, disasters, and bioterrorism. Accessed January 18, 2011, at http://healthyamericans.org/reports/bioterror10/.

U.S. Department of Health and Human Services. (2009a). National health security strategy of the United States of America. Accessed February 21, 2012, at http://www.phe.gov/Preparedness/planning/authority/nhss/strategy/Documents/nhss-final.pdf

U.S. Department of Health and Human Services. (2009b). Interim implementation guide for the national health security strategy of the United States of America. Accessed February 21, 2011, at http://www.phe.gov/Preparedness/planning/authority/nhss/implementationguide/Documents/iig-final.pdf.

U.S. Department of Health and Human Services. (2009c). HHS declares public health emergency for swine flu. Accessed February 25, 2011, at http://www.hhs.gov/news/press/2009pres/04/20090426a.html.

U.S. Department of Health and Human Services. (2014). Global health security agenda: toward a world safe & secure from infectious disease threats. Accessed May 5, 2014, at http://www.globalhealth.gov/global-health-topics/global-health-security/GHS%20Agenda.pdf.

U.S. Department of State. (2007). North American Plan For Animal and Pandemic Influenza. Accessed September 27, 2014 at http://www.spp-psp.gc.ca/eic/site/spp-psp.nsf/vwapj/pandemic-influenza.pdf/$FILE/pandemic-influenza.pdf.

U.S. Department of State. (2012). North American Plan For Animal and Pandemic Influenza. Accessed September 27, 2014 at http://www.phe.gov/Preparedness/international/Documents/napapi.pdf

Weaver, M., Tuckman, J. (2009). Mexican swine flu deaths spark worldwide action. Accessed May 30, 2011, at http://www.guardian.co.uk/world/2009/apr/27/swine-flu-search-outbreak-source.
Weick, K.E., Sutcliffe, K.M. (2011). *Managing the unexpected.* Hoboken, NJ: Wiley.
Zhong, N., Zeng, G. (2006). What we have learnt from SARS epidemics in China. *British Medical Journal, 333*(7564), 389–391.

CHAPTER 3

The Effectiveness of U.S. Public Health Surveillance Systems for Situational Awareness during the 2009 H1N1 Pandemic

MICHAEL A. STOTO

Introduction

In spring 2009, a novel H1N1 influenza virus, now denoted pH1N1, emerged in North America and spread to the rest of the world in less than two months (World Health Organization, 2009). In the United States, where some of the first cases emerged, one of the public health challenges was to track the spread of the new virus and characterize its epidemiologic properties to guide and monitor the effects of response efforts. Existing public health surveillance and laboratory systems rapidly developed a case definition and new testing procedures, but public health laboratories soon became overloaded with samples to be tested, and surveillance definitions and procedures were changed as necessary to handle the load. Later in the year, as the epidemiologic characteristics of pH1N1 emerged, traditional influenza surveillance systems were augmented with new systems tailored to the emerging epidemiology (Brammer et al., 2011). Some of these new systems could be described as syndromic surveillance approaches that, by using prediagnostic data, were thought to have a distinct advantage over the traditional surveillance method in terms of timeliness (President's Council of Advisors on Science and Technology, 2009).

The epidemiology of pH1N1 has been well described elsewhere (Jhung et al., 2011; Swerdlow et al., 2011), and adding to this understanding is not the goal of this chapter. Rather, our purpose is to learn from the 2009 H1N1 pandemic about the strengths and weaknesses of current U.S. public health surveillance systems and to identify implications for measuring public health emergency preparedness. To do this, we focus on two critical issues. First, we address the widely held perception that children and young adults were at "higher risk." Second, we assess the validity and utility of syndromic surveillance systems that were promoted by the President's Council of Advisors on Science and Technology (PCAST) (President's Council of Advisors on Science and Technology, 2009) and other authorities. Both of these issues relate to the ability of public health surveillance systems to provide "situational awareness"—critical information needed to respond to disease outbreaks and other public health emergencies—including numbers of cases and other traditional surveillance data, and information on critical response resources, medical care capacity, environmental threats, and public awareness (Government Accountability Office, 2010a).

We begin with a discussion of the data and methods used in this chapter, including indicators of the information environment during 2009 and how that might have biased the available surveillance data. We then review (1) the evidence regarding differential age-specific risks associated with pH1N1 and (2) surveillance systems' ability to monitor pH1N1 cases accurately over time. The discussion section addresses the limitations of this study, the implications of this analysis regarding both the strengths and weaknesses of current surveillance systems, alternatives that should be considered for the future, and the implications of this analysis for the measurement of public health preparedness.

Background

To provide situational awareness during a public health emergency, public health agencies rely on a collection of public health surveillance systems. Many of these systems are operated by the Centers for Disease Control and Prevention (CDC), and they include systems for virologic surveillance and for tracking outpatient illness, influenza-associated hospitalizations, pneumonia- and influenza-related mortality, influenza-associated pediatric deaths, and the geographic spread of influenza (Brammer et al., 2011). Other data are provided by state and local health departments, and private-sector organizations, as described later.

The primary means for virologic surveillance is the World Health Organization(WHO)-affiliated National Respiratory and Enteric Virus Surveillance System (NREVSS), through which 140 public- and private-sector collaborating laboratories submit weekly information on the total number of respiratory specimens tested for influenza and the number positive by influenza type, subtype, and age group (Brammer et al., 2011).

Outpatient illness surveillance is conducted by the CDC's Influenza-Like Illness Surveillance Network (ILINet). ILINet receives weekly reports from more than 3,300 healthcare providers on the total number of patients seen for any reason and the number of patients with influenzalike illness (ILI), by age group, defined as a temperature of more than 37.8°C and cough and/or sore throat, in the absence of a known cause other than influenza (Brammer et al., 2011). In addition, since late 2009, the CDC has partnered with the International

Society for Disease Surveillance through the Distributed Surveillance Taskforce for Real-Time Influenza Burden Tracking and Evaluation (DiSTRIBuTE) project to gather and analyze aggregate emergency department (ED) surveillance data from a number of state and local jurisdictions, each using its own definition of ILI (Distributed Surveillance Taskforce for Real-Time Influenza Burden Tracking and Evaluation, 2011). Our analysis also uses ED data from an integrated health system operating 18 hospitals in a western state (McDonnell et al., 2012).

The CDC, in collaboration with state health departments and academic centers in 10 states, collects data on laboratory-confirmed influenza-associated hospitalizations in children and adults through the Emerging Infections Program (EIP). This population-based surveillance is conducted in 60 counties that represent 7% of the U.S. population (Brammer et al., 2011). In 2009, the New York State Department of Health supplemented this system with its Sentinel Hospital Program (SHP) (Noyes et al., 2011).

The CDC collects timely, influenza-associated mortality data through two different systems. The 122 Cities Mortality Reporting System receives data from 122 cities throughout the United States on the total number of death certificates received and the number of those for which pneumonia or influenza was listed as the underlying or contributing cause of death. The Influenza-Associated Pediatric Mortality Surveillance System tracks laboratory-confirmed influenza-related deaths among children younger than 18 years based on reports submitted by state, local, and territorial health departments (Brammer et al., 2011). In addition, starting in August 2009, the CDC requested that states submit aggregate data on hospitalizations and deaths from influenza using either a laboratory-confirmed or syndromic case definition through its new aggregate hospitalizations and deaths reporting activity (AHDRA) reporting system.

Another innovation in 2009 was the development and implementation of a module for the CDC's Behavioral Risk Factor Surveillance System (BRFSS) to provide data on ILI in the community. Between September 2009 and March 2010, more than 250,000 adults and children responding to this ongoing, state-based population survey were asked about their own ILI, which was defined as the presence of fever with cough or sore throat the previous month (Centers for Disease Control and Prevention, 2011a).

The geographic distribution of influenza activity across the United States is reported weekly by state and territorial epidemiologists. States report influenza activity as no activity, sporadic, local, regional, or widespread (Brammer et al., 2011). In addition, many of the surveillance data systems described earlier provide regional- or state-level data that are available in the CDC's "Weekly Influenza Surveillance Report FluView."

The final data sources for our analysis come from Google. Google Flu Trends are based on the number of queries using a specific set of flu-related search terms that they have found to be related, in the aggregate, to the number of people who have flu symptoms (Ginsberg et al., 2009). Google Insights for

Search is a more generic tool for quantifying the relative number of Google searches on a certain topic on a weekly basis (Google, 2011). For our analysis we used the number of Internet searches for "swine flu" ("H1N1" was similar during fall 2009, but was uncommon in the spring). We also restricted the analysis to searches for swine flu news items. The information environment, of course, is far more complex than these indices can represent, but they provide an objective general sense of public interest and concern.

Methods

Because there are no data that describe the actual rates of pH1N1 infection in the United States, or its consequences, we adopted a "triangulation" approach (Gilson et al., 2011) in which multiple contemporary data sources, each with different expected biases, are compared to identify time patterns that are likely to reflect biases versus those that are more likely to be indicative of actual infection rates. This public health systems research approach is grounded in the understanding that each of these surveillance systems is a production process. From this perspective, surveillance data are the result of a series of decisions made by patients, healthcare providers, and public health professionals about seeking and providing healthcare and about reporting cases to health authorities. Outpatient, hospital-based, and ED surveillance systems, for instance, all rely on individuals deciding to present themselves to the healthcare system based on their interpretations of their symptoms. Even the number of Google searches and self-reports of ILI in the BRFSS survey can be influenced by searchers' interpretation of the seriousness of their symptoms. Virologic surveillance and systems based on laboratory confirmations all depend on physicians deciding to send samples for testing. Moreover, every element of this decision-making process is influenced by the informational environment (e.g., media coverage, implementation of active surveillance), processing and reacting to the information on an individual level (e.g., the healthcare seeker's self-assessment of risk, incentives for seeking medical attention and self-isolation, the healthcare provider's ordering of laboratory tests), and technical barriers (e.g., communication infrastructure for data exchange, laboratory capacity), all of which change constantly.

Results

The Information Environment

By way of background for the subsequent analyses, Figure 3-1A represents trends in the number of U.S. Google searches for "swine flu" between April 2009 and December 2009 on a scale of 0 to 100. Both the number of general searches (labeled as "Activity index") and news searches ("News index") grew rapidly from zero in mid-April to 100 in the week ending May 2, 2009, corresponding to a rapid set of announcements from the CDC and the WHO about the emergence of the pandemic. Both indices drop off by the end of May. The general searches, but not the news searches, pick up again at the end of August, reaching a peak of 13 on a scale of 0 to 100 at the end of October, and drop off to zero by the end of the year.

Figure 3-1B presents the Google Insights activity index for the United States and for Massachusetts and Georgia populous, and presumably typical states in CDC regions 1 (Northeast) and 4 (South), respectively. In the South, "swine flu" searches peaked at the end of August at 15 and again at 12 in mid-October. In the Northeast, on the other hand, the activity index peaked at 19 at the end of October—higher and a week later than the United States as a whole.

Age-Related Risks of pH1N1

One of the most commonly held perceptions about pH1N1 is that children and young adults are at especially "high risk." For instance, on May 17, 2009, in an article titled "Age of Flu Victims Has Big Implications," *The Washington Post* reported that "perhaps the most worrisome features so far are the number and severity of cases in teenagers and young adults. This was noticed early, and the pattern has not changed much now that there are 5,000 laboratory-confirmed infections and probably more than 100,000 overall. The average age of the confirmed and probable cases is 15 years. Two-thirds are younger than 18" (Brown, 2009). Similarly, an August 2009 PCAST report said that confirmed cases were concentrated in younger age groups, up to 24 years, almost all severe cases were in people younger than 65 years, and the consequences of infection in this epidemic were already known to be far more severe for children and young adults, and seemingly milder for people older than 65 years (President's Council of Advisors on Science and Technology, 2009).

With seasonal influenza, serious illness requiring hospitalization and death are uncommon in children (except for infants) and young adults, so this pattern has important public health implications. Indeed, the fact that the first cases of pH1N1 that came to light in southern California, Mexico, and in New York City were in children and young adults was an important clue that a new pandemic viral subtype had emerged (Cordova-Villalobos et al., 2009). The perception, based on these reports, that children and young adults were "at risk" also led to school closings in spring 2009 (Heymann et al., 2004; Hodge, 2009); the issuance of recommendations for schools, universities, and daycare centers (Centers for Disease Control and Prevention, 2010), and recommendations that children and adolescents be given priority for immunizations (Centers for Disease Control and Prevention, 2009a). The same assumption also influenced recommendations from the WHO (World Health Organization, 2010).

Regarding the other end of the age spectrum, on May 22, 2009, the CDC reported the early results of an antibody study indicating that children had no existing cross-reactive antibody to pH1N1, whereas about one-third of adults older than 60 years had such a reaction. These results were attributed to the

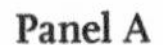

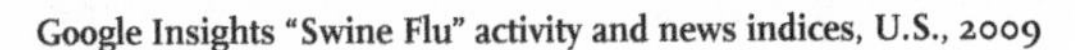

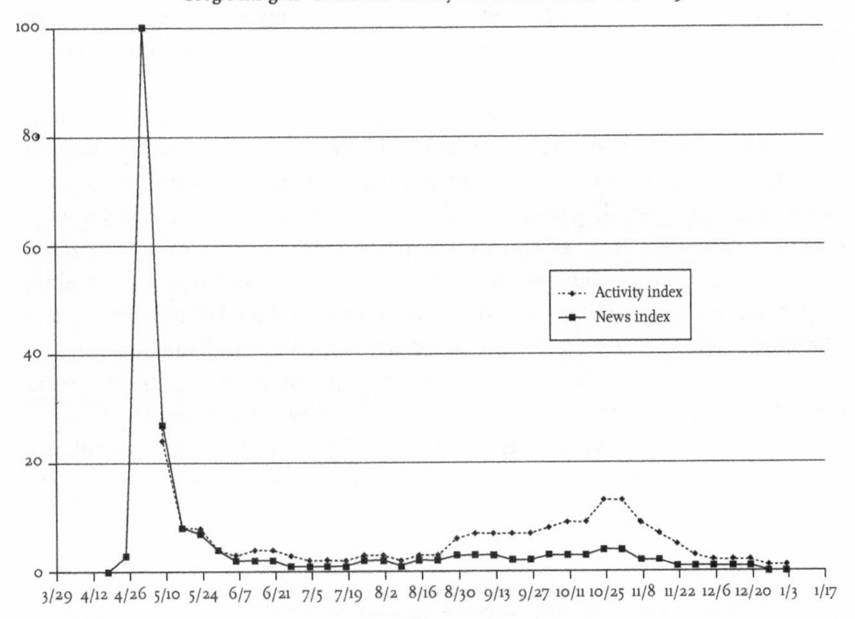

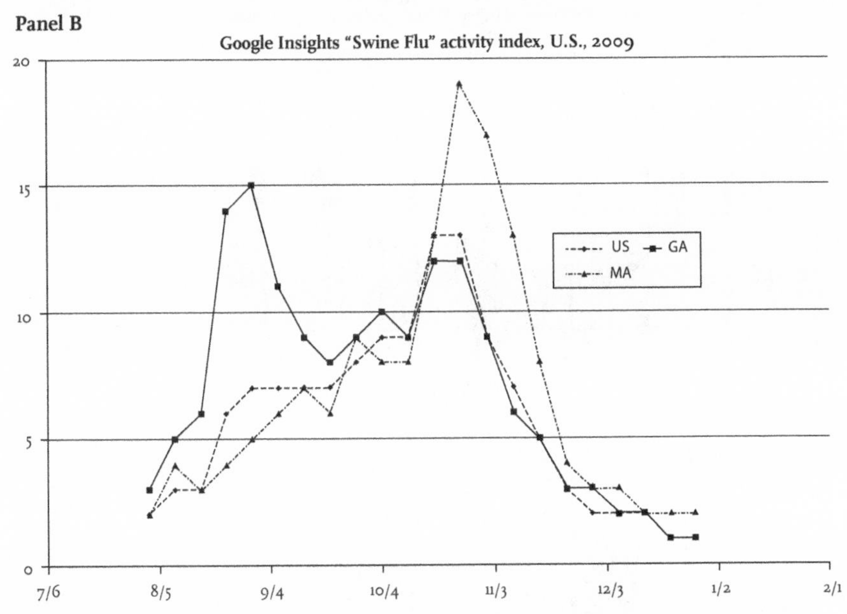

FIGURE 3-1 Google "Swine Flu" indices for the Northeast, South, and entire United States. Panel A. Google Insights "Swine Flu" activity and news indices, U.S., April 12, 2009–January 2, 2010. Panel B. Google Insights "Swine Flu" activity index, U.S., Georgia (GA), and Massachusetts (MA), August 2, 2009–January 2, 2010.

SOURCE: Google Insights search for "swine flu" at http://www.google.com/insights/search/#q=SWINE%20FLU&geo=US&date=1%2F2009%2012m&cmpt=q.doi:10.1371/journal.pone.0040984.g001.

possibility that older people had been previously exposed, either through infection or vaccination, to an influenza A(H1N1) virus that was more closely related to pH1N1 than contemporary seasonal influenza viruses (Centers for Disease Control and Prevention, 2009b).

Typical of the information available early during the pandemic, a report from the CDC published ahead of print by *The New England Journal of Medicine* on May 7, 2009, noted that 60% of 642 confirmed cases were 18 years or younger (Dawood et al., 2009). Similarly, a report of 272 patients who were hospitalized with laboratory-confirmed pH1N1 from April to mid-June 2009 found that 45% were younger than 18 years and 5% were 65 years or older (Jain et al., 2009). Another early study, published in the CDC's *Morbidity and Mortality Weekly Report* in late August, reported that the attack rate was greatest among children 5 to 14 years (147 per 100,000 population)—14 times greater than the rate for adults 60 years and older (Centers for Disease Control and Prevention, 2009c). Shortly afterward, a CDC pediatric deaths surveillance study reported that children younger than 18 years represented 36 of the 477

Panel A

Aggregate hospitalization and death reporting activity (AHDRA) hospitalization and deaths rates per 100,000 population by age group, laboratory-confirmed pH1N1 influenza infection—United States, August 2009–February 2010.

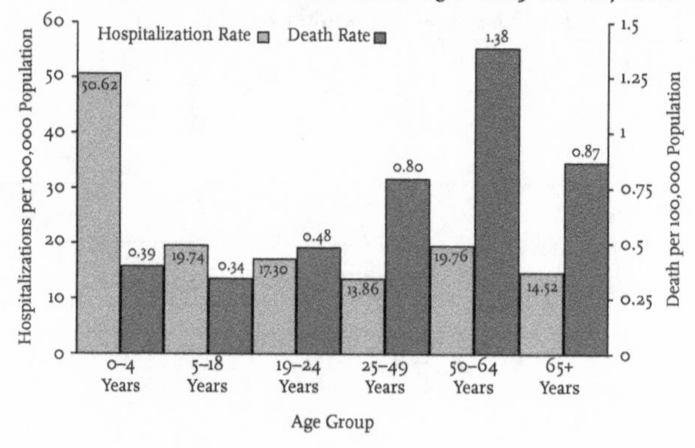

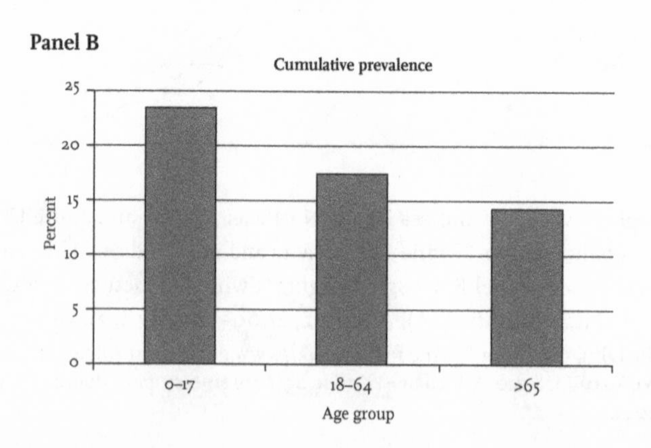

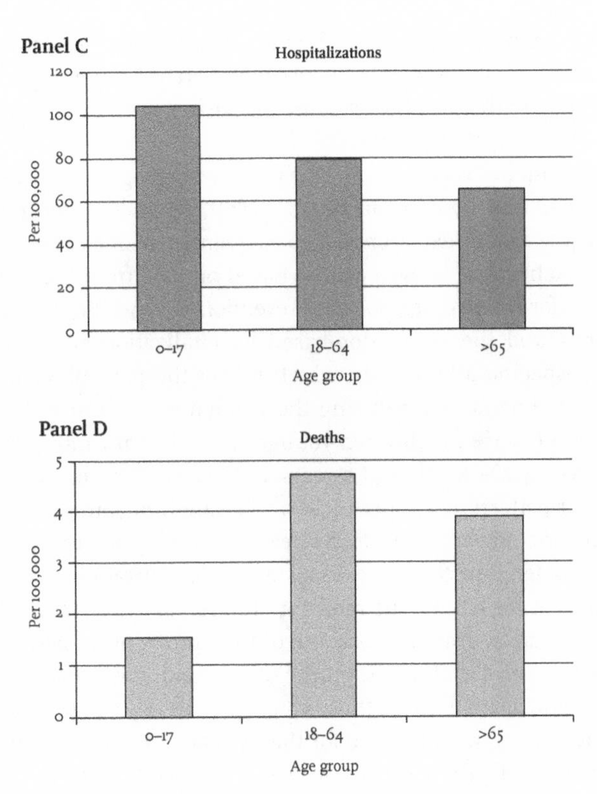

FIGURE 3-2 pH1N1 infection, hospitalization, and death rates. Panel A. Aggregate hospitalization and death reporting activity (AHDRA) hospitalization and death rates per 100,000 population by age group, laboratory-confirmed pH1N1 influenza infection—United States, August 2009–February 2010.

SOURCE: Jhung et al., 2011. Panel B, C & D. 2009 H1N1-Related Deaths, Hospitalizations and Cases, U.S. April 2009–January 16, 2010. Author's calculations based on CDC EIP program estimates: Updated CDC estimates of 2009 H1N1 influenza cases, hospitalizations and deaths in the United States, April 2009–April 10, 2010 Available from: http://www.cdc.gov/h1n1flu/estimates_2009_h1n1.htm. doi:10.1371/journal.pone.0040984.g002

laboratory-confirmed pH1N1 deaths through early August (Centers for Disease Control and Prevention, 2009d).

National, population-based hospitalization and mortality rates did not become available until after the CDC established AHDRA in August 2009. Using data from the states reporting laboratory-confirmed cases, the CDC reported that the greatest rates of hospitalization were observed among the 0- to 4-year-old age group, which had rates two to three times greater than those observed in the other age groups (Figure 3-2A). In addition, the majority of hospitalizations (>70%) reported were in patients younger than 50 years, and fewer than 10% were in patients 65 years or older (Jhung et al., 2011). Using data from AHDRA, the CDC reported that the age distribution of laboratory-confirmed pH1N1 influenza-associated death rate was markedly different from that seen in typical influenza seasons, when the majority of deaths occur in the elderly population, 86% of pH1N1 deaths reported to AHDRA were in persons under 65 years of age, with the highest rates found in persons aged 50–64 years (Figure 3-2C) (Jhung et al., 2011).

To understand the risks properly, one must first recognize that there are two different risks in question: incidence (the risk that someone becomes infected) and severity (the risk of experiencing consequences such as severe illness that requires hospitalization, or even death). Based on data from the CDC EIP program (Centers for Disease Control and Prevention, 2009e), Figure 3-2B presents the attack rate and the population-based hospitalization and death rates by age. The age-specific attack rates, which reflect the percentage of the population infected at some point during the pandemic, do bear out the elevated risk to children (23.4% for children younger than 18 years and 17.5% for adults 18–64 years vs. 14.2% for those 65 years and older). The hospitalization rates show a similar pattern: 104.0 per 100,000 for children younger than 18 years, 79.2 per 100,000 for adults 18 to 64 years, and 65.4 per 100,000 for those 65 years and older. Although the attack and hospitalization rates are greater for children than for adults, the rates for children are less than twice that for seniors—not quite as dramatic as some of the figures presented at the beginning of this section. Death rates, on the other hand, are substantially greater for adults 18 to 64 years than for those younger than 18 years (4.72 per 100,000 vs. 1.56 per 100,000), with the rate for the 65-years-and-older population at an intermediate level of 3.88 per 100,000.

These rates, presented in Figure 3-2B–D; however, are all based on certain assumptions that must be examined. The basis for the estimates is the number of influenza-associated hospitalizations reported in the CDC's EIP program, which covers 62 counties in 10 states, not the number of pH1N1 cases, hospitalizations, and deaths reported to state and local health officials (individual case reporting was discontinued in May 2009 when laboratory capacity proved insufficient to handle the surge in number of potential cases). Reed and colleagues (2009) estimated these multipliers based on a variety of data relating to both seasonal and pH1N1 influenza, but assumed they are the same for every age group and constant over time (however, they account for the change in testing recommendations on May 12). The number of incident cases is estimated as a constant multiple of the number of confirmed cases, which explains why the estimated age-specific attack and hospitalization rates have similar patterns. The multipliers are based on estimates of the fraction of influenza cases in which health care is sought, specimens are tested, and the tests are positive (Reed et al., 2009).

However, by mid-May, the number of clinical samples being submitted to state labs for testing became overwhelming, and the CDC and state health departments recommended viral testing only if it would affect the patient's care. Furthermore, states no longer reported individual confirmed and probable cases to the CDC (Lipsitch et al., 2009a). Moreover, as case counts grew, aggregate reporting replaced individual case reports in most jurisdictions, and most symptomatic cases were not tested, confirmed, or reported, and the proportion tested varied geographically and over time (Lipsitch et al., 2011). Combined with the perceptions that children were at greater risk and older adults less so, it is possible that children and young adults with ILI would be more likely to seek care and to be tested, whereas older adults were less likely to be tested. Population-based BRFSS data suggest that between September 2009 and March 2010, health care was sought by 56% of children with self-reported ILI, compared with 40% of adults (Centers for Disease Control and Prevention, 2011a), and it is possible that the differential was stronger earlier in the outbreak, when fears about the risks for children were more common.

Regarding the attack rate, BRFSS survey data suggest that between September 2009 and March 2010, the average monthly proportion of children younger than 18 years who reported having experienced ILI in the preceding 30 days was 28.4%, compared with 8.1% in adults (Centers for Disease Control and Prevention, 2011b). These percentages vary by month, but at their peak in November (referring to illness in October and November), they were 35.9% for children and 20.4% for adults. No national data are available for the spring wave, but a survey conducted in New York City in mid-June found self-reported ILI prevalence rates of 20% and 22% in children 0 to 4 years and 5 to 17 years, respectively, versus 10% and 6% in adults 18 to 64 years and 65 years and older, respectively (Hadler et al., 2010).

With respect to hospitalizations and deaths, the patterns in Figure 3-2C based on EIP data are similar to those based on the AHDRA surveillance system summarized in Figure 3-2A. In reporting the AHDRA rates, Jhung and colleagues (2011) make the point that the age distributions are markedly different than those for seasonal influenza. These CDC estimates do not, however, show that children have a greater risk of dying than adults. Indeed, if reckoned in terms of the case fatality rate—the proportion of individuals who die of the disease—the risks would be skewed even more toward older groups because the denominator (the number infected) is less. Moreover, after the announcement of the CDC antibody study suggesting that older adults have some residual protection against H1N1 viruses, it is possible that seniors with ILI might not have been tested and their subsequent pH1N1-related death not classified as such. Correcting for such an effect, about which there is no statistical evidence, would increase the pH1N1-associated death rate in the 65-years-and-older age group.

Given concerns about the perceived severity of pH1N1 for children, parents might have been more likely to seek medical care for their children than in previous years or compared with adults with the same symptoms. McDonnell and colleagues (2012) find evidence of this, at least for the spring wave, in an analysis of data from an integrated hospital system operating 18 hospital EDs. During the week beginning April 27, 2009, the number of pediatric (18 years or younger) ED visits increased 19.7% from the previous week, compared with 1.0% for adult patients. In addition, the proportion of pediatric ED patients admitted to the hospital decreased 5.6 percentage points, from 23.2% to 17.6%, whereas the adult admission rates were decreased only 0.6 percentage points, from 13.3% to 12.7% (McDonnell et al., 2012). In another study done by Dugas and colleagues (2012), the Google Flu Trends Web search queries were correlated with weekly visits to the pediatric ED but not the adult ED during the three waves of pH1N1 peaks. Because pH1N1 was very much in the news during this week, but there were not likely to be many actual cases in the hospital system's population, these findings suggest that the increase in pediatric ED cases represents parent overreaction.

A similar effect can be seen in ED use and hospital admission rates in New York City (Farley, 2009). As shown in Figure 3-3A, pediatric ED visits with ILI as a chief complaint peaked in late April, after the news about pH1N1 cases in high school students who had traveled to Mexico and their classmates, and rose sharply around May 15, when the global pandemic was prominent in the news. Figure 3-3B, however, indicates that laboratory-confirmed hospital admissions did not peak until May 26, suggesting that some ED visits earlier in the month reflected parental concern rather than pH1N1 infection.

A comparison of data from EIP coverage areas in New York state with an alternative SHP surveillance system established to monitor pH1N1, however, shows the opposite effect. Analyzing data from October 1, 2009, through March 31, 2010, Noyes and colleagues (2011) noted the age distribution of confirmed cases was very different in the two surveillance systems: children comprise 59% of SHP admissions but only 27% of EIP admissions. These figures suggest that children might be at a greater risk of pH1N1-related hospitalization that the CDC EIP estimates suggest. However, the two surveillance systems differ in a number of ways that might affect this comparison; they cover different counties within the state, and the SHP includes data from a single surveillance hospital in a given area only compared with the comprehensive coverage of the EIP. Perhaps more important, according to the authors, is the dependence on provider-driven testing practices. The EIP's nationally defined protocol might have missed patients presenting with atypical clinical presentations or whose rapid influenza test (which is known to have a low sensitivity for pH1N1) was a false negative. The SHP, on the other hand, tested all patients admitted with ILI (Noyes et al., 2011). It is also possible these factors differed between children and adults. Another dimension is the time period covered. The CDC EIP estimates refer to April 2009 through January 16, 2010, with most cases distributed in roughly equal parts between the spring wave (April through July) and the fall wave (August through November). The New York analysis, on the other hand, covers October 1, 2009, through March 31, 2010, and finds that the SHP data include a sustained number of ILI admissions in December and January.

Thus, the picture about the age-specific risks of pH1N1 that emerges from these analyses is mixed. With respect to the risk of infection per se, it does appear that children were more likely than adults to report ILI in population-based surveys, but these suggest the ratio is closer to 2:1 than 14:1

Panel A

Rate of Influenza-like Illness (ILI) Syndrome Visits (based on chief complaint) to NYC Emergency Departments by Age Group
April 01, 2009–July 06, 2009

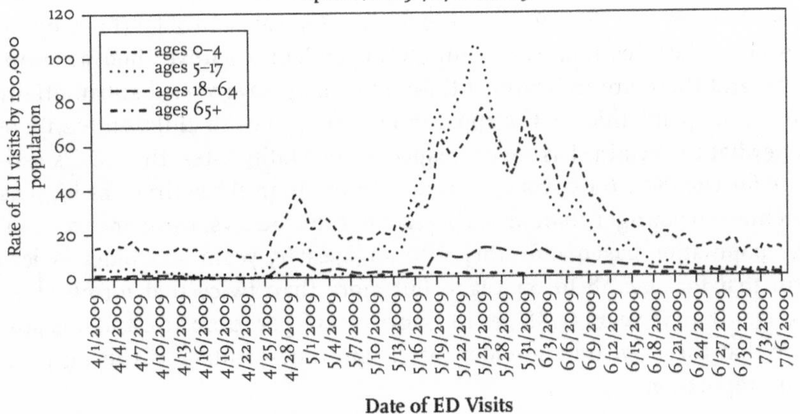

Panel B

Laboratory Confirmed H1N1 Hospital Admissions and Emergency Department (ED) Visits for Influenza-like Illness (ILI) in NYC
April 26–July 06, 2009

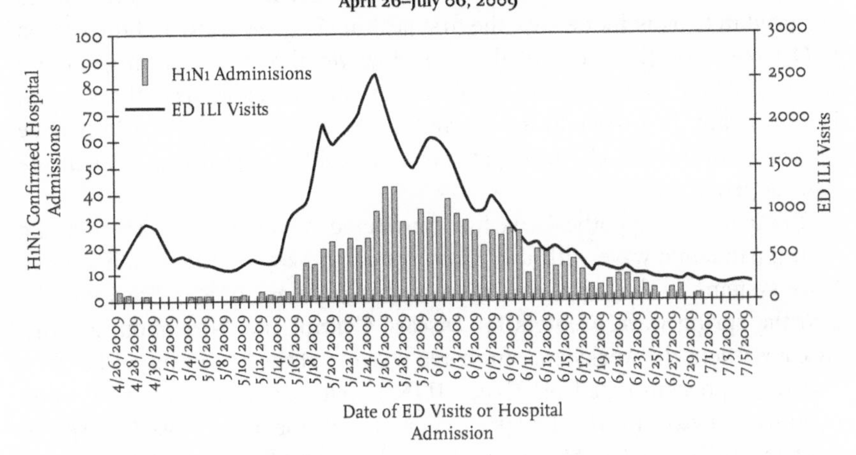

FIGURE 3-3 Influenza-related emergency department visits and hospitalizations. Panel A. Rate of ILI syndrome visits (based on chief complaint) to New York City emergency departments by age group, April 1, 2009–July 6, 2009.
Panel B. Laboratory-confirmed H1N1 hospital admissions and emergency department (ED) Visits for ILI in New York City, April 1, 2009–July 6, 2009.
SOURCE: New York City Department of Health and Mental Hygiene Health Alert #27: Pandemic (H1N1) 2009 influenza update, revised reporting requirements and testing procedures. Available from: http://www.nyc.gov/html/doh/downloads/pdf/cd/2009/09md27.pdf. doi:10.1371/journal.pone.0040984.g003.

(to cite an extreme example [Centers for Disease Control and Prevention, 2009c]). The age-specific rate of hospitalization for pH1N1 influenza also seems to be greater for children than adults, falling from 104.0 per 100,000 for ages 0 to 17 years to 64.4 per 100,000 for ages 65 years and older (Figure 3-2). However, these estimates are highly dependent on unverified assumptions, and there are indications these rates may have varied substantially during the pandemic, so the apparently greater rates in children (<2:1) are somewhat uncertain. Last, with respect to mortality rates, the CDC's estimate for the 18-to-64-years age group is more than three times as high as for children younger than 18 years (4.72 per 100,000 vs. 1.56 per 100,000). The population-based mortality rate for ages 65 years and older is less than that for ages 18 to 64 years, but more than twice that for children younger than 18 years (3.88 per 100,000 vs. 1.56 per 100,000), and it is possible that the 65-years-and-older rate is an underestimate resulting from underreporting.

Monitoring pH1N1 Cases over Time

It is generally accepted that pH1N1 influenza activity in the United States occurred in two distinct waves: the first peaking in June 2009 and the second in October 2009 (Brammer et al., 2011). However, the specific timing of these waves, and how the timing may have varied in different regions of the country, is less certain. In particular, trends and patterns in surveillance data may be related to awareness—both by patients and healthcare providers—about the risks of pH1N1.

To explore this hypothesis, we first considered surveillance reports from the spring pandemic wave with data from two of the key near-real-time surveillance systems as they appeared at the end of June 2009, about two months into the spring wave (Centers for Disease Control and Prevention, 2009f). By convention, the weeks are numbered starting at the beginning of January. Figure 3-4 presents data from CDC's ILINet system, reflecting the proportion of outpatient visits for ILI. The proportion of visits for ILI increased sharply in week 17, which ended on May 2, 2009, to 2.8%, a level that exceeds the national baseline and is more characteristic of the winter months.

Figure 3-5, which displays the number and percentage of respiratory specimens in the United States testing positive for influenza reported by WHO-/NREVSS-collaborating laboratories, also shows a dramatic increase in the number of positive specimens—represented by the height of the bar—for week 17. These peaks correspond temporally to a rapid series of announcements, starting on Tuesday, April 21, of human-to-human transmission in California of a new viral subtype, of a major outbreak in Mexico, of confirmed cases in New York City students who had traveled to Mexico, confirmation of worldwide spread of the new virus leading to an increase in the WHO's pandemic alert level, and closing of approximately 300 U.S. schools. Note that Figure 3-3 shows a similar peak at the end of April in New York City hospital ED visits for ILI.

Percentage of Visits for Influenza like Illness (ILI) Reported by the US Outpatient Influenza like Illness Surveillance Network (ILINet), National Summary 2008–09 and Previous Two Seasons

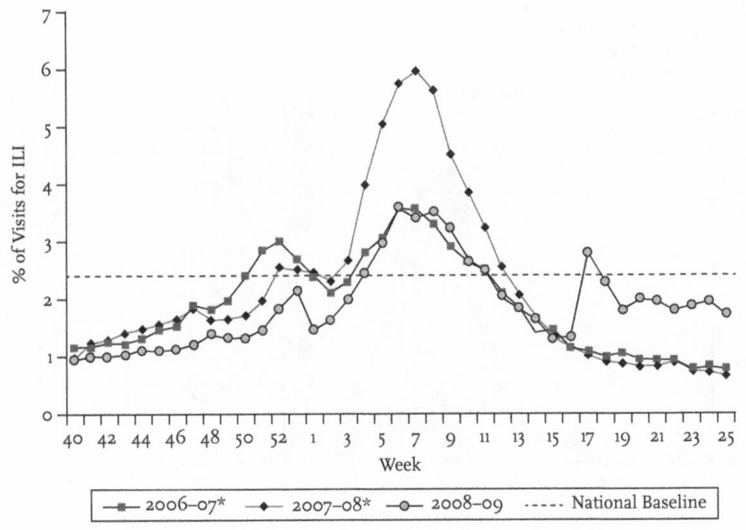

* There was no week 53 during the 2006–07 and 2007–08 seasons, therefore the week 53 data point for those seasons is an average of weeks 52 and 1.

FIGURE 3-4 Outpatient influenza like illness surveillance. Percentage of visits for ILI Reported by the U.S. Outpatient Influenza-like Illness Surveillance Network (ILINet), National Summary 2008–09 and Previous Two Seasons.

SOURCE: CDC Flu View, 2008–2009 Influenza Season Week 25 ending June 27, 2009. Available from: http://www.cdc.gov/flu/weekly/weeklyarchives2008-2009/weekly25.htm. doi:10.1371/journal.pone.0040984.g004.

One possible explanation for these peaks is they reflect the rapid spread of ILI throughout the United States. It is also possible, however, they reflect increased concern about the pandemic, leading people to seek health care for symptoms they might otherwise treat themselves, and physicians to send clinical samples in for testing. Indeed the Google Insights activity index, as shown in Figure 3-1, grew from 0 to 100 during this time, and never rose to more than 15 throughout the rest of 2009.

Moreover, a closer examination of Figure 3-5 shows that it is the number of samples submitted, not the number of positive tests, that accounts for the sharp increase in week 17. Of the 3,911 samples tested during week 16, 7.1% were positive for influenza. During week 17, the number of samples submitted grew to 30,020, but only 12.3% were positive for influenza. And excluding the specimens that were determined to be influenza A but subtyping was not done, at most 4.6% of the samples submitted during week 17 were possibly pH1N1 (i.e., either determined to be novel H1N1 or "unsubtypable" influenza A). As shown by the black line in Figure 3-5, the proportion positive for influenza grows to about 40% in June, but the maximum proportion of samples

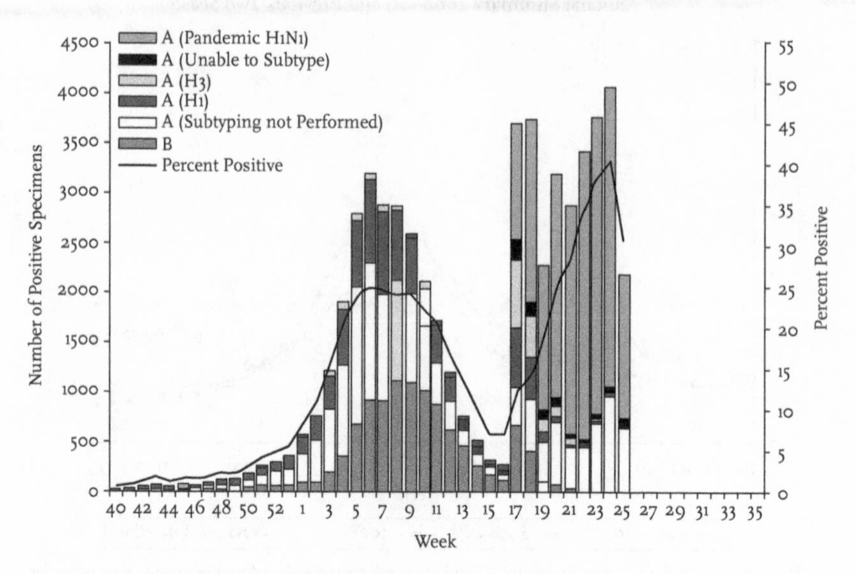

FIGURE 3-5 Laboratory-confirmed influenza cases reported to CDC by U.S. WHO/NREVSS collaborating laboratories, national summary, 2008–09.
SOURCE: CDC Flu View, 2008–2009 Influenza Season Week 25 ending June 27, 2009. Available from: http://www.cdc.gov/flu/weekly/weeklyarchives2008-2009/weekly25.htm. doi:10.1371/journal.pone.0040984.g005.

submitted that might be pH1N1 never exceeds 35% (based on the author's calculations and not shown in the figure). Because the proportion of submitted samples that can possibly be pH1N1 was so low during weeks 17 and 18, it seems likely that the sharp increase depicted in Figure 3-5 does not represent rapid spread of the pandemic virus in the U.S. population, but rather increased awareness on the part of patients in seeking care and physicians in sending clinical samples for testing.

The fall wave presents an opportunity to assess the ability of surveillance systems to monitor regional trends during pH1N1. In particular, it was widely noted that the fall wave began earlier in the South and later in the Northeast. This pattern can be seen clearly in the ILINet data in Figure 3-6, and also in percent of samples submitted to WHO/NREVSS that were positive for influenza (not shown). The patterns in Google Flu Trends data, thought to be a proxy for the number of people with flu symptoms, for the same period (but using Georgia and Massachusetts as proxies for the regions, because the data are available for selected states and not by region) are remarkably similar. However, DiSTRIBuTE project ED surveillance data from the same states (which are only available starting in October) display a somewhat different pattern. In both Georgia and Massachusetts, the difference between the maximum and minimum is much less than in either the ILINet or Google Flu Trends data. The

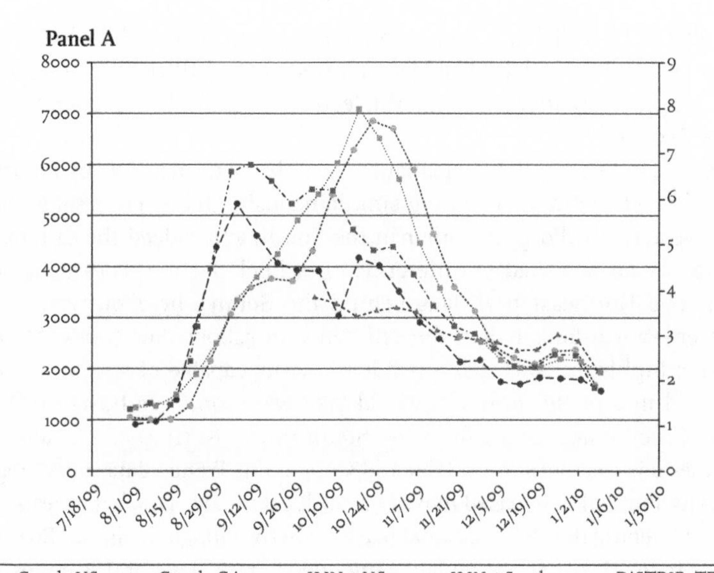

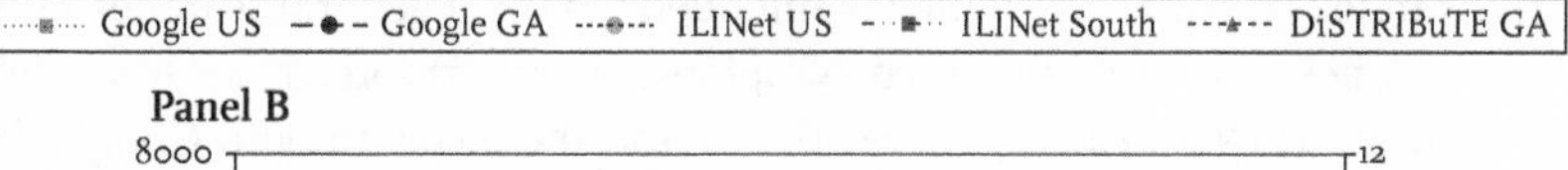

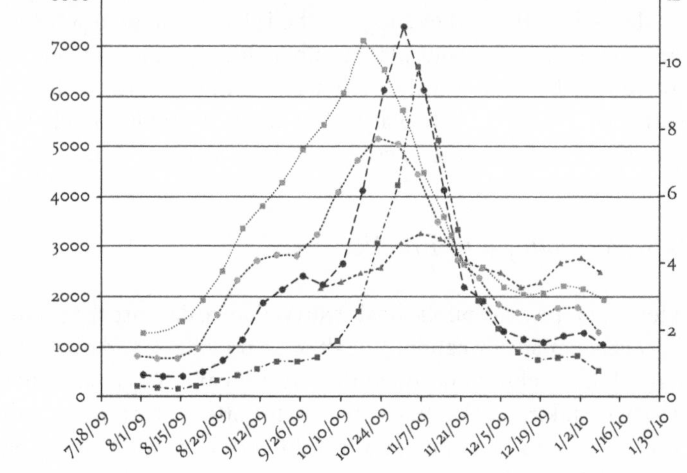

FIGURE 3-6 Influenzalike illness surveillance for the Northeast, South, and entire United States. Panel A. Percentage of visits for influenza-like illness (ILINet), U.S. and South, July 31, 2009–January 8, 2010; Google Flu Trends index, U.S. and Georgia (GA), August 2, 2009–January 10, 2010; scaled DiSTRIBuTE ILI trends, Georgia (GA), October 3, 2009–January 9, 2010. Panel B. Percentage of visits for influenza-like illness (ILINet), U.S. and Northeast (NE), July 31, 2009–January 8, 2010; Google Flu Trends index, U.S. and Massachusetts (MA), August 2, 2009–January 10, 2010; scaled DiSTRIBuTE ILI trends, Massachusetts (MA), October 3, 2009–January 9, 2010.

SOURCES: Author's calculations based on CDC, Google, and DiSTRIBuTE data available from: http://www.cdc.gov/h1n1flu/cdcresponse.htm, http://www.google.org/flutrends/ and http://isdsdistribute.org/moreinfo.php.doi:10.1371/journal.pone.0040984.g006.

Georgia DiSTRIBuTE data drop throughout the entire period, as do the ILINet or Google Flu Trends data. The Massachusetts DiSTRIBuTE data, on the other hand, peak shortly after either the ILINet or Google Flu Trends data, and again in late December.

There are two possible explanations for the patterns seen in Figure 3-6, both of which could be operating simultaneously. One hypothesis is that the fall wave actually did peak earlier in the South, and indeed the difference in timing has been related to differences in school starting dates (Chao et al., 2010). The Northeast peak lags behind the South's by about two months, however—much longer than the difference in school start times. Moreover, it seems highly unlikely that a pandemic virus capable of spreading around the world in a matter of weeks would take two months to travel up the east coast of the United States from the South to the Northeast. The alternative hypothesis is that both the ILINet and Google Flu Trends data reflect regional concerns about pH1N1, based in part on the local media. This hypothesis is supported by seeing the same regional patterns in the Google Insights "Swine Flu" activity index (Figure 3-1B), which is intended to reflect general searches rather than searches based on one's own symptoms. Furthermore, a two-week delay between the ILINet peak in the Northeast and the peaks in both Google data sources for Massachusetts further suggests the ILINet peak represents people seeking care out of concern about pH1N1 rather than symptoms alone. Thus, although there could be some real differences in timing between the South and the Northeast, it seems likely that ILINet and Google Flu Trends data, at least in part, reflect regional differences in concerns about pH1N1.

Implications for Policy and Practice

From a systems perspective, public health surveillance data are the product of a series of decisions made by patients, healthcare providers, and public health professionals about seeking and providing health care and about reporting cases or otherwise taking action that comes to the attention of health authorities. All these decisions are potentially influenced by what these people know and think. Outpatient, hospital-based, and ED surveillance systems, for instance, all rely on individuals deciding to present themselves to obtain health care, and these decisions are based in part on their interpretations of their symptoms. Even the number of Google searches and self-reports of ILI in the BRFSS survey can be influenced by individuals' interpretation of the seriousness of their symptoms. Virologic surveillance and systems based on laboratory confirmations depend on physicians deciding to send specimens for testing. Every element of this decision-making process is potentially influenced by the informational and policy environment (e.g., media coverage, current case definitions and practice recommendations, implementation of active surveillance), processing and reacting to information on an individual level (e.g., healthcare seeker's self-assessment of risk, incentives for seeking medical attention and self-isolation, healthcare provider's ordering of laboratory tests), and technical barriers (e.g., communication infrastructure for data exchange, laboratory capacity). Because all these factors change over time, so did the biases in the surveillance data, and, as a result, the U.S. public health systems' ability to characterize and track the pH1N1 was unreliable.

Although this analysis is limited by the lack of a gold standard—in this case, definitive knowledge of the actual number of pH1N1 cases and the characteristics of the individuals who were affected—a triangulation approach that compares multiple data systems, each with different expected biases over time, strongly suggests that children and young adults are overrepresented in many pH1N1 surveillance systems, especially in the spring wave. In other words, children and young adults may not have been "at risk" to the extent that some thought, but rather the perception they were led to surveillance results that supported this perception. Furthermore, because ILINet, ED surveillance data, and other syndromic surveillance systems that depend on counts of people seeking care, especially for children, are influenced by the information environment, some apparent trends and geographic differences were, in part, reflections of what people thought was happening rather than actual numbers of cases. Comparing data from the spring and fall wave of pH1N1 in Wales, Keramarou and colleagues (2011) find a similar effect, with relatively more ILI visits in the spring, when media activity was intense, and fewer in the fall, when media activity waned). Chowell and colleagues (2011) also note that, in Mexico, the median age of laboratory-confirmed ILI cases was 18 years overall in 2009, but increased to 31 years during the fall wave. In France, ILI cases peaked during the first week of September (week 36), but according to virologic and clinical data, the pandemic started in mid-October (week 44). Casalegno and colleagues (2011) noted that many of the early ILI cases were actually rhinovirus and other noninfluenza viruses, and attributed the September increase in pediatric ILI cases to massive media coverage at the start of the school year and the general level of anxiety at that time.

Of course, epidemiologists recognize these potential biases and typically note them and present their analysis of the available data with appropriate caveats. But, especially when the crisis is acute and the need for information urgent, what seems like subtle methodological points to policymakers and the public can become lost easily. Even straightforward points can be confused. For instance, the dramatic increase in week 17, shown in the height of the bar in Figure 3-5 seems consistent with the alarmist headlines at that time and can be misinterpreted easily as a sudden increases in pandemic cases. In fact, as the analysis (and even just a careful reading of the graph) shows, this increase reflects mainly an increase in the number of samples submitted for testing rather than the percentage positive for pH1N1.

Confusion about whether children and young adults were more "at risk" for pH1N1 is compounded by different ideas about the meaning of risk. This term can mean the probability that one is infected, develops symptoms, requires hospitalization, or dies. Furthermore, the risk of severe consequences can be figured in terms of those who are infected or develop symptoms, or in terms of everyone in some demographic group. Careful analysis of the data suggests that children and young adults do seem to have been more likely than older people to have been infected with pH1N1. On the other hand, the relative proportions of infected cases—or of the population—who die or require hospitalization may be greater for older adults. The pH1N1 surveillance literature uses nearly all the possible definitions of risk, often with little clarification regarding which one is intended, and this further confuses public understanding of the situation. Minor differences among surveillance systems regarding standard age groupings, for instance, and differences in standard data presentation formats also add to the confusion.

The tendency to report cumulative case counts, especially during the early days of the pandemic, also complicated the interpretation of the data. By definition, cumulative case counts can only increase—they are not reduced as people regain their health or die after a course of illness—even if the incidence of new cases peaks. Cumulative counts also increase as new cases that occurred before epidemiologists were aware of the outbreak are discovered. Perhaps because case counts are a feature of other types of disasters, policymakers expect them in disease outbreaks, but presenting the data in this way can lead to misunderstandings.

This analysis benefits from hindsight and is not intended as a criticism of the epidemiologists who had the much more difficult challenge of interpreting the data as the pandemic was emerging and spreading throughout the population. Indeed, the goal is not to question the epidemiology of pH1N1, but rather to learn from the U.S. experience about the performance of critical surveillance systems. In addition, this analysis adopts an outsiders' perspective—that is, we are not aware of all the information—or the pressures—that epidemiologists faced during the pandemic. Although in some ways this is a limitation, in other respects it allows us to question some of the assumptions that, in the press of time and events, the public health officials dealing with pH1N1 may not have had the luxury of making.

The U.S. public health surveillance response to pH1N1 offers much to admire. Together with surveillance activities in Mexico, and benefiting from advances in laboratory capacity and notification systems introduced the previous decade, epidemiologists identified and characterized a new pathogen relatively quickly, allowing the CDC and, shortly afterward, the WHO to issue alerts about the emergence of a new pandemic strain, triggering a rapid global public health response to pH1N1 (Cordova-Villalobos et al., 2009). These alerts triggered pandemic influenza plans that had been prepared in recent years, which focused initially on surveillance activities, including the development of a case definition and testing procedures, and nonpharmaceutical control measures. A variety of existing influenza surveillance systems were supplemented with newly developed ad hoc systems to provide timely information to guide policymakers and to monitor the public health response (Brammer et al., 2011).

However, although not definitive, our analysis of the of the public health surveillance systems that provided situational awareness in the United States calls into question two aspects of the conventional wisdom about the 2009 H1N1 pandemic. In particular, children and young adults might not have experienced greater risks from severe consequences as some thought. Furthermore, apparent patterns in the timing and relative size of the spring and fall waves, and of geographic differences in the timing of the fall wave, seem to depend in large part on perceptions of what was happening. Although the extent of the biases suggested by this analysis cannot be known precisely, the analysis identifies underlying problems with surveillance systems—in particular, their dependence on patient and provider behavior, which is influenced by a changing information environment—that could limit situational awareness in future public health emergencies.

These problems are particularly germane for syndromic surveillance systems, which are highly dependent on individuals' decisions to stay home from school, to self-treat, or to seek health care, and thus on changes in the information environment. The earliest appearance of the pandemic did not trigger a quantitative alert in any of these systems, either in Mexico or in the United States (Lipsitch et al., 2011). Lipsitch and colleagues (2011) report both instances in which syndromic surveillance was thought to be effective for situational awareness and others in which it was misleading. Our analysis of the pH1N1 experience, and another comparison of syndromic surveillance systems in fall 2011 at two universities (Zhang, 2011), did not support the PCAST report's enthusiastic endorsement of this approach for situational awareness (President's Council of Advisors on Science and Technology, 2009).

It should also be noted that the analysis described in Chapter 2 shows that syndromic surveillance played an important role in detecting the pH1N1 outbreak, but a different one than is commonly used to justify these systems. Syndromic surveillance systems are typically used to detect outbreaks before conventional surveillance systems to enable a rapid public health response. Because pH1N1 emerged in the winter, there were too few cases to be detected against the background of the normal flu season. However, when Mexican public health authorities became aware of severe respiratory illness cases, syndromic surveillance systems provided positive confirmation that the virus had spread widely throughout Mexico (Zhang, 2013).

This analysis has implications for the ongoing redesign of the CDC BioSense program, which was mandated originally in the Public Health Security and Bioterrorism Preparedness Act of 2002 to establish an integrated national public health surveillance system for early detection and rapid assessment of potential bioterrorism-related illness (Centers for Disease Control and Prevention, 2011b). Current redesign efforts focus on building a network of syndromic surveillance systems and a community of surveillance practitioners who share data and interpretations, including enhancements to the data acquisition process to improve data quality and timeliness (Government Accountability Office, 2010a). In this context, as in other information technology discussions, data quality and timeliness refer to the transfer of information from the source to the point of analysis, and efforts to ensure that data from hospitals or other healthcare providers are transmitted quickly and without loss of fidelity to BioSense analysts. The proposed enhancements do not address the biases identified in this chapter, which affect the quality of epidemiologic information—as opposed to the data—that BioSense produces.

Similarly, the Global Health Security Agenda announced in February 2014 seeks to build capacity by developing, strengthening, and linking global networks for real-time biosurveillance (Department of Health and Human Services, 2014). Such capacities are clearly important, but the 2009 H1N1 experience reminds us that real-time biosurveillance systems may contain inaccurate information about epidemiologic risks. So, as noted in Chapter 2, to ensure that it is meeting its goals, the Global Health Security Agenda must track not only capacities (laboratory, reporting networks), but also capabilities, such as the ability to consolidate and make sense of rapidly emerging information to characterize epidemiologic risks (Stoto, 2014).

Our analysis is not intended as a criticism of the epidemiologists charged with the immense challenge of tracking the impact of a new pathogen. Rather, this analysis shows how fundamentally difficult the surveillance challenge is, and sheds light on the adequacy of existing surveillance systems for such efforts. As with most novel pathogens, the emergence of pH1N1 was characterized by uncertainty that took weeks to months to resolve. Epidemiologists familiar with the emergence of novel pathogens compare the rapidly evolving facts and scientific knowledge rightly to the "fog of war,"(Stoto et al., 2005), and the United Kingdom's Pandemic Influenza Preparedness Programme has shown how it should be factored into public health preparedness planning (Pandemic Influenza Preparedness Team, 2011). Many emergency preparedness professionals, however, still think in terms of single cases triggering a response in hours or days, and this thinking is reflected in such key public health preparedness documents as the CDC's *2011 Public Health Preparedness Capabilities: National Standards for State and Local Planning* (Division of State and Local Readiness in the Office of Public Health Preparedness and Response, 2011). A more appropriate response would be a plan to step up surveillance efforts early during the event to fill in the uncertainties apparent in the original data.

Moreover, to the extent that future public health crises are characterized by similar unknowns, this analysis of the 2009 H1N1 experience identified a root cause that is likely to be problematic in the future: surveillance systems that depend on patients and providers taking action—to seek care, to send samples for testing, and so on. These actions depend, to some extent, on what people hear in the media and official reports, creating an inherent circularity that is difficult to disentangle. This problem is most prominent in surveillance systems based on reported cases, but also affects everything from syndromic surveillance systems that monitor individuals' decisions to seek health care to virologic surveillance systems that depend on physicians submitting specimens to be tested. This is yet another example of how case-based surveillance systems can lead to biased statistical data (Stoto, 2008). Similarly, Lipsitch and colleagues (2009a, 2011) and Garske and colleagues (2009) show how biased case ascertainment, especially early during the pH1N1 pandemic, led to overestimating the case fatality rate.

The optimal solution is to develop population-based surveillance systems that are less dependent on individuals' and their physicians' decisions, and thus less sensitive to the circular effect of the media environment. Lipsitch and colleagues (2009b), for instance, have suggested identifying well-defined population cohorts at high risk for pH1N1 infection and ensuring that everyone in that group is tested to avoid biases resulting from physician decisions about who should be tested. Kok and Dywer (2011) review a number of possible designs, and Lipsitch and colleagues (2011) describe their beneficial effects. Another possibility is to make more timely use of ongoing, national population-based surveys such as the CDC's BRFSS. This survey used in 2009 to provide monthly data on the proportion of the population with influenzalike symptoms, but the results were not published until long after the pandemic wave had passed (Centers for Disease Control and Prevention, 2011a). New York City mounted a more limited but also more timely telephone survey in May 2009 and June 2009 (Hadler et al., 2010). With proper planning and statistical techniques, the same survey could be used to produce more timely data. Ultimately, a population-based seroprevalence survey, such as those deployed in the United Kingdom (Miller et al., 2010) and Hong Kong (Cowling et al., 2010), would provide the least biased data on who is at risk for infection, and temporal and geographic patterns. The benefits of such studies, however, are tempered by practicalities of obtaining informed consent, the unavailability and limitations of early serologic tests, and the costs, so Lipsitch and colleagues (2011) concluded that a large-scale prepandemic investment would be needed to improve current influenza serologic assay technology sufficiently so that valid serologic tests could be developed quickly at the start of the next pandemic.

Other problems sprang from common difficulties in presenting scientific information clearly to policymakers and the public. Epidemiologists were aware of the distinction between the risk of pH1N1 infection and its consequences, yet policymakers developed immunization strategies and priorities predicated on the assumption that children were at high risk of its consequences. Presumably this also reflects a general concern for and need to protect children, but surely population perceptions about children being "at risk" contributed to this. One might argue that epidemiologists cannot control how their data are used, but the standard definition of public health surveillance is the "ongoing, systematic collection, analysis, and interpretation of health-related data essential to the planning, implementation, and evaluation of public health practice, closely integrated *with the timely dissemination of these data to those responsible for prevention and control*" (emphasis added) (Thacker and Berkelman, 1988, p. 164).

Beyond considerations of needed surveillance system improvements, this analysis also has implications for how to measure preparedness. For instance, the CDC's and the Trust for America's Health's most recent state-by-statement assessments of public health preparedness focus on ensuring that state and local public health laboratories have the capacity to respond rapidly, identify or rule out particular known biological agents, and increase the workforce and laboratory throughput needed to process large numbers of samples during an emergency (Office of Public Health Preparedness and Response, 2010; Trust for America's Health, 2010). None of these measures would have ensured that public health surveillance systems could have avoided the biases identified in this analysis and tracked accurately who was at risk for pH1N1 and monitored the development of the pandemic over time and in different geographic areas. Nor did syndromic surveillance or other approaches to harnessing the vast amounts of data in electronic medical records avoid problems with bias in 2009, nor could they be expected to do so in the future. Although these capacities are clearly necessary, they are not sufficient. Rather, assessing the nation's level of preparedness requires measures of the systems capability to track an outbreak and characterize its risks accurately, and to communicate this information clearly to policymakers.

In addition to its substantive contributions, this analysis illustrates the quality improvement approach called for in the U.S. National Health Security Strategy (U.S. Department of Health and Human Services, 2010a). Emphasizing processes (chains of events that produce specific outcomes) and systems of people and information, the quality improvement approach refers to a range of specific practices that include procedures and system changes based on their effects on measurable outcomes, reduce unnecessary variability in outcomes while preserving system differences that are critical to the specific environment, promote continuous improvement rather than one-time initiatives, and support critical event/failure mode analysis. In general, our analysis is an example of an effort "to collect data on performance measures from real incidents . . . analyze performance data to identify gaps, [and] recommend and apply programs to mitigate those gaps," an approach called for in the National Health Security Strategy implementation guide (U.S. Department of Health and Human Services, 2010b).

Learning about public health systems' emergency response capabilities is challenging because actual events are unique, and both the epidemiologic facts and the context varies from one community to another. In other words, there is no replication—a centerpiece of the scientific method. In this context, to address the lack of a gold standard to describe the actual trends in the rate of pH1N1 infection and its consequences over time, we adopted a "triangulation" approach that compares multiple data sources, each with different likely biases. We focused specifically on two time periods, the month of May when the spring peak occurred and the fall wave, which started at the end of August and continued through November. In the fall, we also focused on the South and the Northeast regions of the United States, which had the earliest and latest fall peaks, respectively. Statistical calculations were limited to simple data transformations to ease comparability and graphical analysis. This type of analysis is necessarily qualitative and contextual; rather than serving as a recipe for doing this in other settings, this analysis should be seen as an example that illustrates the concept. Similar analyses of other events will require a different approach.

Acknowledgments and Disclosures

This research was conducted with funding support awarded to the Harvard School of Public Health under cooperative agreements with the U.S. CDC (grant no. 5P01TP000307-01). The author is grateful for comments from John Brownstein, Melissa Higdon, Tamar Klaiman, John Kraemer, Larissa May, Christopher Nelson, Hilary Placzek, Ellen Whitney, Ying Zhang, the staff of the CDC Public Health Surveillance Program Office, and others who commented on presentations. The data and conclusions have been previously published in:

- Stoto, M. A. (2012). The effectiveness of U.S. public health surveillance systems for situational awareness during the 2009 H1N1 pandemic: a retrospective analysis. *PLoS One*, 7(8), e40984.

References

Brammer, L., Blanton, L., Epperson, S., Mustaquim, D., Bishop, A. (2011). Surveillance for influenza during the 2009 influenza A (H1N1) pandemic: United States, April 2009–March 2010. *Clinical Infectious Diseases*, 52(Suppl 1), S27–S35.

Brown, D. (2009). Age of flu victims has big implications. *The Washington Post*. Accessed November 22, 2011, at http://www.washingtonpost.com/wp-dyn/content/article/2009/05/16/AR2009051601850.html.

Casalegno, J.S., Frobert, E., Escuret, V., Bouscambert-Duchamp, M., Billaud, G. (2011). Beyond the influenza-like illness surveillance: the need for real-time virological data. *Eurosurveillance*, *16*(1), 19756.

Centers for Disease Control and Prevention. (2009a). 2008–2009 Influenza season week 25 ending June 27, 2009. Accessed November 22, 2011, at http://www.cdc.gov/flu/weekly/weeklyarchives2008-2009/weekly25.htm.

Centers for Disease Control and Prevention. (2009b). 2009 H1N1 vaccination recommendations. Accessed November 22, 2011, at http://www.cdc.gov/h1n1flu/vaccination/acip.htm.

Centers for Disease Control and Prevention. (2009c). 2009 Pandemic influenza A (H1N1) virus infections: Chicago, Illinois, April–July 2009. *MMWR Morbidity and Mortality Weekly Report*, *58*(33), 913–918.

Centers for Disease Control and Prevention.(2009d). Serum cross-reactive antibody response to a novel influenza A (H1N1) virus after vaccination with seasonal influenza vaccine. *MMWR Morbidity and Mortality Weekly Report*, *58*(19), 521–524.

Centers for Disease Control and Prevention. (2009e). Surveillance for pediatric deaths associated with 2009 pandemic influenza A (H1N1) virus infection: United States, April–August 2009. *MMWR Morbidity and Mortality Weekly Report*, *58*(34), 941–947.

Centers for Disease Control and Prevention. (2009f). Updated CDC estimates of 2009 H1N1 influenza cases, hospitalizations and deaths in the United States, April 2009–April 10, 2010. Accessed November 22, 2011, at http://www.cdc.gov/h1n1flu/estimates_2009_h1n1.htm.

Centers for Disease Control and Prevention. (2010). CDC guidance for state and local public health officials and school administrators for school (K–12) responses to influenza during the 2009–2010 school year. Accessed November 22, 2011, at http://www.cdc.gov/h1n1flu/schools/schoolguidance.htm.

Centers for Disease Control and Prevention. (2011a). About BioSense. Accessed November 22, 2011, at http://www.cdc.gov/biosense/index.html.

Centers for Disease Control and Prevention. (2011b). Self-reported influenza-like illness during the 2009 H1N1 influenza pandemic: United States, September 2009–March 2010. *MMWR Morbidity and Mortality Weekly Report, 60*(2), 37–41.

Chao, D.L., Halloran, E.M., Longini, I.M. (2010). School opening dates predict pandemic influenza A (H1N1) outbreaks in the United States. *Journal of Infectious Diseases, 202*(6), 877–880.

Chowell, G., Echevarrã-Zuno, S., Viboud, C., Simonsen, L., Tamerius, J. (2011). Characterizing the epidemiology of the 2009 influenza A/H1N1 pandemic in Mexico. *PLoS Medicine, 8*(5), e1000436.

Cordova-Villalobos, J.A., Sarti, E., Arzoz-Padres, J., Manuell-Lee, G., Mendez, J.R. (2009). The influenza A(H1N1) epidemic in Mexico: lessons learned. *Health Research Policy and Systems, 7*, 21.

Cowling, B.J., Chan, K.H., Fang, V.J., Lau, L.L., So, H.C. (2010). Comparative epidemiology of pandemic and seasonal influenza A in households. *The New England Journal of Medicine, 362*(23), 2175–2184.

Dawood, F.S., Jain, S., Finelli, L., Shaw, M.W. (2009). Emergence of a novel swine-origin influenza A (H1N1) virus in humans. *The New England Journal of Medicine, 360*(25), 2605–2615.

Department of Health and Human Services. (2014). Global health security agenda: toward a world safe & secure from infectious disease threats. Accessed May 5, 2014, at http://www.globalhealth.gov/global-health-topics/global-health-security/GHS%20Agenda.pdf.

Distributed Surveillance Taskforce for Real-Time Influenza Burden Tracking and Evaluation. (2011). About DiSTRIBuTE. Accessed November 22, 2011, at http://isdsdistribute.org/moreinfo.php.

Division of State and Local Readiness in the Office of Public Health Preparedness and Response. (2011). Public health preparedness capabilities: national standards for state and local planning. Accessed November 22, 2011, at http://www.cdc.gov/phpr/capabilities/.

Dugas, A.F., Hsieh, Y.H., Levin, S.R., Pines, J.M., Mareiniss, D.P. (2012). Google FluTrends: correlation with emergency department influenza rates and crowding metrics. *Clinical Infectious Diseases, 54*(4), 463–469.

Farley, T. (2009). 2009 New York City Department of Health and Mental Hygiene Health alert #27: pandemic (H1N1) 2009 influenza update, revised reporting requirements and testing procedures. Accessed November 22, 2011, at http://www.nyc.gov/html/doh/downloads/pdf/cd/2009/09md27.pdf.

Garske, T., Legrand, J., Donnelly, C.A., Ward, H., Cauchemez, S. (2009). Assessing the severity of the novel influenza A/H1N1 pandemic. *British Medical Journal, 339*, b2840.

Gilson, L., Hanson, K., Sheikh, K., Agyepong, I.A., Ssengooba, F. (2011). Building the field of health policy and systems research: social science matters. *PLoS Medicine, 8*(8), e1001079.

Ginsberg, J., Mohebbi, M.H., Patel, R.S., Brammer, L., Smolinski, M.S. (2009). Detecting influenza epidemics using search engine query data. *Nature, 457*(7232), 1012–1014.

Google. (2011). Google Insights for Search. Accessed November 22, 2011, at http://www.google.com/insights/search/#.

Government Accountability Office. (2010a). Efforts to develop a national biosurveillance capability need a national strategy and a designated leader. Accessed March 1, 2012, at http://www.gao.gov/new.items/d10645.pdf.

Government Accountability Office (GAO). (2010b). Public health information technology: additional strategic planning needed to guide HHS's efforts to establish *Geo L* Jelectronic situational awareness capabilities. Accessed November 22, 2011, http://www.gao.gov/new.items/d1199.pdf.

Hadler, J.L., Konty, K., McVeigh, K.H., Fine, A., Eisenhower, D. (2010). Case fatality rates based on population estimates of influenza-like illness due to novel H1N1 influenza: New York City, May-June 2009. *PLoS One, 5*(7), e11677.

Heymann, A., Chodick, G., Reichman, B., Kokia, E., Laufer, J. (2004). Influence of school closure on the incidence of viral respiratory diseases among children and on health care utilization. *Pediatric Infectious Disease Journal, 23*(7), 675–677.

Hodge, J.G. (2009). The legal landscape for school closures in response to pandemic flu or other public health threats. *Biosecurity and Bioterrorism, 7*(1), 45–50.

Jain, S., Kamimoto, L., Bramley, A.M., Schmitz, A.M., Benoit, S.R. (2009). Hospitalized patients with 2009 H1N1 influenza in the United States, April–June 2009. *The New England Journal of Medicine, 361*(20), 1935–1944.

Jhung, M.A., Swerdlow, D., Olsen, S.J., Jernigan, D., Biggerstaff, M. (2011). Epidemiology of 2009 pandemic influenza A (H1N1) in the United States. *Clinical Infectious Diseases, 52*(Suppl 1), S13–S26.

Keramarou, M., Cottrell, S., Evans, M.R., Moore, C., Stiff, R.E. (2011). Two waves of pandemic influenza A(H1N1) 2009 in Wales: the possible impact of media coverage on consultation rates, April–December 2009. *Eurosurveillance, 16*(3), 19772.

Kok, J., Dywer, D.E. (2011). How common was 2009 pandemic influenza A H1N1? *The Lancet Infectious Diseases, 11*(6), 423–424.

Lipsitch, M., Finelli, L., Heffernan, R.T., Leung, G.M., Redd, S.C. (2011). Improving the evidence base for decision making during a pandemic: the example of 2009 influenza A/H1N1. *Biosecurity and Bioterrorism, 9*(2), 89–115.

Lipsitch, M., Hayden, F.G., Cowling, B.J., Leung, G.M. (2009a). How to maintain surveillance for novel influenza A H1N1 when there are too many cases to count. *The Lancet, 374*(9696), 1209–1211.

Lipsitch, M., Riley, S., Cauchemez, S., Ghani, A.C., Ferguson, N.M. (2009b). Managing and reducing uncertainty in an emerging influenza pandemic. *The New England Journal of Medicine, 361*(2), 112–115.

McDonnell, W.M., Nelson, D.S., Schunk, J.E. (2012). Should we fear "flu fear" itself? Effects of H1N1 influenza fear on ED use. *American Journal of Emergency Medicine, 30*(2), 275–282.

Miller, E., Hoschler, K., Hardelid, P., Stanford, E., Andrews, N. (2010). Incidence of 2009 pandemic influenza A H1N1 infection in England: a cross-sectional serological study. *The Lancet, 375*(9720), 1100–1108.

Noyes, K.A., Hoefer, D., Barr, C., Belflower, R., Malloy, K. (2011). Two distinct surveillance methods to track hospitalized influenza patients in New York State during the 2009–2010 influenza season. *Journal of Public Health Management and Practice, 17*(1), 12–19.

Office of Public Health Preparedness and Response. (2010). 2010 report: public health preparedness: strengthening the nation's emergency response state by state. Accessed November 22, 2011, http://www.bt.cdc.gov/publications/2010phprep/pdf/complete_PHPREP_report.pdf.

Pandemic Influenza Preparedness Team. (2011). UK influenza pandemic preparedness strategy 2011: strategy for consultation. Accessed November 22, 2011, at http://www.dh.gov.uk/en/Consultations/Liveconsultations/DH_125316.

President's Council of Advisors on Science and Technology. (2009). Report to the president on U.S. preparation for 2009-H1N1 influenza. Accessed November 22, 2011, at http://www.whitehouse.gov/assets/documents/PCAST_H1N1_Report.pdf.

Reed, C., Angulo, F.J., Swerdlow, D.L., Lipsitch, M., Meltzer, M.I. (2009). Estimates of the prevalence of pandemic (H1N1) 2009, United States, April–July 2009. *Emerging Infectious Diseases, 15*(12), 2004–2007.

Stoto, M.A. (2008). Public health surveillance in the 21st century: achieving population health goals while protecting individuals' privacy and confidentiality. *Georgetown Law Journal, 96*(2), 703–719.

Stoto, M.A. (2014). Biosurveillance capability requirements for the Global Health Security Agenda: lessons from the 2009 H1N1 pandemic. *Biosecurity and Bioterrorism, 12*, 225–230.

Stoto, M.A., Dausey, D.J., Davis, L.M., Leuschner, K., Lurie, N. (2005). Learning from experience: the public health response to West Nile virus, SARS, monkeypox, and hepatitis A outbreaks in the United States. Accessed January 21, 2013, at http://www.rand.org/content/dam/rand/pubs/technical_reports/2005/RAND_TR285.pdf.

Swerdlow, D.L., Finelli, L., Bridges, C.B. (2011). 2009 H1N1 influenza pandemic: field and epidemiologic investigations in the United States at the start of the first pandemic of the 21st century. *Clinical Infectious Diseases, 52*(Suppl 1), S1–S3.

Thacker, S.B., Berkelman, R.L. (1988). Public health surveillance in the United States. *Epidemiologic Reviews, 10*, 164–190.

Trust for America's Health. (2010). Ready or not 2010: protecting the public's health from disease, disasters, and bioterrorism. Accessed November 22, 2011, at http://healthyamericans.org/assets/files/TFAH2010ReadyorNot%20FINAL.pdf.

U.S. Department of Health and Human Services. (2010a). National health security strategy of the United States of America. Accessed November 22, 2011, at http://

www.phe.gov/Preparedness/planning/authority/nhss/strategy/Documents/nhss-final.pdf.
U.S. Department of Health and Human Services. (2010b). Interim implementation guide for the national health security strategy of the United States of America. Accessed November 22, 2011, at http://www.phe.gov/Preparedness/planning/authority/nhss/implementationguide/Documents/iig-final.pdf.
World Health Organization. (2009). Pandemic (H1N1) 2009: update103. Accessed November 22, 2011, at http://www.who.int/csr/don/2010_06_04/en/index.html.
World Health Organization. (2010). WHO regional office for Europe guidance for influenza surveillance in humans. Accessed November 22, 2011, at http://www.euro.who.int/__data/assets/pdf_file/0020/90443/E92738.pdf.
Zhang, Y., May, L., Stoto, M.A. (2011). Evaluating syndromic surveillance systems at institutions of higher education: a retrospective analysis of the 2009 H1N1 influenza pandemic at two universities. *BMC Public Health*, *11*, 591.
Zhang, Y., Lopez-Gatell, H., Alpuche-Aranda, C., Stoto, M.A. (2013). Did advances in global surveillance and notification systems make a difference in the 2009 H1N1 pandemic?–A retrospective analysis. *PLoS ONE*, *8*, e59893.

CHAPTER 4

Variability in School Closure Decisions in Response to 2009 H1N1

TAMAR KLAIMAN, JOHN D. KRAEMER,
AND MICHAEL A. STOTO

Introduction

As concern about pandemic influenza in the United States grew in recent years, school closings were seen increasingly as a means of "social distancing" capable of slowing the spread of disease through the population (Ferguson, 2006). Thus, when the H1N1 pandemic emerged suddenly in 2009, it was not surprising that more than 726 K–12 schools in the United States closed, affecting 368,282 students (Cauchemez et al., 2009; Stein and Wilgorn, 2009). However, school closure can cause lost instruction time and substantial economic losses for both families and educational facilities (Lempel et al., 2009), and community upheaval. Because the decision to close schools is rife with challenges, clarifying and considering how to balance the multiple goals and objectives before a disease outbreak is an important component of public health emergency preparedness.

Analysis of the 2009 H1N1 pandemic in the United States shows there was extensive variation across the country in expressed rationales, decision triggers, and decision-making authority for school closures. As a result, decisions were often inconsistent, contributing to a sense that the government did not know how to respond, and perhaps was ineffective in meeting public health goals. From a systems improvement perspective, excess variation in health system structures and processes is a cause for concern, indicating possible inefficiencies and opportunities to improve the system (Institute of Medicine, 2008; Lurie et al., 2004). Adopting this perspective, the goal of this analysis is to identify the critical issues that arose during the spring 2009 H1N1 outbreak, to analyze sources of variation, and to identify lessons learned to assist school districts and public health systems to improve their school closure decision-making process.

In particular, we describe three key issues that challenged decision makers during the 2009 H1N1 pandemic: (1) clarifying goals, (2) clarifying authority and the decision-making process, and (3) dealing with uncertainty in preparing and issuing official guidance. Although we refer to a number of specific decisions that were made, our purpose is not to critique those decisions per se, but rather to use them to identify problems that are likely to arise in future pandemics and other public health emergencies and to learn from them to improve public health systems' capabilities. Similarly, we do not presume to say what school closing policies should be, but rather focus on the lessons learned from the 2009 experience to strengthen public health systems' response to future events.

Methods

Many aspects of the 2009 H1N1 pandemic were well described in the media, on the Internet, and in scientific publications, so we have based this analysis primarily on monitoring contemporaneous key sources and Lexis-Nexis and Internet searches. In particular, we identified media reports via Google alerts and Lexis-Nexis using the search terms "swine flu," "H1N1," and "school closure" (and appropriate truncated and extended variations of these search terms). We included local and national media sources in the analysis, and we accepted overlapping stories in multiple sources to gain a full picture of events taking place. As researchers subsequently published studies on the 2009 H1N1 pandemic in the academic literature, we supplemented our analysis with a review of this literature to develop as comprehensive a picture as possible of school closure decision making. Our focus was on events during spring 2009, but we consider some distinctions with the fall in the discussion that follows.

At least two members of the research team read each media report and noted key issues that arose. In addition, we observed conference calls and meetings between health departments and school officials in the Boston and Washington, DC, metropolitan areas, and we held informal interviews with decision makers and community members as feasible. Many interviews were conducted ad hoc during flu clinics or meetings, because decision makers did not have time for extensive formal interviews.

We organized the data collected from media reports and interviews into major themes, which we then vetted with public health researchers, practitioners, and education officials to ensure we captured the key issues and did not exclude any obvious concerns. These data were then compared for consistency with articles in the academic literature when they became available. Although these methods cannot tell us the frequency with which specific issues arose, we are confident we have identified and developed at least a basic understanding of the key public health issues.

School Closings during the 2009 H1N1 Outbreak

Timing and Extent of School Closings

School closures during the pandemic's first wave occurred in several phases. Initially, schools were closed on a somewhat ad hoc basis. After the Centers for Disease Control and Prevention (CDC) issued preliminary guidance on April 26, schools with 2009 H1N1 cases generally closed for at least seven days. On May 1, the CDC changed its guidance to suggest 14 days of closure, and most schools with cases closed with the intent to remain shuttered for 14 days. However, CDC guidance changed again on May 5 to say that closure was, in general, not necessary. By the end of the outbreak, most schools were that closed remained shut for three days or less (Rebmann et al., 2013). After May 5, most schools did not close after a case was identified, with the notable exception of the New York City school system, which continued closing schools into June to protect particularly vulnerable children. A timeline of major school closure events is provided in Box 4-1.

Rationale for School Closure

Three different rationales for closing schools during a public health emergency emerged in the 2009 H1N1 pandemic: (1) limiting spread of the virus in the community, (2) protecting vulnerable children, and (3) reacting to staff shortages or children kept at home because of infection or parents' fears of infection.

At the outset, in the United States, as in Europe and some Asian countries (Cauchemez et al., 2014; Sypsa and Hatzakis, 2009), the most common rationale for school closure was to limit spread of the pH1N1 virus in the community. This is based on the idea that schools provide an ideal context for spread of infectious diseases because children are more susceptible to infection, less likely to adopt behavioral changes that reduce disease spread, and more likely to sustain person-to-person contact for lengthy periods. Closing schools, therefore, may limit spread among children and their families, and the general community, and can be an important component of a community's "social distancing" efforts (Cauchemez et al., 2009). Closing schools, for instance, was an important component of Mexico's highly regarded social distancing efforts in response to the 2009 H1N1 pandemic (Lacey and McNeil, 2009). Although rigorous data on the health effects of school closure in Mexico are not available, it was the most visible intervention the country took to combat the emergent pandemic, and public health policy experts generally agree that it was a prudent step (Stern and Markel, 2009). U.S. school administrators and public health officials typically justified the costs of school closure on the same grounds (Chan and Sulzberger, 2009; Ferguson, 2006; Germann et al., 2006; Heymann et al., 2004).

Evidence of the impact of school closure on the spread of influenza, however, is limited and mixed. Historical analyses and epidemiologic modeling studies for influenza and other respiratory diseases suggest that social distancing measures, especially if implemented early during an outbreak and

Box 4-1 TIMELINE OF SCHOOL CLOSURES

- *April 23, 2009*: The first suspected 2009 H1N1 cases in a school in the United States are identified at St. Francis Preparatory School in New York City. Eight confirmed cases were reported on April 26 (Dawood et al., 2009).
- *April 24, 2009*: All schools in Mexico City—serving about seven million students—are closed as a social distancing measure to slow the spread of 2009 H1N1 (Lacey and McNeil, 2009).
- *April 25, 2009*: Byron Steele High School in Cibolo, Texas, is the first school in the United States closed because of 2009 H1N1. The following day, all schools in the Schertz–Cibolo–Universal City independent school district are closed by the Texas Department of State Health Services (Hsu, 2009).
- *April 26, 2009*: School officials close St. Francis Preparatory School to disinfect the school. The same day, the CDC recommends closing schools for seven days when a case is identified (Dawood et al., 2009).
- *May 1, 2009*: The CDC recommends that schools close for up to 14 days if a case of 2009 H1N1 is identified (De la Torre, 2009).
- *May 5, 2009*: The CDC changes its guidance to recommend that schools generally do not need to close and families should, instead, keep ill children home for at least seven days (Stephens, 2009).
- *June 2, 2009*: New York City closes its final school in response to 2009 H1N1. New York continued school closures well after the CDC ceased recommending closure, with the justification that closure would protect particularly vulnerable students from within-school transmission (Bosman, 2009).
- *August 7, 2009*: The CDC recommends against school closures in most cases, instead recommending that ill children remain at home, as part of its comprehensive guidance for schools to use during the fall semester (Seid et al., 2007).

sustained, can reduce substantially both the total number of cases and the peak attack rate (Cauchemez et al., 2009; Ferguson, 2006; Hatchett et al., 2007; Longini et al., 2005; Markel et al., 2007). On the other hand, the most recent systematic review found only 19 studies with primary empirical data on the impact of school closure per se, many of which had significant methodological challenges (Cauchemez et al., 2009). Some mathematical models suggest that school closure has a limited impact on cumulative case counts, because children not attending school are free to transmit infection to their families and others in the community (Cauchemez et al., 2009). Other modeling studies suggest that combining school closure with sequestering children in the home may curb pandemic spread and peak incidence, possibly reducing the extent to which healthcare resources may be overwhelmed or buying time for vaccination (Germann, 2006), although some models suggest schools would have to be closed for two months to achieve these results (Lee et al., 2010).

Differences are attributable in large part to assumptions underlying the models, reflecting uncertainties about epidemiology and student behavior that may be better understood as more data become available. At a minimum, though, it is clear that the effectiveness of school closure depends on students not congregating in large numbers in other settings, and this proved to be a challenge in 2009 (Bosman, 2009). Epidemiologic data on the actual effect of school closure on influenza transmission in 2009 are limited. However, one study of rates of acute respiratory infection in Dallas found a slower increase in acute respiratory infection cases than in adjacent communities while Dallas' schools were closed, with rates becoming similar after they reopened (Copeland et al., 2012).

Although advocated as a social distancing measure that imposes less societal costs than workplace closures or public disruptions, it became evident during the spring 2009 H1N1 pandemic wave that school closures imposed substantial costs in some instances. Parents complained of the difficulty of finding childcare or of the financial costs associated with finding someone to take care of their children or staying home (Institute of Medicine, 2008). Data from New York City suggest both that economic hardship reduced the effectiveness of school closure and imposed greater burdens on poorer families, with almost twice as many children from single-wage families leaving the house (30%) than dual-wage families (17%) (Borse et al., 2001). This is consistent with Australian research that found that, although most families reported only mild or moderate inconvenience, one in seven reported severe disruptions resulting from school closure (Effler et al., 2010). One study from Chicago found only 18% of households affected by school closures reported missing work (Jarquin et al., 2011), and a nationwide study in the United States found that although 30% of families affected by school closure either lost pay or had a child miss free or reduced-price school lunches, only 3% called the disruption severe (Steelfisher et al., 2010). However, this study only reported aggregate results, and policymakers—when weighing the likely adverse effects of school closure against its benefits—require data that are disaggregated to show the effect on marginalized groups. One of the few studies to disaggregate found that Australian parents without paid leave were three times more likely to report losing pay (Kavanagh et al., 2012). Because these parents were likely lower paid, nonsalaried employees, it can be expected that the relative importance of lost pay was greater for them than other parents.

New York City officials originally based their decision to close schools one at a time on the need to balance public health interests "with the child-care and educational needs of families" (Hartocollis and Hernandez, 2009, p. 13). These officials noted, however, that closures were compromised as a control measure if "the kids don't go to school and instead go to the shopping mall or go to the park" (Chan and Sulzberger, 2009, p. 14), as library officials in Queens reported a large number of children congregating after their schools were closed (Hartocollis and Hernandez, 2009). Indeed, formal studies of students in Boston and Pittsburgh have documented this behavior. High school students in the Boston's Winsor School, a private girls' school in Boston that closed from May 20 to 26 after a sudden increase in absenteeism, reported the average number of days during this period on which they participated in the following activities: shopping, 1.47 days; visiting a friend, 2.21 days; using public transport, 1.89 days; eating out, 2.44 days; and outdoor activities, 3.42 days (Miller et al., 2010). During a one-week closure of an elementary school in southwestern Pennsylvania that closed during this period, 69% of students reported having visited at least one location outside their home (Gift et al., 2010), and these findings are broadly consistent with research from Australia, although school closures were implemented there earlier during the pandemic when there was greater public apprehension about pH1N1 (McVernon et al., 2011).

There is, however, some evidence that school closure reduced student contacts, including research by Miller and colleagues (2010) who found a reduction in classmate contacts for students of a closed Boston school, although community contacts continued at a substantial rate. At the same time, Jackson and colleagues (2011) found that students whose school in the United Kingdom closed as a result of pH1N1 reported 65% fewer contacts—defined as people to whom the student spoke—when schools were closed (an average of 25 per day) than when open (an average of 71 per day), with most of the reduction being among classmates and not the general public.

As data emerged to suggest that school-age children experienced a greater attack rate than other age groups, and an unusually high rate of complications from the 2009 H1N1 pandemic (Babwin, 2009), protecting children—especially those who may be particularly vulnerable to complications—became a justification for school closure during the 2009 outbreak. In New York City, where officials continued closing schools even after the CDC stopped recommending it, Mayor Michael Bloomberg eventually clarified that school closure would not slow transmission and that closure "has absolutely nothing to do with the spread of the disease" (Chan and Sulzberger, 2009, p. 14). Rather, the rationale for closures shifted to preventing secondary cases among particularly vulnerable school contacts (Bosman, 2009).

The third rationale was purely practical. Staff shortages, whether a result of actual illness or concerns about infection, or children kept at home because parents feared they would become infected, simply made it impossible to keep schools open. We did not observe this rationale in the spring 2009 H1N1 pandemic; however, closure resulting from very high absenteeism became common in the fall resurgence. For example, several Connecticut schools closed in October because of high student absenteeism. "You can't teach with one- to two-thirds of the class absent," explained the superintendent of a district with closed schools (Merritt, 2009). During the last week of October 2009, about 350 schools were closed nationwide, a high proportion of which appeared to be in response to high absenteeism (Babwin, 2009). In some instances, it created significant public confusion when some schools were closed because of absenteeism but others stayed open even though they had H1N1 cases (Awofisayo et al., 2013).

Triggers for School Closings

Modeling studies consistently show that, to be effective, school closure to limit communitywide transmission requires an early trigger, such as on recognition of the first case in a community (Glass and Barnes, 2007). These results reflect the assumption that influenza transmission often occurs before patients develop symptoms, so there can be a substantial number of infections before a sizable number are identified. Detection of a novel strain usually occurs after it is well established in a locale, so the communitywide benefit of school closures is likely diminished substantially at that point (Cauchemez et al., 2009). Indeed, in 2009, transmission was often not identified in a locale until clusters had already been detected in schools (Dawood et al., 2009).

pH1N1 cases are defined for epidemiologic purposes as "suspected," "probable," or "laboratory confirmed," and the initial pH1N1 case definitions emphasized contact with other known cases (Centers for Disease Control and Prevention, 2009). In particular, a suspected case, based on symptoms, became a probable case if there were other cases in a child's school. As such, these definitions created a degree of circularity, because suspected cases in a school were sometime enough to make others into probable cases.

Most U.S. schools did not close in the spring until a probable case surfaced or greater than normal rates of influenzalike illness were observed at the school (Klaiman et al., 2009; New York City Government, 2009). In New York City, a Catholic high school with students who had recently returned from Mexico became an early focal point for infections and was closed shortly after cases were confirmed, but after at least eight children were ill. In Texas, however, the Fort Worth school district closed all 144 schools after one confirmed and three other suspected school-age cases were reported (Hsu, 2009). In Montgomery County, Maryland, school officials closed a public high school after a single probable case was identified. At the same time, other Maryland schools with probable cases remained open after consulting local health officials, although this decision appears to have been driven by the belief that transmission within the schools had not occurred and secondary cases were unlikely (Glod and de Vise, 2009).

We did not observe schools adopting formal thresholds for closure (e.g., a certain percentage of students identified as ill or absent) in the United States, although these were used in Japan in spring 2009 (Cowling et al., 2008). Similarly, Taiwan used what was termed a "2-3-5 strategy" to dismiss a class for a minimum of five days when two or more students from the same class were confirmed with a pH1N1 infection within three days (Hsueh et al., 2010). Because Taiwan's schools are structured such that students are in the same classroom with the same students for all courses (with teachers rotating between classes), public health authorities believed that dismissal of particular classes within a school would achieve public health goals with minimal social costs (Ferguson, 2006).

Authority and Decision-Making Process for School Closures

Much of the variation in school closure decisions in 2009 was a result of differences from one jurisdiction to another in whom the legal and practical authority for making decisions was vested. Depending on the jurisdiction, the legal authority to close schools in response to a public health threat may rest with school or health officials, either at the state or local level. In addition, in some jurisdictions, closure authority changes if an emergency has been declared, potentially in different ways depending on the form of the declared emergency (Hodge, 2009). Many states include school closure measures in their pandemic plans (Hsu, 2009; Klaiman et al., 2009), but the plans are often vague about who has the authority to make the decision to close schools. It is not surprising, therefore, that there was substantial variation in decisions to close schools during April 20009 and May 2009, and that there was conflict between authorities in some jurisdictions.

In Cibolo, Texas, the first American jurisdiction to close schools, the decision was made by state health officials (Maloney, 2009). In Fort Worth, Texas, on the other hand, local school officials made the decision to close schools districtwide, on the basis of advice from the local health department (Roser and Bloom, 2009). In Montgomery County, Maryland, shortly after health officials decided to close schools, the school superintendent protested the decision in a memo to the county school board stating, "We do not believe that this is the right decision given the lack of compelling evidence for continued closure provided to us by state and county health officials" (Institute of Medicine, 2008).

In New York City, public schools were closed by the city schools chancellor in consultation with the New York City Department of Health and Mental Hygiene (New York City Government, 2009). In addition, the local Roman Catholic archdiocese closed some schools independently on suspicion of 2009 pH1N1 cases (Stein and Wilgorn, 2009). It is unclear whether city officials had the authority to order private schools closed, but they did recommend closure (Klaiman et al., 2009).

In some instances, public health and school officials faced contradictory concerns. One frequent issue that arose dealt with laws mandating the number of instruction days that schools must provide to receive state funding. In several states, schools that closed for public health purposes risked losing state education funding or incurring significant costs by extending the school year. States responded to this issue in different ways. Rhode Island law authorizes the state education commissioner to issue waivers of the instruction days requirement for schools closed because of emergencies, and such waivers were granted to schools closed for 2009 pH1N1 (Reynolds, 2009). New York law authorized waivers for schools closed resulting from weather and other disruptions, but not epidemics (Medina, 2009). The state legislature responded by passing a law authorizing a waiver similar to that in Rhode Island (New York Assembly Bill A.B. 8710 §1., 2009). Tennessee's legislature passed a similar bill (Jackson, 2009). Connecticut law authorized a waiver for "extreme circumstances," which the state education commissioner decided did not include closures for influenza, and the state legislature did not enact a proposed statutory exemption. Closed Connecticut schools had to reschedule classes to ensure they met for 180 instruction days (De la Torre, 2009). State education officials in Alabama similarly indicated that any school closed for influenza would lose a portion of its state funding if it did not reschedule enough classes to meet the minimum number of instruction days (Doyle, 2009).

The potential for substantial confusion about school closure authority continues to persist. Potter and colleagues (2012) identified variability regarding whether state or local officials have legal authority to close schools. More concerning, seven states grant this authority either to multiple officials or to no specific person, making closure decisions considerably more complicated. Based on computational models, Potter and colleagues (2012) concluded that granting authority to local officials (something barred in 14 states) may be preferable because it allows local disease transmission to be taken into account.

Official Guidance

Early during the spring outbreak, state and local health departments followed CDC guidance that districts "consider adopting school dismissal." This guidance was influenced primarily by early reports suggesting a high case fatality rate from 2009 pH1N1 and that youth may be at greater than average risk. The CDC's initial guidance also suggested that schools with cases stay closed for 14 days (Ruane and Glod, 2009), reflecting concerns about the risks of reopening while disease was still being transmitted. Such "guidance," often transmitted through state and local health departments, carries substantial weight in local decision making. In part because state and local officials do not have the same epidemiologic knowledge as the CDC, guidance is often regarded as a recommendation, and local officials are often very hesitant to act contrary to CDC guidance, even if they do not believe it takes full account of local circumstances (Stoto et al., 2013).

The CDC subsequently revised its guidance, announcing that schools closed under the prior guidance could reopen, but included the caveat that "decisions about school closure should be at the discretion of local authorities based on special circumstances and local considerations, including public concern and the impact of school absenteeism and staffing shortages" (U.S. Department of Health and Human Services, 2009).

When additional data showed that the novel 2009 pH1N1 was not especially severe, the CDC again revised its recommendation to keeping ill children at home (U.S. Department of Health and Human Services, 2009). Some schools, however, continued closing "to be on the safe side" (Stolarz and Williams, 2009).

Officials were often frustrated by frequent changes in CDC guidance. For example, shortly after the CDC increased its closure recommendation from 7 to 14 days, a Fort Worth, Texas, official stated, "The CDC is changing its plans and guidance on a daily basis" (Weiss, 2009). However, especially at the beginning of a disease outbreak, knowledge about disease severity, transmissibility, and the extent to which people with various underling conditions are at increased risk of complications is based necessarily on limited data. It should not be surprising for this information and the resulting guidance to be revised as more cases accumulate. Indeed in the CDC's August 2009 school closure guidance, the agency notes that although it did not currently recommend closure, this could change if the disease's severity increased (Centers for Disease Control and Prevention, 2009).

The CDC's August 2009 school closure guidance suggests that local authorities make school closure decisions by balancing "the risks of keeping the students in school with the social disruption that school dismissal can cause" (Centers for Disease Control and Prevention, 2009). The guidance notes that "the potential benefits of preemptively dismissing students from school are often outweighed by negative consequences," but also that "school dismissals may be warranted, depending on the disease burden and other conditions." Recognizing that the severity may change, the CDC issued alternate guidance to be followed in the event of more serious disease (Centers for Disease Control and Prevention, 2009).

Results

The Institute of Medicine describes a "public health system" as "a complex network of individuals and organizations that have the potential to play critical roles in creating the conditions for health" (Institute of Medicine, 2002, p. 28). In the context of emergency preparedness, this includes "communities, health-care delivery systems, employers and business, the media, homeland security and public safety, academia, and the governmental public health infrastructure" (Institute of Medicine, 2008, p. 10). The emergence of the novel H1N1 pandemic in 2009 clearly showed unnecessary variation in the way that school closings were handled, suggesting problems in the public health *system* that must be addressed.

To address these problems, we have adopted a systems improvement approach (Lotstein et al., 2008; Seid et al., 2007), seeking to identify and reduce unnecessary *variability* in processes and outcomes while preserving system differences that are critical to the specific environment (Berwick, 1996). This approach views a system's activities explicitly as defined processes—that is, chains of events that produce specific outcomes; a focus on changes that allow complex, intertwined systems of people and information to work more effectively; changes made based on their effects on measurable outcomes; and the encouragement of continuous improvement rather than one-time initiatives. Systems improvement efforts use specific activities such as learning collaboratives, process analysis, and critical event or failure mode analysis. From this perspective, our analysis of school closings is an example of learning from a critical event about the nature and causes of variation in important aspects of the public health system's performance.

Although the CDC does not currently recommend large-scale school closure, questions about whether, when, and how to do so are likely to arise in the future, whether for pH1N1 or some other pathogen. Because closure decisions require local public health concerns to be balanced with broader societal concerns, public health and school officials should consider the challenges inherent in closure and develop realistic plans to address them. Our analysis of the events of 2009 suggests three issues that require attention. First, as an outbreak develops, the goals of school closing should be clarified and specific measures adapted to the goals. Second, as part of planning and preparedness efforts, the legal and practical authority to close schools should be clarified. Last, decision makers should expect uncertainty and act accordingly.

Clarify Goals and Forms of School Closing

As indicated earlier, three different and conflicting rationales for closing schools emerged in the 2009 H1N1 pandemic: (1) limiting spread of the virus in the community, (2) protecting vulnerable children, and (3) reacting to staff shortages or children kept at home because parents feared they would become infected. The rationale matters because it drives considerations such as whether to close schools at all, the nature and extent of closure, and the triggers for closure and reopening. In addition, closure decisions require effective balancing of potential benefits and consequences, and this cannot be done without a clear idea of what benefits are desired. In practice, there is evidence that the purpose of school closures may have been unclear even to those involved in closures. For example, surveys of principals (Shi et al., 2014) and teachers (Dooyema et al., 2014) in Michigan found that high percentages listed both proactive and reactive reasons for school closure.

CDC guidance recognized the potential costs and difficulties of closure, calling for a careful balancing between potential benefits from closure and the potential "negative consequences, including students being left home alone, health workers missing shifts when they must stay home with their children, students missing meals, and interruption of students' education" (Centers for Disease Control and Prevention, 2009). Officials considering closure must weigh not only the total amount of disruption, but also the extent to which social costs will be borne disproportionately by certain segments of society, such as those who depend on school lunches to meet nutritional needs. Closure, if adopted, should be necessary to achieving goals that cannot be achieved effectively through lesser alternatives, such as requiring ill students to stay home or granting liberal absences. It is unclear to what extent school and health officials balanced hardships from closure against health protection, but such balancing played a role in the CDC's decision to stop advising that schools close when it determined that pH1N1 was less dangerous than initial reports suggested. Indeed, mathematical models produced after the pandemic suggested that the societal costs of extended school closure—especially of the multimonth duration believed necessary to affect community-level transmission markedly—would have imposed much greater societal costs than benefits (Brown et al., 2011; Xue et al., 2012).

School closure can take a variety of forms (Cauchemez et al., 2009). One end of the spectrum is full closure—neither educational nor administrative functions continue and school personnel do not arrive for work. Alternatively, classes can be dismissed, but some or all administrative functions may continue in partial closures. Partial closures may also allow schools to continue providing meals or other social services during the period of class dismissal (Berkman, 2008), and continue to hold social events such as proms, and academic gatherings such as Scholastic Aptitude Test or American College Testing testing services. However, partial closure that allows students to congregate may defeat its purpose. During spring 2009, it appears the great majority of closures were full and were conducted preemptively.

There are a variety of alternatives to closure that schools might consider. One of these is currently endorsed by the CDC for most instances: requiring ill students to remain home to avoid infecting others (Centers for Disease Control and Prevention, 2009). In addition, schools could reduce the likelihood that children with underlying conditions predisposing them to complications of pH1N1 will be exposed by authorizing a liberal absence policy for those students. A school basing its closure decision largely on the goal of ameliorating public fears might relax attendance requirements for all students.

However, because public schools are funded based on student attendance levels, some schools may choose to close during times of high absenteeism to make up classes later in the year. Alternatively, they could attempt to overcome concerns about students missing class material by instituting online teaching, which at least one school in Maryland attempted (de Vise, 2009). Indeed, the U.S. Department of Education (2009) has suggested a variety of offsite continuity of instruction tools, including the use of electronic media to teach children who are at home, although it is unclear how many teachers are prepared for distance teaching.

If the goal is to protect particularly vulnerable students, schools may wish to defer to parents' decisions about the costs and benefits of a vulnerable student missing school, and allow parents broader license to consult medical professionals and to keep their children home preemptively. Other officials may prefer a blunter option—such as closure—on the grounds that parents may lack information to weigh risks and benefits. In addition, closing schools later during an outbreak may still serve to protect vulnerable children and staff from complications if within-school intensity of transmission is high.

Clarify Legal Authority for School Closure

As described earlier, school closure decisions in 2009 were often inconsistent among neighboring jurisdictions and over time. This may have contributed to a sense that the government did not know how to respond, and perhaps was ineffective in meeting public health goals. Similar problems were seen during the 1918–1919 pandemic when, as Stern and colleagues (2009, p. w1076) report, "ill-defined lines of authority among governmental branches contributed to the eruption of interagency conflict in U.S. cities . . . [and] confusion about authority and jurisdiction helped lead to distrust in health officials and political leaders." The 2009 and the 1918–1919 experiences suggests that, at the very least, officials must consider in advance who has the authority to close schools and identify what goals they wish to accomplish through a potential closure. Although these lessons were learned nearly 100 years ago in a previous H1N1 influenza pandemic, they seem to have been lost.

Inconsistencies of this sort can be particularly obvious in a region such as the Washington, DC, metropolitan area, which includes two states and the District of Columbia, plus numerous local jurisdictions, but one media market. In such settings, and even in isolated jurisdictions, it seems important to be sure that reasons for differences in decisions be communicated clearly to the public.

Regardless of who has the formal authority to close schools in a jurisdiction, the 2009 experience shows that it is helpful to solicit input from a range of stakeholders, such as local and state health and school officials, students, their parents, and school staff. Broader inclusion of stakeholders both improves the likelihood that decisions are made with full information and promote consideration of benefits and costs that will accrue to different affected groups. Coordination of this sort also helps to ensure the credibility of the message (Maher, 2009). The New York school closures described earlier, for instance, conveyed a sense of a unified city government decision, announced jointly by the top-ranking school and health officials, and press announcements also frequently included Mayor Michael Bloomberg.

Expect Uncertainty

Decisions about whether and how to close schools logically depend on epidemiologic information about who is likely to be infected, the severity of illness in those infected, and periods of infectiousness. Infectious disease outbreaks, however, are often characterized by scientific uncertainty (Stoto et al., 2005), and the 2009 H1N1 pandemic was no different. In many instances, planning activities had assumed a pandemic with different transmission and severity characteristics than actually developed (Hoffman, 2013). Changing and variable case definitions led to uncertain understanding of the epidemiologic risks, which in turn led to frequent changes in official guidance. In addition, health departments often lacked critical health systems information. For example, in a survey conducted by the National Association of County and City Health Officials for a 10-week period in 2009, up to half of the health departments lacked data on school closures and absenteeism in any given week, and 73% to 88% lacked information from universities in their jurisdictions (Cantey et al., 2013). This uncertainty made all the decisions regarding school closing more difficult. In particular, information emerged during the spring to suggest the pH1N1 infection was less severe than most pandemic planning assumptions, and children were more likely to be infected and experience severe consequences. Each of these factors influenced decisions about whether and how to close schools.

If the 2009 H1N1 pandemic is any guide to the future, public health and other officials should expect and plan for uncertainty about the facts and frequent changes in official guidance that is based on a constantly evolving epidemiologic knowledge base. This begins with acknowledging the uncertainty and requires flexibility in policies and procedures, such as consideration of variations of school closing and alternatives as discussed earlier. During the 2009 H1N1 pandemic, for instance, the goal of Acting CDC Director Richard Bessor was to "tell everything we knew, everything we didn't know, and what we were doing to get the answers" (Maher, 2009, p. 152). Unfortunately, this lesson has only been learned in part in the years since the 2009 pandemic, with recommendations for school closure procedures—although well intended—often relying on information about case counts, severity, and transmissibility that will likely not exist during a pandemic's critical, early stages (Halder et al., 2010). See Chapter 3, for instance, for a discussion of the impact of early assumptions about children being at "greater risk" during the 2009 H1N1 pandemic.

In particular, because pandemic influenza has and will likely always continue to affect communities differently, in both social and epidemiologic terms, monitoring the situation at the local level plays an important role in closure decisions. Communities will experience varying levels of transmission, and some populations have more people who are highly susceptible to complications than others. Wealthier communities may be able to keep schools closed because parents have childcare alternatives, whereas communities with more disadvantaged populations may depend on schools for a variety of resources, such as childcare and school lunches. The 2009 experience suggests that local school and health officials must monitor the situation in their communities and work together closely to integrate local information with state and federal guidance.

Planning for uncertainty includes development of systems to track the epidemic and its consequences, and to evaluate the impact of control efforts—that is, to provide "situational awareness." It also requires a degree of humility in presenting decisions to both senior policymakers and the public, stating clearly the basis on which decisions were made and noting the likelihood that they can, or are likely to, change. More important, it also requires clear communication to the public about the rationale for decisions, particularly when different contexts justify what may otherwise be perceived to be contradictory decisions (Awofisayo et al., 2013).

Implications for Policy and Practice

A careful analysis of the 2009 H1N1 pandemic finds extensive variation across the United States in expressed rationales, decision triggers, and decision-making authority for school closures. This led to decisions that were often inconsistent from one locale to another and over time, contributing to a sense that the government was unsure how to respond and was perhaps ineffective. From a systems improvement perspective, however, such excess variation is a cause for concern, indicating possible inefficiencies and opportunities to improve the system.

Because school closure decisions require local public health concerns to be balanced with broader societal concerns, analysis of the 2009 H1N1 pandemic suggests three issues public health and school officials should consider in planning for and making school closure decisions in the future. First, the goal of school closing should be made clear, and specific measures should be tailored to the goal and modified over time as evolving knowledge requires. Second, legal and practical authority to close schools should be clarified in advance as part of planning and preparedness efforts. Last, decision makers should expect uncertainty and maintain situational awareness, be flexible in policies and procedures, and act with humility.

Acknowledgments and Disclosures

This chapter was developed in collaboration with a number of partnering organizations, and with funding support awarded to the Harvard School of Public Health Center for Public Health Preparedness under cooperative agreements with the U.S. CDC (grant no. 5P01TP000307-01; Preparedness and Emergency Response Research Center). The content of these publications and the views and discussions expressed in this chapter are solely those of the authors and do not necessarily represent the views of any partner organizations, the CDC, or the U.S. Department of Health and Human Services, nor does mention of trade names, commercial practices, or organizations imply endorsement by the U.S. government. The authors thank Melissa Higdon and Mikhaila Richards for their assistance with this manuscript.

References

Awofisayo, A., Ibbotson, S., Smith, G. E., Janmohamed, K., Mohamed H., Olowokure, B. (2013). Challenges and lessons learned from implementing a risk-based approach to school advice and closure during the containment phase of the 2009 influenza pandemic in the West Midlands, England. *Public Health, 127*(7), 637–643.

Babwin, D. (2009). Swine flu prompts hundreds of schools to close. Associated Press State and Local Wire.

Berkman, B. E. (2008). Mitigating pandemic influenza: the ethics of implementing a school closure policy. *Journal of Public Health Management and Practice, 14*(4), 372–378.

Berwick, D. (1996). A primer on leading the improvement of systems. *British Medical Journal, 312*, 619–622.

Borse, R. H., Behravesh, C. B., Dumanovsky, T., Zucker, J. R., Swerdlow, D., Edelson, P. (2001). Closing schools in response to the 2009 pandemic influenza A H1N1 virus in New York City: economic impact on households. *Clinical Infectious Diseases, 52*(Suppl 1), S168–S172.

Bosman, J. (2009). Flu closings failing to keep schoolchildren at home. *New York Times*, May 21, 2009, Section A, 27.

Brown, S. T., Tai, J. H. Y., Bailey, R. R., Cooley, P. C., Wheaton, W. D., Potter, M. A. (2011). Would school closure for the 2009 H1N1 influenza pandemic have been worth the cost? A computational simulation of Pennsylvania. *BMC Public Health, 11*, 353.

Cantey, P. T., Chuk, M. G., Kohl, K. S., Herrmann, J., Weiss, P., Graffunder, C. M. (2013). Public health emergency preparedness: lessons learned about monitoring of interventions from the National Association of County and City Health Officials survey of nonpharmaceutical interventions for pandemic H1N1. *Journal of Public Health Management and Practice, 19*(1), 70–76.

Cauchemez, S., Ferguson, N. M., Wachtel, C., Tegnell, A., Saour, G., Duncan, B., Nicoll, A. (2009). Closure of schools during an influenza pandemic. *The Lancet Infectious Diseases, 9*, 473–481.

Cauchemez, S., Van Kerkhove, M. D., Archer, B. N., Cetron, M., Cowling, B. J., Grove, P., Hunt, D., et al. (2014). School closures during the 2009 influenza pandemic: national and local experiences. *BMC Infectious Diseases, 14*(1), 207.

Centers for Disease Control and Prevention. (2009). Technical report for state and local public health officials and school administrators on CDC guidance for school (K–12) responses to influenza during the 2009-2010 school year. Available online at http://www.cdc.gov/h1n1flu/schools/schoolguidance.htm

Chan, S., Sulzberger, A. G. (2009). Mayor says more school closings won't stop swine flu's spread. *New York Times*, May 26, 2009, Section A, 14.

Copeland, D. L., Basurto-Davila, R., Chung, W., Kurian, A., Fishbein, D. B., Symanowski, P. (2013). Effectiveness of school closure for pandemic influenza A (H1N1) on acute respiratory illnesses in the community: a natural experiment. *Clinical Infectious Diseases, 56*(4), 509–516.

Cowling, B. J., Lau, E. H., Lam, C. L., Cheng, C. K., Kovar, J., Chan, K. H. (2008). Effects of school closures, 2008 winter influenza season, Hong Kong. *Emerging Infectious Diseases, 14*(10), 1660–1662.

Dawood, F. S., Jain, S., Finelli, L., Shaw, M. W., Lindstrom, S., Garten, R. J. (2009). Emergence of a novel swine-origin influenza A (H1N1) virus in human. *The New England Journal of Medicine, 361*, 2605–2615.

De la Torre, V. (2009). No break for school in Granby; 180-day year stands. *Hartford Courant*, June 5, 2009.

de Vise, D. (2009). The three R's thrive in swine flu outbreak; Internet facilitates lessons during closure. *The Washington Post,* May 7, 2009, Section Metro, B04.

Dooyema, C. A., Copeland, D., Sinclair, J. R., Shi, J., Wilkins, M., Wells, E., Collins, J. (2014). Factors influencing school closure and dismissal decisions: influenza A (H1N1), Michigan 2009. *Journal of School Health, 84*(1), 56–62.

Doyle, N. (2009). State orders schools here to make up days missed because of swine flu. *Huntsville Times Online.* May 7, 2009. Available online at http://blog.al.com/breaking/2009/05/state_orders_schools_here_to_m.html.

Effler, P. V., Carcione, D., Giele, C., Dowse, G. K., Goggin, L., Mak, D. B. (2010). Household response to pandemic (H1N1) 2009-related school closures, Perth, Western Australia. *Emerging Infectious Diseases, 16*(2), 205–211.

Ferguson, N. M., Cummings, D. A. T., Fraser, C., Cajka, J. C., Cooley, P. C., Burke, D. S. (2006). Strategies for mitigating an influenza pandemic. *Nature, 442,* 448–452.

Germann, T. C., Kadau, K., Longini, I. M., Macken, C. A. (2006). Mitigation strategies for pandemic influenza in the United States. *Proceedings of the National Academy of Sciences of the United States of America, 103,* 5935–5940.

Gift, T. L., Palekar, R. S., Sodha, S. V., Kent, C. K., Fagan, R. P. (2010). Household effects of school closure during pandemic (H1N1) 2009, Pennsylvania, USA. *Emerging Infectious Diseases, 16*(8), 1315–1317.

Glass, K., Barnes, B. (2007). How much would closing schools reduce transmission during an influenza pandemic? *Epidemiology, 18,* 623–638.

Glod, M., de Vise, D. (2009). Hundreds of schools, mostly in Texas, shut; Rockville High will close; many classrooms emptier. *The Washington Post,* May 1, 2009, Section A, A06.

Halder, N., Kelso, J. K., Milne, G. J. (2010). Developing guidelines for school closure interventions to be used during a future influenza pandemic. *BMC Infectious Disease, 10,* 221.

Hartocollis, A., Hernandez, J. C. (2009). Fears of swine flu close three more schools. *New York Times,* May 16, 2009, Section A, 13.

Hatchett, R. J., Mecher, C. E., Lipsitch, M. (2007). Public health interventions and epidemic intensity during the 1918 influenza pandemic. *Proceedings of the National Academy of Sciences of the United States of America, 104*(18), 7582–7587.

Heymann, A., Chodick, G., Reichman, B., Kokia, E., Laufer, J. (2004). Influence of school closure on the incidence of viral respiratory diseases among children and on health care utilization. *The Pediatric Infectious Disease Journal, 23,* 675–676.

Hodge, J. G. (2009). The legal landscape for school closures in response to pandemic flu or other public health threat. *Biosecurity and Bioterrorism, 7*(1), 45–50.

Hoffman, L. M. (2013). The return of the city-state: urban governance and the New York City H1N1 pandemic. *Sociology of Health & Illness, 35*(2), 255–267.

Hsu, S. S. (2009). Strategy on flu under revision. *The Washington Post,* August 4, 2009, A01.

Hsueh, R., Lee, P., Chiu, A. W., Yen, M. (2010). Pandemic (H1N1) 2009 vaccination and class suspensions after outbreaks, Taipei City, Taiwan. *Emerging Infectious Diseases, 16*(8), 1309–1311.

Institute of Medicine. (2002). *The future of the public's health in the 21st century.* Washington, DC: National Academies Press.

Institute of Medicine. (2008). *Research priorities in emergency preparedness and response for public health systems: a letter report.* Washington, DC: National Academies Press.

Jackson, A. (2009). Local events, swine flu waiver. *The Jackson Sun,* May 22, 2009, 2.

Jackson, C., Mangtani, P., Vynnycky, E., Fielding, K., Kitching, A., Mohamed, H. (2011). School closures and student contact patterns. *Emerging Infectious Diseases,* 17(2), 245–247.

Jarquin, V. G., Callahan, D. B., Cohen, N. J., Balaban, V., Wang, R., Beato, R. (2011). Effect of school closure from pandemic (H1N1) 2009, Chicago, Illinois, USA. *Emerging Infectious Diseases,* 17(4), 751–753.

Kavanagh, A. M., Mason, K. E., Bentley, R. J., Studdert, D. M., McVernon, J., Fielding, J. E. (2012). Leave entitlements, time off work and the household financial impacts of quarantine compliance during an H1N1 outbreak. *BMC Infectious Diseases, 12,* 311.

Klaiman, T. A., Ibrahim, J., Hausman, A. (2009). Do state written pandemic plans include federal recommendations? A national study. *Journal of Homeland Security and Emergency Management, 6*(1), 44.

Lacey, M., McNeil, D. G. (2009). Fighting deadly flu outbreak, Mexico shuts schools for millions. *New York Times,* April 25, 2009, Section A, 4.

Lee, B. Y., Brown, S. T., Cooley, P., Potter, M. A., Wheaton, W. D., Voorhees, R. E. (2010). Simulating school closure strategies to mitigate an influenza epidemic. *Journal of Public Health Management and Practice, 16*(3), 252–261.

Lempel, H., Hammond, R. A., Epstein, J. M. (2009). *Economic cost and health care workforce effects of school closures in the U.S.* Working paper. Washington, DC: Brookings Institution.

Longini, I. M., Nizam, A., Xu, S., Ungchusak, K., Hanshaoworakul, W., Cummings, D. A. (2005). Containing pandemic influenza at the source. *Science, 309*(5737),1083–1087.

Lotstein, D., Seid, M., Ricci, K., Leuschner, K. (2008). Using quality improvement methods to improve public health emergency preparedness: PREPARE for pandemic influenza. *Health Affairs, Web Exclusive, 27*(5), w328–w329.

Lurie, N., Wasserman, J., Stoto, M., Myers, S., Namkung, P., Fielding, J., Valdez, R. B. (2004). Local variation in public health preparedness: lessons from California. *Health Affairs, Supplement Web Exclusives,* w341–353.

Maher, B. (2009). Swine flu: crisis communicator. *Nature, 463*(7278), 150–152.

Maloney, R. (2009). Swine flu shuts down Steele High School. *Herald-Zeitung,* April 26, 2009.

Markel, H., Lipman, H. B., Navarro, J. A., Sloan, A., Michalsen, J. R., Stern, A. M. (2007). Nonpharmaceutical interventions implemented by U.S. cities during the 1918–1919 influenza pandemic. *Journal of the American Medical Association, 298*(6), 644–654.

McVernon, J., Mason, K., Petrony, S., Nathan, P., LaMontagne, A. D., Bentley, R. (2011). Recommendations for and compliance with social restrictions during implementation of school closures in the early phase of the influenza A (H1N1) 2009 outbreak in Melbourne, Australia. *BMC Infectious Diseases, 11,* 257.

Medina, J. (2009). Flu takes toll at schools that the city keeps open. *New York Times,* May 23, 2009, Section A, 14.
Merritt, G. E. (2009). Schools close as resurgent swine flu hits hard. *Hartford Courant.* Available online at http://articles.courant.com/2009-10-28/news/schools-swine-flu-1028.art_1_snow-days-swine-flu-schools.
Miller, J. C., Danon, L., O'Hagan, J. J., Goldstein, E., Lajous, M. (2010). Student behavior during a school closure caused by pandemic influenza A/H1N1. *PLoS One,* 5, e10425.
New York City Government. (2009). Health Commissioner Frieden and Schools Chancellor Klein announce city will close two more schools in response to increased flu-like symptoms. May 20, 2009. Accessed on November 13, 2014 at http://www.nyc .gov/html/doh/html/pr2009/pr029-09.shtml.
Potter, M. A., Brown, S. T., Cooley, P. C., Sweeney, P. M., Hershey, T. B., Gleason, S. M. (2012). School closure as an influenza mitigation strategy: how variations in legal authority and plan criteria can alter the impact. *BMC Public Health, 12,* 977.
Rebmann T., Elliott, M. B., Swick, Z., Reddick, D. (2013). US school morbidity and mortality, mandatory vaccination, institution closure, and interventions implemented during the 2009 influenza A H1N1 pandemic. *Biosecurity and Bioterrorism, 11*(1), 41–48.
Reynolds, M. (2009). Swine flu could cut school's session. *The Providence Journal-Bulletin,* June 13, 2009, Section Local, 3.
Roser, M. A., Bloom, M. (2009). Spread of flu virus may be slowing. *Austin American-Statesman,* May 2, 2009, A1.
Ruane, M. E., Glod, M. (2009). D.C. area schools consider options for dealing with flu closures. *The Washington Post,* May 4, 2009, Section A, A05.
Seid, M., Lotstein, D., Williams, V. L., Nelson, C., Leuschner, K. J., Diamant, A., Stern, S., Wasserman, J., Lurie, N. (2007). Quality improvement in public health emergency preparedness. *Annual Review of Public Health, 28,* 19–31.
Shi, J., Njai, R., Wells, E., Collins, J., Wilkins, M., Dooyema, C., Sinclair, J., Gao, H., Rainey, J. J. (2014). Knowledge, attitudes, and practices of nonpharmaceutical interventions following school dismissals during the 2009 influenza A H1N1 pandemic in Michigan, United States. *PLoS One,* 9(4), e94290.
Simpson, C. (2009). U.S. declares public health emergency over swine flu outbreak. *Wall Street Journal,* April 26, 2009, Section Business.
Steelfisher, G. K., Blendon, R. J., Bekheit, M. M., Liddon, N., Kahn, E., Schieber, E. A. (2010). Parental attitudes and experiences during school dismissals related to 2009 influenza A (H1N1): United States, 2009. *MMWR Morbidity and Mortality Weekly Report,* 59(35), 1131–1134.
Stein, R., Wilgoren, D. (2009). Fort Worth shutters all schools; WHO warns of a likely pandemic. *Washington Post,* April 30, 2009.
Stern, A. M., Cetron, M. S., Markel, H. (2009). Closing the schools: lessons from the 1918–19 U.S. influenza pandemic. *Health Affairs, 28*(6), 1066–1078.
Stern, A. M., Markel, H. (2009). What Mexico taught the world about pandemic influenza preparedness and community mitigation strategies. *Journal of the American Medical Association, 302*(11), 1221–1222.

Stolarz, C., Williams, C. (2009). Swine flu tests schools. *The Detroit News*, May 5, 2009.

Stoto, M. A., Dausey, D. J., Davis, L. M., Leuschner, K. J., Lurie, N., Myers, S., Olmsted, S. S., Ricci, K. A., Ridgely, M. S., Sloss, E. M., Wasserman, J. (2005). *Learning from experience: the public health response to West Nile virus, SARS, monkey pox, and hepatitis A outbreaks in the United States.* Santa Monica, CA: RAND technical report.

Stoto, M. A., Nelson, C., Higdon, M., Kraemer, J. D., Hites, L., Singleton C. (2013). Lessons about the state and local public health system response to the 2009 H1N1 pandemic: a workshop summary. *Journal of Public Health Management and Practice, 19*(5), 428–435.

Sypsa, V., Hatzakis, A. (2009). School closure is currently the main strategy to mitigate influenza A(H1N1): a modeling study. *Eurosurveillance, 14*(24), 19240.

U.S. Department of Education. (2009). Lead and manage my school: H1N1 flu information. May 10, 2012. Available online at http://www2.ed.gov/admins/lead/safety/emergencyplan/pandemic/index.html.

U.S. Department of Health and Human Services. (2009). Statement by HHS Secretary Kathleen Sebelius and by Acting CDC Director Dr. Richard Besser Regarding the Change in CDC's School and Child Care Closure Guidance. May 5, 2009. Available online at http://www.hhs.gov/news/press/2009pres/05/20090505a.html.

Weiss, J. (2009). Advice puzzles schools; North Texas districts struggle with changes. *The Dallas Morning News*. Accessed on December 2010 at dallasnews.com.

Xue, Y., Kristiansen, I. S., de Blasio, B. F. (2012). Dynamic modeling of costs and health consequences of school closure during an influenza pandemic. *BMC Public Health, 12*, 962.

CHAPTER 5 Wearing Many Hats

Lessons about Emergency Preparedness and Routine Public Health from the H1N1 Response

MATTHEW W. LEWIS, EDWARD W. CHAN,
CHRISTOPHER NELSON, ANDREW S. HACKBARTH,
CHRISTINE A. VAUGHAN, ALONZO PLOUGH,
AND BRIT K. OIULFSTAD

Introduction

Although the 2009 H1N1 pandemic influenza virus affected many people, it did not have the severe health consequences that were feared initially or that had been part of the federal pandemic influenza planning scenarios. This relative lack of severity and a number of other issues created the somewhat unexpected challenge of forcing the public health system simultaneously to mount a long-term, large-scale response while also maintaining most routine functions. In this respect, the 2009 H1N1 pandemic was typical of many public health emergencies that—unlike less common events such as earthquakes, hurricanes, or explosive attacks—emerge slowly and continue over a long period of time. Thus, although much of the policy debate surrounding public health emergency preparedness has focused on doomsday scenarios such as aerosolized anthrax (Centers for Disease Control and Prevention Office of Public Health Preparedness and Response, 2008) or nuclear detonations (Homeland Security Council, 2005), pH1N1 provides important lessons on the challenges involved in balancing routine and emergency public health functions.

These challenges were abundantly evident in Los Angeles County Department of Public Health's (LACDPH) 2009 pH1N1 response. In most important respects, the LACDPH's response was a success, delivering almost 200,000 doses of vaccine to the public and coordinating with more than 3,600 community partners to deliver an additional 3.4 million doses. The LACDPH also received and distributed antivirals and personal protective equipment from the federal Strategic National Stockpile, issued more than 20 pH1N1 health alert notifications via the California Health Alert Network, and ran a large public information campaign. Throughout all of this, the LACDPH maintained a broad range of routine public health services in infectious disease control, chronic disease preventions, maternal and child health, HIV/AIDS, community health clinics, and many other services.

This chapter describes some of the challenges the LACDPH faced during the pH1N1 response associated with simultaneous operation of emergency and routine operations. Although the challenges described are wide ranging, they all stem from the need to work concomitantly within two organizational structures: the "routine" structure used for daily LACDPH operations and the "emergency" structure prescribed by the Incident Command System (ICS) used by all first-responder organizations from fire to police and (increasingly) to governmental public health agencies. The general challenges encountered related to division of labor, channels of input in decision making, workload, and the timeliness and execution of decisions. These general challenges and specific examples described are drawn from an independent after-action report (AAR) of the pH1N1 response commissioned by the LACDPH and conducted by a team led by the RAND Corporation, which also included strong partnership and involvement from LACDPH staff. Such structured reviews are often conducted by military, emergency management, fire, and, increasingly, public health organizations. The chapter concludes with a set of recommendations adopted by the LACDPH that are potentially relevant to other health departments, particularly those operating in large, complex, metropolitan contexts.

Methods

Given the practical purposes of an AAR, our objectives in conducting this review were to (1) gather input from a broad array of stakeholders; (2) identify the most important issues (i.e., problems) in the response, and the root causes of each; (3) identify and vet proposed solutions with senior leaders; and (4) elicit implementation priorities from organizational leadership and identify next steps. Because there is little methodological consensus on how best to conduct an AAR of a large-scale public health operation, we reviewed AAR approaches used in a variety of sectors, such as wildfire fighting (Wildland Fire Lessons Learned Center, 2005), U.S. Army training and operations (U.S. Army, 1993), and transportation accident reviews. From this review, and working closely with LACDPH personnel, we developed a multiphase, qualitative exploratory approach in the tradition of Grounded Theory Method. With this approach, data are collected without clear hypotheses, patterns in the data are coded and categorized, and from these categories key themes are identified and a theory to account for the patterns is derived, or reverse engineered (Charmaz, 2006; Glaser and Strauss, 1977). The analysis was conducted between February 2010 and July 2010.

Phase I: Identify Candidate Themes

We used a large-sample survey to elicit major themes from a broad group of stakeholders. This Web-based, anonymous survey—administered on a voluntary basis to all 4,000 of LACDPH employees and 800 registered volunteers—elicited lessons from 405 of 600 core staff, including both junior and senior LACDPH staff, and staff from volunteer organizations involved in the 2009 pH1N1 response. Via free-response write-in sections, these respondents noted both areas of successes and areas of "perceived challenges" in the response. There were a total of 425 challenges described that we coded into 73 types for later discussion and clarification.

Phase II: Identify the Most Salient Problems and Themes

We next conducted 14 focus groups with key ICS branches and sections involved in the response. Each focus group involved 7 to 12 people and focused on priority types of "perceived challenges" identified by the survey and additional issues raised in the groups. These groups provided an open forum for discussion and used diagramming to elicit root causes and potential corrective actions.

Phase III: Refine and Prioritize Root Causes and Solutions

We conducted interviews with 19 individuals who held key leadership roles during the response. The interviews focused on priorities identified earlier and additional issues raised by interviewees. They also included additional attempts to identify root causes and to discuss the feasibility of potential improvements.

Phase IV: Disseminate Findings of the Study among Key Audiences, Prioritize Corrective Actions, and Prepare for Implementation

We summarized the findings of the review and presented them to the LACDPH executive leadership in the form of a "change conference." The findings were also documented in a written report that was shared broadly within the LACDPH and was submitted as an action report/improvement plan to the Homeland Security Exercise and Evaluation Program. Table 5.1 provides a timeline for key events.

This study was approved and monitored by RAND's Human Subjects Protection Committee (Table 5-1).

TABLE 5-1 Timeline of Events

DATE	EVENT
April 24, 2009	California Department of Health call to local public health officials to prepare for pH1N1 response; LACDPH senior officials participate
April 26, 2009	LACDPH activates its Department Operations Center (DOC) the same day that the Department of Homeland Security declares a national public health emergency
April 28, 2009	LACDPH declares a local public health emergency
May 5, 2009	Announcement released that school closures should be evaluated on a case-by-case basis
May 8, 2009	DOC deactivated
Spring 2009	Planning for the fall influenza season
August 1, 2009	LACDPH initial planning meeting to begin scheduling POD sites among other planning items
Early October 2009	POD sites are planned to open, but the first sites are canceled as a result in a delay in receiving the vaccine
October 22, 2009	DOC activated
October 23, 2009	The first POD sites open
Mid November 2009	Nearly half the planned for POD sites canceled

DOC, departmental operations center; LACDPH, Los Angeles County Department of Public Health; POD, point of dispensing.

Results

Operating in Two Cultures, Two Organizational Structures

During routine functioning, most large, metropolitan health departments operate through major service area divisions and programs to implement largely categorically funded activities. There are also, typically, a variety of cross-program collaborations and overall direction set by the director/health officer, with an executive team composed by major division and program directors.

In contrast, response organizations typically use the ICS, a special form of organization to structure emergency operations. The ICS, the use of which is required by federal public health preparedness grants, is characterized by a hierarchical chain of command, use of common terminology to describe key positions of authority, clearly delineated management sections (e.g., command, finance, logistics, operations, planning), modular organizational structures, management by objectives, and use of well-defined emergency response functional roles (Bigley and Roberts, 2001; Qureshi et al., 2005). The goal is to create a standardized set of interoperable organizational "building blocks" shared across the full spectrum of response organizations that can facilitate ad hoc coordination among individuals and organizations that do not normally work together. Figure 5-1 illustrates the key ICS management sections.

Several aspects of the ICS diverge from the usual operating mode and day-to-day culture of public health departments, and thus can present challenges for health departments. In particular, the functions covered by the ICS "sections" (e.g., command, finance, logistics, operations, planning) often cut across routine organizational departments or business units in public health departments, creating friction between routine and emergency organizational structures. Moreover, although informal communications might be entirely appropriate during normal times, the need to manage emergencies often requires strict adherence to a clear chain of command and clearly prescribed channels of communication among responders.

Similarly, the ICS tends to operate according to different decision-making norms than routine public health organizations. Although routine public health culture usually favors deliberation, consensus, and heavy reliance on scientific evidence, emergency response often requires relatively rapid decision making based on incomplete, ambiguous, and changing information (Parker et al., 2010). Although decisions in the pH1N1 response were not always rapid, officials had months to plan for vaccine and antiviral delivery operations; it required a great deal of decision making under uncertainty. For example, it was not known until very late what type of vaccines would be available for distribution, in what quantities, to whom they could be administered, and when they would be delivered.

"Going into ICS" is usually an important marker of when a health department or other entity is in "response mode," and the decision to move out of ICS usually marks the final stages of a response. During a very severe, high-velocity incident (e.g., a massive bioterrorism attack), there would be little question about the need to suspend routine operations and launch emergency organizational processes immediately. The fact that pH1N1 was both less severe and less fast paced than other emergencies created considerably more ambiguity about how to balance routine and emergency priorities.

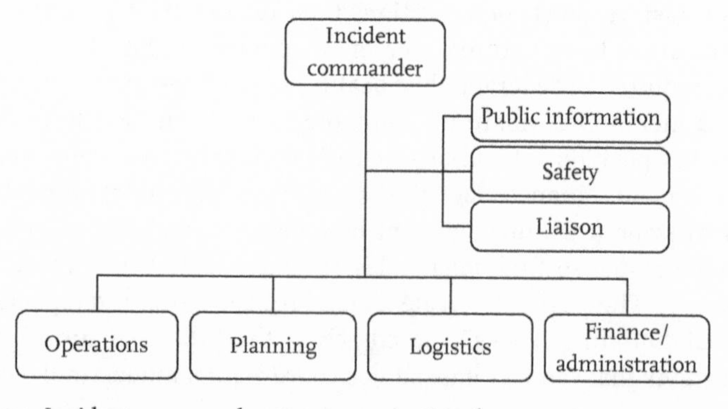

FIGURE 5-1 Incident command system organizational structure.

The remainder of the chapter describes how these tensions between routine and emergency organization, culture, and decision-making norms manifested themselves during the 2009 pH1N1 response, and offers concrete recommendations for managing those tensions in the future.

Planning during Normal Operations versus Planning in ICS

The tension between routine and emergency organizational structures arose with regard to planning the sites for points of dispensing (PODs), the facilities (often schools, community centers, armories, and so on) where vaccines were to be provided to the general public. There were differences in the criteria used to select POD sites from routinely used sites (e.g., seasonal flu vaccine clinics) that arose from the needs of emergency mass delivery of vaccines, especially the ability to handle the large traffic flows involved in a mass vaccination. Some officials and staff sought out the routine sites, which typically involve much lighter traffic flows, on the grounds that doing so would help maintain buy-in from the important community partners (e.g., community centers, churches) who operate those facilities. In some cases, this resulted in delays in decisions about which PODs to open, occasional late decisions to cancel planned PODs, and some PODs that did not perform with the required high throughput.

It is not clear that one perspective was right and the other wrong. Both sought to achieve important goals. The challenge, therefore, lay in developing a shared set of expectations within the LACDPH about to what extent emergency versus routine organizational structures and norms prevailed, and how the two should be balanced at any point in time.

Implementing Chain of Command and Communication Channels

As noted earlier, routine public health decision making is often characterized by extensive deliberation, with a wide range of individuals communicating with each other. Emergency ICS management structures, in contrast, emphasize more formalized communication channels and a clear chain of command as a way to manage information in a fast-paced environment. This strategy ensures that those ultimately responsible for decisions have access to a wide variety of appropriately filtered and aggregated information sources.

A particular manifestation of the tensions between routine and emergency organizational structures and norms was the lack of a clear and shared understanding regarding the channels that staff outside the formal ICS chain of command could use to provide input to decisions. For instance, our data showed instances in which senior LACDPH leaders, with no formal role in the ICS structure, would share ideas for improving POD operations with subordinates who did have formal roles in the response. This had the unintended consequence of circumventing the formal chain of command. These instances reportedly caused confusion among response staff, who sometimes needed to bypass standard ICS processes to accommodate the requests of non-ICS staff. Such instances often required improvisation, assumption of a substantial amount of additional work, or both. Again, the point is not that there was a right and a wrong perspective. Rather, given the moderate intensity and long duration of pH1N1, there was often a lack of clarity about whether routine versus emergency structures and norms should prevail, and how they might be balanced effectively.

Managing Workload to Match Response

The prolonged nature of the pH1N1 response operations created problems for many of the LACDPH staff who were part of the ICS. They were tasked throughout the course of several months with continuing their day-to-day responsibilities and also executing their roles within the ICS concomitantly. An ICS best practice is to release participating staff from some or all of their day-to-day responsibilities, depending on the scale of the incident. Because of the moderate severity and ongoing nature of the pH1N1 response, this did not always happen, occasionally resulting in heavy ICS staff workloads and reduced staff capacity to contribute to response activities. Although there was extensive staff involvement with the response planning and execution, many (approximately 50% of staff participated in some role) AAR participants felt that one root cause of this problem was that the authority to suspend staff's day-to-day responsibilities during an emergency lay with staff members' day-to-day managers, who might have felt less responsibility to accommodate ICS response objectives than their (continuing) day-to-day objectives.

Another observation was that, although there were guidelines for what would trigger "going into" ICS, there were no well-articulated guidelines for when to end the ICS structure and response. As the response continued in time, there did not appear to be a set of conditions in place that would help define when the response could be "stood down," and who would make that call.

Articulating and Executing Decisions

Perhaps because of the largely unresolved tensions described earlier between routine and emergency organizational structures and norms, a common theme in interviews and focus groups was that some decisions were influenced from outside the ICS structure and LACDPH, and were not always clearly articulated and widely distributed to stakeholders. The extant doctrine, practices, and personnel policies did not support the chain of command appropriately nor include input from many stakeholders to the ICS decision-making processes. An example was decisions by LACDPH leaders regarding implementing potentially beneficial changes to POD operations that were made "on the ground" during POD operations. Although well intentioned, they did not flow through the ICS chain of command either at the POD or the LACDPH operations center, and hence were reportedly disruptive to local operations.

Implications for Policy and Practice

The tensions observed during the pH1N1 response between routine and emergency public health operations are perhaps not surprising. For decades, the primary focus of governmental public health agencies has been health promotion and disease prevention. This is reinforced by the categorical funding constraints that govern much of routine, day-to-day departmental operations. Although public health has always responded to acute incidents (e.g., outbreaks of food-borne disease), responding to large-scale, high-intensity incidents over prolonged periods in a way that involves collaboration with a broad group of partners is a relatively recent addition to its portfolio of responsibility. However, the reality of public health practice today is that all public health department employees must be competent to shift rapidly to, and to perform, emergency response operations. Introducing preparedness into public health can be compared with a merger and acquisition process in which an existing enterprise must absorb and integrate a new enterprise with a different culture and practices. Like most such processes, there are inevitable tensions; all the more so given that the national preparedness "call to arms" after 9/11 fell on a weakened public health infrastructure (Institute of Medicine 2003; Lurie et al., 2006). Although particular severe and acute public health emergencies might require exclusive focus on emergency response, most incidents are less acute and require that health departments engage concomitantly in routine and emergency functions.

This chapter discussed some of these tensions as they were manifest in the pH1N1 response. Although we focused on the LACDPH's 2009 pH1N1 response, these challenges apply to most local health departments, particularly those in large, complex metropolitan areas. The remainder of the chapter presents recommendations for addressing these challenges that emerged from the LACDPH's after-action review and subsequent improvement plan.

Develop/Refine Escalating Continuity of Operation Plans with Clear Triggers for Balancing Emergency and Routine Operations

A common theme in our findings is that moderate-severity incidents that require major responses for significantly long time periods, such as pH1N1, can lead to ambiguity about when, how quickly, and to what extent to transition between routine and emergency operations. To help achieve greater clarity, health departments and their partners should work collaboratively to identify clear and progressively escalating Continuity of Operation (COOP) plans with clear trigger conditions. As the level of the required response increases, emergency response activities should increase and day-to-day responsibilities should decrease. The final authority to trigger COOP plans should reside at a higher level of leadership than both routine supervisors and incident response leadership (e.g., the responsibility of the health officer), so that the priorities of both may be assessed fairly. Our analysis concluded that phased COOP plans and triggers—allowing a smooth transition from periods with low resource demands to those with higher resource demands—would add a useful dimension of flexibility to this process.

Provide Coaching on ICS and Crisis Decision Making

To help public health officials negotiate the tensions between routine and emergency organizational structures and norms, we recommend the creation of two new roles (which could be played by one and the same individual). The first is a trained, experienced coach or mentor to support public health emergency decision making (see, for example, Fielden [2005]). Supported by existing decision-making assessment tools, this person would have the skills to recognize and counter common weaknesses in individual and group decision making, and would monitor decision processes for quality and would provide feedback and guidance in real time. This person would also be responsible for documenting decisions, including rationales, critical decision points, assent/dissent, and so forth.

The second role is that of an ICS mentor to support appropriate use of ICS rules and best practices. Most LACDPH staff rarely get the opportunity to practice the ICS, and the hierarchical command and control structure of the ICS runs against the prevailing culture of consensus building in public health. Response participants would likely benefit from the support of an ICS expert acting in the role of ICS coach or mentor who can give advice, especially to leaders, in real time. This person would help decision makers adapt ICS principles to the realities, nuances, and strengths of public health in ways that balance fidelity to the doctrine with the need for flexibility.

This position might have a number of specific responsibilities, including (1) providing input on the potential value of observed departures from ICS rules, (2) providing regular feedback to the Incident Commander on areas for improvement, and (3) developing and maintaining ICS-related checklists, job action sheets, or other job aids for key ICS positions. Providing this sort of real-time support and mentoring could help address concerns about maintaining the chain of command, creating appropriate divisions of labor, and helping to ensure proper execution of decisions. It could also help decision makers make decisions that strike a balance between timeliness and accuracy.

Create a Rapid Process Improvement Cell and Processes

To provide real-time feedback on balancing routine and emergency operations, we recommend creating a "process improvement" cell in the central ICS structure to carry out this important activity. This recommendation includes embedding a person in the planning cell of local POD ICS structures who would be responsible for documenting local innovations and reporting those back to the central process improvement cell. Local activities and innovations that arise from local expertise would be captured and communicated back to the central process improvement cell regularly. There, the promising and potentially scalable local innovations could be refined, piloted, and possibly distributed to PODs that might benefit.

Schedule Regular Opportunities to Practice Crisis Decision Making

Good decision making is notoriously difficult to describe in explicit terms and often has a know-it-when-you-see-it quality. Development of such "tacit" skills and knowledge is usually best facilitated through regular opportunities to practice (Seely-Brown and Duguid, 1991; Wenger, 2000). Thus, public health organizations need to practice crisis decision making actively under realistic scenarios, limited/inaccurate information, and even exaggerated time pressures to understand how to streamline normal decision-making processes while still maintaining quality. They also need to practice balancing routine and emergency decision making, and "cross-training" in different ICS sections to understand more completely the challenges and responsibilities of other sections. By actually making decisions, as opposed to training on scenarios for which decisions are a forgone conclusion, staff will develop a better understanding regarding the tradeoffs of decisional speed and accuracy, and know how to make decisions outside of their organizations' normal timelines most effectively.

Our review of the LACDPH's 2009 pH1N1 response yielded several valuable lessons on how the tailoring and implementation of the ICS and crisis decision making can be improved. The addition of new sections and roles to the ICS would help to tailor the LACDPH for public health emergency response capture, vet, pilot, and distribute best practices, and to enhance crisis decision making. Anecdotal reports suggest that many other state and local health departments experienced the same challenges and could benefit from the same recommendations. Learning these lessons and developing workable ways to address them should be a priority as the nation continues to bring emergency preparedness into the mainstream of public health practice.

Acknowledgments and Disclosure

The authors thank Catherine Knox, Michael Contreras, Karen Ricci, and Donna White for support of this research.

References

Bigley, G., Roberts, K.. (2001). The incident command system: high-reliability organizing for complex and volatile task environments. *Academy of Management Journal*, *44*(6), 1281–1299.

Centers for Disease Control and Prevention Office of Public Health Preparedness and Response. (2008). Cities Readiness Initiative (CRI) funding. Accessed July 29, 2011, at http://www.bt.cdc.gov/cdcpreparedness/coopagreement/08/cri.asp.

Charmaz, K. (2006). *Constructing grounded theory: a practical guide through qualitative analysis.* Thousand Oaks, CA: Sage Publications.

Fielden, S. (2005). *Literature review: coaching effectiveness: a summary.* U.K. National Health Service Leadership Centre. Accessed February 5, 2013, at http://literacy.kent.edu/coaching/information/Research/NHS_CDWPCoachingEffectiveness.pdf.

Glaser, B. G., Strauss, A. (1977). *Discovery of grounded theory: strategies for qualitative research.* Los Angeles, CA: Aldine Publications.

Homeland Security Council. (2005). *National planning scenarios: executive summaries, version 20.2.* Washington, DC: Homeland Security Council.

Institute of Medicine. (2003). *The future of the public's health in the 21st century.* Washington, DC: National Academy Press.

Lurie, N., Wasserman, J., Nelson, C. (2006). Public health preparedness: evolution or revolution? *Health Affairs, 25,* 935–945.

Parker, A., Nelson, C., Shelton, S., Lewis, M. (2010). *Defining, measuring, and improving crisis decision-making in public health.* Santa Monica, CA: RAND Corporation.

Qureshi, K., Gebbie, K. M., Gebbie, E. N. (2005). *Public Health Incident Command System: a guide for the management of emergencies or other unusual incidents within public health agencies,* vol. 1, 1st ed. New York.

Seely-Brown, J., Duguid, P. (1991). Organizational learning and communities-of-practice: toward a unified view of working, learning, and innovation. *Organization Science, 2,* 40–57.

U.S. Army. (1993). *A leaders guide to after-action reviews.* Training circular 25–20. Washington, DC: Headquarters, Department of the Army.

Wenger, E. (2000). Communities of practice and social learning systems. *Organization, 7*(2), 225–246.

Wildland Fire Lessons Learned Center. (2005). *Conducting effective after action reviews.* Tucson, AZ: National Advanced Fire & Resource Institute.

CHAPTER 6

Variation in the Local Management of Publicly Purchased Antiviral Drugs during the 2009 H1N1 Influenza Pandemic

JENNIFER C. HUNTER, DANIELA C. RODRÍGUEZ,
AND TOMÁS J. ARAGÓN

Background

On April 26, 2009, the U.S. government declared a public health emergency in response to the threat posed by the 2009 H1N1 influenza virus, A(H1N1) pdm09 (Centers for Disease Control and Prevention, 2009). With no vaccine immediately available, this declaration led the Centers for Disease Control and Prevention (CDC) to ship large quantities of medical provisions from the strategic national stockpile (SNS) to state health departments around the nation in an effort to mitigate and control outbreaks of the novel virus. Included in this shipment were 11 million regimens of antiviral drugs (two neuraminidase inhibitors: oseltamivir and zanamivir), which were later accompanied by new federal guidance on the recommended clinical use of these drugs during the pandemic (Centers for Disease Control and Prevention, 2010; Centers for Disease Control and Prevention, 2011b). These events prompted state and local health departments to make decisions regarding how and where publicly purchased antivirals would be used in their communities to treat ill persons and to slow the spread of disease.

The large-scale deployment of antivirals during the H1N1 influenza response presents a unique opportunity to study the local public health implementation of plans and protocols to support medical countermeasure dispensing. As one of the CDC public health emergency preparedness capabilities, *medical countermeasure dispensing* is defined as, "the ability to provide medical countermeasures (including vaccines, antiviral drugs, antibiotics, antitoxin, etc.) in support of treatment or prophylaxis . . . to the identified population in accordance with public health guidelines and/or recommendations" (U.S.

Department of Health and Human Services, 2008, p. 71). The H1N1 influenza pandemic offered a highly unusual situation in which state and local health departments across the country carried out this function concomitantly during a prolonged event of national significance. Before 2009, local, state, and federal public health agencies had developed plans to help anticipate and address the antiviral drug needs of their community during an influenza pandemic. This "natural experiment" provides a nearly ideal situation for studying variations in practice.

The need for the public health management of antiviral drugs during an influenza pandemic did not take public health officials by surprise. Before 2009, public health agencies and community partners had been engaged actively in preparedness activities in anticipation of antiviral use during an influenza pandemic. Among those efforts were the large-scale purchase of antiviral drugs at the state and federal levels and the development of plans to use these medications appropriately to treat influenza illness and to reduce the impact of a pandemic (U.S. Government Working Group, 2009). However, given few opportunities to observe real-world response to an influenza pandemic, the preparedness community's understanding of state and local readiness for implementing a large-scale antiviral program has been limited. As a result, prepandemic assessments have reached wide-ranging conclusions regarding this preparedness capacity.

In 2008, a federal assessment of pandemic influenza state operating plans found that "there are very few gaps in State readiness for antiviral drug distribution" (U.S. Government Working Group, 2009, p. 26). Just one year later, the U.S. Department of Health and Human Services Office of the Inspector General reported notable gaps in antiviral plans at the local level, despite high scores in antiviral preparedness at the state level (U.S. Department of Health and Human Services, 2009a, 2009b). Although these reports may, at first, seem contradictory, the findings illuminate the differences in the roles, responsibilities, and capacities of health departments at the state and local levels. For many states, including California, the primary responsibility for managing local antiviral drug activities resides with local health departments (LHDs) to enable local control, planning, and implementation (California Department of Health Services, 2006; Centers for Disease Control and Prevention, 2008, 2009). Therefore, evaluations at the state level may have provided an incomplete assessment of the capacities required to implement this pandemic response function fully.

Given the expected importance of antiviral drugs as an influenza pandemic control measure, particularly before the availability of vaccine, and the infrequent opportunity to assess the ability of public health departments to meet community members' demand for this medical countermeasure, the 2009 H1N1 influenza response provided a valuable learning opportunity. Although the demand for antiviral drugs during the 2009 H1N1 influenza response was not as dramatic as had been predicted in many prepandemic planning scenarios (U.S. Department of Health and Human Services, 2008), this analysis nevertheless provides an illustration of how LHDs drew on their previous work to ensure antiviral drugs were available, as needed, in their community. We also show how the H1N1 pandemic tested antiviral planning assumptions and forced LHDs to respond creatively to new and unexpected challenges. The purpose of this chapter is twofold. First, we describe the range of implementation strategies used by LHDs in California to manage publicly purchased antiviral drugs, and identify related challenges experienced by health departments and their community partners. We focus on publicly purchased antiviral drugs because of the unprecedented deployment of these medications from the SNS to health departments around the nation, and because of the unique role of governmental public health in making decisions regarding how and where publicly purchased antivirals would be used in their communities to treat ill persons and to slow the spread of disease. Second, we assess the strengths and limitations of the research methods used in this study for the purpose of informing future research in public health emergency preparedness and response.

Methods

This research used a mixed-methods approach. First, a multidisciplinary focus group of pandemic influenza planners from key stakeholder groups in California was convened to generate ideas and identify critical themes related to the local implementation of antiviral activities during the H1N1 influenza response. These qualitative data informed the development of a Web-based survey, which was distributed to all 61 LHDs in California, for the purpose of assessing experiences of LHDs from a representative sample of local health agencies in California.

Phase I: Focus Group

The first phase consisted of a teleconference-based focus group, comprised of members of the California Pandemic Influenza Vaccine and Antiviral (PIVA) Advisory Group. This statewide advisory group of pandemic planners and experts had convened before the 2009 H1N1 pandemic for the purpose of providing the California Department of Public Health with recommendations regarding vaccine and antiviral implementation before an influenza pandemic (Hunter et al., 2009; California Department of Public Health, 2009b). All PIVA Advisory Group members were invited to participate in the focus group via e-mail, and were provided with an agenda that included an overview of focus group topics before the teleconference. The focus group topics included questions about antiviral acquisition, dispensing, and use. Also included were questions regarding challenges that were faced in these areas.

The focus group took place by phone in July 2010 and lasted 120 minutes. Twenty-three advisory group members participated in the teleconference, including representatives from state and local public health departments, federal agencies, private-sector associations, academic institutions, hospitals, law enforcement agencies, and nongovernmental organizations. The focus group was led by two facilitators. Notes were taken by the facilitators and an additional note taker, and were transcribed and merged into one document for review before being provided to focus group participants for participant validation. The focus group notes were reviewed to distill any relevant information that could be used to improve and strengthen the survey.

Phase II: Web-Based Survey

During the second phase of the study, a Web-based survey was distributed to all 61 LHDs in California. This survey covered, in greater detail, the same antiviral topics discussed in the focus group informed by focus group input, literature reviews, prepandemic planning with the PIVA Advisory Group, experiences of study personnel, and pilot testing with practice-based and academic-based experts. LHD involvement in the planning, coordination, and implementation of activities related to publicly purchased antivirals (i.e., those purchased by state or federal entities) were assessed in the following survey domains:

- Acquisition, distribution, allocation, dispense, and use of antivirals
- The tracking and monitoring of the use of antivirals
- Communications with other organizations regarding antivirals
- Challenges faced by LHDs in any of the aforementioned areas

All LHDs in the state of California were recruited for participation in the survey, with the goal of obtaining a representative sample of LHD experiences managing antivirals during the H1N1 influenza response. A complete list of current LHD health officers and SNS coordinators for each of the 61 LHDs in California (58 county health departments and three independent municipal health departments) was obtained from the California Department of Public Health. Based on the focus group discussion, persons in these two functional roles were expected to be most knowledgeable about the antiviral response at the local level.

The survey invitation was distributed to health officers and SNS coordinators for all 61 LHDs, along with a short description of the survey goals, via e-mail from the office of the principal investigator of Cal PREPARE, a CDC preparedness and emergency response research center at the University of California, Berkeley. Recipients were instructed to forward the survey to the person in their department who was most informed about the health department's H1N1 influenza antiviral response, and to submit one response for their health department. Survey data collection took three weeks in August 2010 and September 2010. Two reminders were sent to invited participants via e-mail to increase response rates.

Survey data were downloaded from the Web survey provider and merged with county demographic data. Demographic data for the LHD catchment areas were collected from publicly available sources to classify LHDs by population size and to make comparisons of responding and nonresponding agencies (National Association of County and City Health Officials, 2008). Health departments were classified into one of three population size categories based on the number of individuals served, adopting a categorization convention used by the National Association of County and City Health Officials: (1) small LHDs, fewer than 50,000 people; (2) medium LHDs, between 50,000 people and 499,999 people; and (3) large LHDs, 500,000 people or more (California Emergency Management Agency, 2009). A descriptive analysis of the survey results is presented here, with quotations from the focus group and responses to open-ended survey questions, to illustrate salient issues.

Results

These results describe the data obtained from LHD staff through the Web-based survey.

Sample Demographics

Sixty-one LHDs were invited to participate in this study. Forty-four local health departments completed the survey, resulting in a 72% response rate. These counties represent 74% of the population of California. Participating agencies did not differ statistically from nonparticipating agencies with respect to the size of population served by the health department or median household income. There was a borderline significant difference in the geographic distribution of responding counties, with the lowest participation in the southern region (46%) compared with the inland region (81%) and the coastal region (76%) (U.S. Census Bureau, 2000).

The most widely represented functional role for respondents was SNS coordinators, with more than half of participants identifying themselves as such. Other common functional roles were emergency preparedness coordinator/director and health officer. Nearly all respondents stated they were very knowledgeable about their LHD's antiviral activities during 2009 H1N1. Survey respondents who indicated they knew only "a little" about their LHD's antiviral response were not allowed to complete the survey. Two respondents fell into this category and were not included in the overall response rate.

Acquiring, Distributing, and Allocating Antivirals

Acquiring Antivirals

All LHDs received antivirals from state or federal stockpiles, with a few LHDs receiving antivirals from a local cache or purchasing antivirals directly from the commercial or retail market as well. In this report, those antivirals purchased by state or federal government agencies for public use are referred to as "publicly purchased antivirals" or "state and federal stockpiles."

Distributing Antivirals

Twenty-eight LHDs reported distributing publicly purchased antivirals to other organizations for dispensing to the public, which accounts for 64% of respondents. The organizations and agencies that received antiviral drugs from LHDs are presented in Table 6-1. Of those cited most frequently were clinics, hospitals, and pharmacies (71%, 64%, and 54%, respectively). Although many LHDs distributed antivirals to hospitals, others found that

TABLE 6-1 Number of LHDs That Distributed Antivirals to Other Organizations for Dispensing to Public (n = 28)

	SIZE OF POPULATION SERVED BY LHD							
	SMALL (<50,000)		MEDIUM (50,000–499,999)		LARGE (500,000+)		ALL LHDs	
ORGANIZATION/ENTITY	N	%	N	%	N	%	N	%
Public clinics/health centers	2	50	11	69	7	88	20	71
Private hospitals	0	0	10	63	8	100	18	64[†]
Retail pharmacies	3	75	8	50	4	50	15	54
Public hospitals	2	50	3	19	8	100	13	46
Private clinicians	0	0	5	31	4	50	9	32
Tribal health clinic/hospitals	1	25	4	25	3	38	8	29
Prisons	0	0	1	6	4	50	5	18
College/universities	0	0	4	25	1	13	5	18
Direct to patient*	0	0	3	19	2	25	5	18
Skilled nursing facilities/long-term care facilities	1	25	1	6	2	25	4	14
Military bases	0	0	0	0	0	0	0	0
Airports	0	0	0	0	0	0	0	0
Other	1	25	3	19	1	13	5	18
Total	4		16		8		28	

Of the 28 LHDs that distributed publicly purchased antivirals to other organizations for dispensing to the public, Table 6-1 summarizes the number and proportion of LHDs that reported distributing antivirals to each type of organization or entity, stratified by size of population served by LHD.
LHD, local health department.
*Direct-to-patient methods include household delivery and pickup, and health department.
[†]Statistically significant difference with respect to population size served by LHDs (Fisher's exact test, $p < .05$).
LHD, local health department.

hospital pharmacies were unable to accept publicly purchased antivirals, as described by one survey respondent: "We contracted with [a chain retail pharmacy] for this service since hospitals could not accept public antivirals into their pharmacies." Receiving organizations classified under "Other" include HIV care providers, addiction programs, homeless centers, and children's homes.

Allocating Antivirals

LHDs selected organizations to dispense publicly purchased antivirals for the following reasons: to reach the uninsured or underinsured (89%), to reach severely ill persons (61%), to reach medically at-risk persons such as pregnant women (57%), and/or because the organization was well known in the community (61%). LHDs also noted that dispensing sites were chosen based on storage capacity or the ability of a pharmacy to reconstitute antiviral suspension correctly for children.

The number of antivirals allocated to these dispensing sites was determined based on the characteristics of the patient population served (41%), requests for antivirals (37%), number of persons served by a medical or treatment facility (33%), and/or epidemiologic data and patient volume (26%).

Eight of the 28 LHDs that distributed antivirals to other organizations for dispensing to the public reported they required facilities to show that antivirals were not commercially available before they could receive publicly purchased antivirals (28%). This strategy was based on the rationale that publicly purchased antivirals should be used only as a last resort after the commercial and retail markets had been depleted.

Antiviral Dispensing, Use, and Shortages

Antiviral Dispensing

Thirty-one LHDs reported that publicly purchased antivirals were dispensed for patient use in their jurisdiction (70%). Although approximately 90% dispensed fewer than 250 doses of publicly purchased antivirals, other LHDs reported that more than 10,000 doses were dispensed to the public. Small LHDs most commonly reported that no doses of publicly purchased antivirals were dispensed (ranging between 0 doses and 250 doses), whereas medium and large health departments most commonly noted that between one dose and 250 doses of publicly purchased antivirals were dispensed—ranging from zero to 1,000 doses for medium LHDs and zero to more than 10,000 doses for large LHDs. For those LHDs reporting that publicly purchased antivirals were not dispensed in their jurisdiction, many reported they had few influenza cases, and demand for antivirals was low. Others indicated their strategy was to use publicly purchased antivirals when shortages were reported in the local commercial market, which did not occur in their communities.

All LHDs that distributed publicly purchased antivirals to dispensing sites required those organizations to agree to certain terms of dispensing. Eighty-six percent of these 28 LHDs required dispensing sites to track antiviral use and to report it to the health department. Providing antivirals free of charge to the uninsured or underinsured and providing antivirals free of charge to all were required by 61% and 50% of these LHDs, respectively. Other requirements noted by respondents included returning unused antivirals to the LHD, following current recommendations for use, requesting documentation from recipients to ensure eligibility, and using temperature-controlled storage.

Antiviral Use

Potential uses of antiviral drugs include treatment, preexposure prophylaxis, and postexposure prophylaxis. Of the 31 LHDs reporting that publicly purchased antivirals were dispensed in their community, most allowed publicly purchased antivirals to be used for treatment (90%) and for postexposure prophylaxis (77%), whereas a minority allowed dispensing sites to use these antivirals for preexposure prophylaxis (26%). It should be noted that eight LHDs noted that allowable uses were determined by dispensing site; when we control for the participants who marked this option exclusively, all health departments approved antivirals to be used for treatment. The target groups for treatment and prophylaxis are presented in Tables 6-2 and 6-3. In addition, several LHDs further specified that restrictions on populations eligible for publicly purchased antivirals for treatment were lifted when antivirals were not commercially available. Regarding prophylaxis, LHDs noted that publicly purchased antivirals were dispensed to uninsured or underinsured persons, children, and household members of ill persons early in the pandemic to slow transmission of the virus.

To determine eligibility to receive publicly purchased antivirals, 24 of the 31 LHDs reporting that publicly purchased antivirals were dispensed for patient use in their jurisdiction instituted verification procedures. Fifty-four percent of these LHDs reported using pharmacists or dispensing sites to determine eligibility status, 46% reported that physicians provided proof of eligibility, and 25% indicated that patients self-reported their eligibility status. Six LHDs did not require any eligibility verification.

Antiviral Shortages

Of all LHD respondents, 26 indicated their communities experienced shortages of at least one type of antiviral drug (60%). Shortages were primarily of the pediatric formulation of oseltamivir followed by the adult formulation of oseltamivir (reported by 96% and 38% of LHDs with shortages, respectively). No shortages of zanamivir or peramivir were reported.

Antiviral Tracking and Monitoring

LHDs were asked about their ability to track the movement of antivirals from stockpile sites to recipients. Of the 28 health departments that

TABLE 6-2 Target Groups for Treatment with Publicly Purchased Antivirals (n = 28)

	SIZE OF POPULATION SERVED BY LHD							
	SMALL (<50,000)		MEDIUM (50,000–499,999)		LARGE (500,000+)		ALL LHDs	
ELIGIBLE GROUPS	N	%	N	%	N	%	N	%
Uninsured or underinsured persons	3	75	11	69	3	38	17	61
Any ill person	2	50	3	19	5	63	10	36
Persons at high risk for medical complications of influenza (e.g., pregnant women)	1	25	5	31	1	13	7	25
Persons in an occupation-based target group (e.g., healthcare workers)	1	25	4	25	0	0	5	18
Other	0	0	3	19	1	13	4	14
Don't know/unable to answer	0	0	0	0	0	0	0	0
Total	4		16		8		28	

Of the 28 LHDs reporting that publicly purchased antivirals could be used for treatment, Table 6-2 summarizes the groups eligible for antiviral treatment with publicly purchased antivirals, stratified by size of population served by LHDs.
*Statistically significant difference with respect to population size served by LHDs (Fisher's exact test, $p < .05$).
LHD, local health department.

distributed antivirals, nearly all were able to track the federal/state stockpile to their health department (93%), and from the health department to the dispensing sites (100%). Most LHDs were able to track from dispensing sites to recipients (71%).

Twenty-four LHDs received antiviral use data from dispensing sites with varying degrees of frequency. Half these LHDs received antiviral use reports weekly or more frequently. Some health departments received basic use data, such as number of courses dispensed or lot numbers, whereas others received more specific data, including demographic information, intended use of antivirals (e.g., treatment, post-exposure prophylaxis, PEP), or reason that public stockpiles were use (e.g., shortages, uninsured recipient). These data were used primarily for making allocation decisions, monitoring, planning for future antivirals, reaching target populations, and providing data to other agencies. Use data were received primarily by fax, but also by e-mail, phone calls, face-to-face meetings, and mail.

TABLE 6-3 Target Groups for Prophylaxis with Publicly Purchased Antivirals (n = 25)

	SIZE OF POPULATION SERVED							
	SMALL (<50,000)		MEDIUM (50,000–499,999)		LARGE (500,000+)		ALL LHDs	
ELIGIBLE GROUP	N	%	N	%	N	%	N	%
Household members of persons with H1N1 influenza	3	100	10	77	4	44	17	68
Persons at high risk for medical complications of influenza (e.g., pregnant women)	3	100	4	31	5	56	12	48
Healthcare workers	2	67	4	31	3	33	9	36
Other first responders	2	67	1	8	1	11	4	16
Household members of healthcare workers	1	33	0	0	1	11	2	8
Other	0	0	3	23	3	33	6	24
Don't know/unable to answer	0	0	2	15	2	22	4	16
Total	3		13		9		25	

Of the 25 LHDs reporting that publicly purchased antivirals could be used for pre- or post-prophylaxis, Table 6-3 summarizes the groups eligible for prophylaxis with publicly purchased antivirals, stratified by size of population served by LHD.
*Statistically significant difference with respect to population size served by LHDs (Fisher's exact test, $p < .05$).
LHD, local health department.

Communications

The most common mechanisms LHDs used for communicating with other organizations participating in the antiviral response were e-mail (56%), blast fax (53%), phone calls (49%), and in-person/face-to-face meetings (42%). Other commonly cited communications mechanisms were teleconference (33%), websites (30%), and the California Health Alert Network (21%). The remaining LHDs indicated that communication with other agencies around antivirals did not occur in their jurisdiction or was not applicable to their health department's response.

LHDs also used various mechanisms to inform the public about where eligible persons could obtain antivirals. Around half the LHDs indicated the health department (57%) or the clinician (45%) was the source of information for these individuals. Others relied on pharmacists (32%), the media (16%), or employers (7%). The remaining LHDs did not communicate with the public because they perceived antiviral need to be low.

Only six LHDs found there were stakeholder groups with whom they had to establish communications for the antiviral response that had not been planned originally. These stakeholder groups included smaller clinics, retail pharmacies, certain minority populations, community clinics, local school districts, community-based organizations, state correctional facilities, and indigent populations.

Antiviral Challenges for LHDs

LHDs were asked about antiviral challenges faced and feedback received during the H1N1 influenza response. In terms of challenges, LHDs were asked to identify issues that were problematic early and later during the pandemic response. "Early" was defined as April to June 2009; "later" was defined as July 2009 onward. These challenges are presented in Figure 6-1.

Changes in antiviral guidance and multiple sources of information about antivirals presented a serious challenge to LHDs. This was the most widely cited issue both early and late in the pandemic, and was described as "very challenging" by more than one-third of health departments. One LHD noted, "Changing guidance made it difficult to determine appropriate recipients." Other participants indicated that state and federal antiviral guidance during H1N1 differed from what they had anticipated, particularly with respect to the target population for stockpiled antivirals. This discrepancy required their

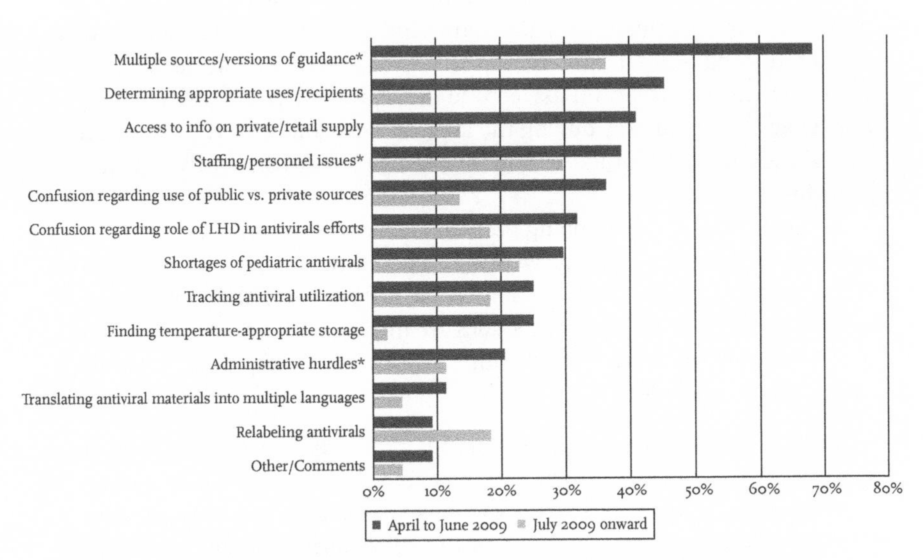

FIGURE 6-1 Antiviral challenges reported by local health departments (LHD) by time period (n = 44). Proportion of LHDs reporting each antiviral challenge, by time period (April–June 2009 and June 2009 onward). *Issues reported to be "very challenging" by 40% or more respondents of those LHDs reporting a challenge. SOURCE: © 2012 Hunter et al; Open Access content.

health departments to revise their planned activities to support this strategy. Several respondents indicated the following:

> The drugs from the SNS were originally intended to [be] used only when the drugs were no longer available through the commercial market. During the H1N1 epidemic the state required that we make the drugs available to people who were unable to afford the meds.

> The state's late decision to make the SNS antivirals available on a compassionate basis . . . created a great deal of trouble for my department.

> . . . had this event been more widespread, guidance from the state could have caused considerable issues related to the first responder community.

Shortages of pediatric antivirals and staffing issues at the LHDs also remained significant challenges for LHDs throughout the pandemic. The staffing issues were highlighted by one respondent:

> H1N1 served as a "dry run" for a more severe pandemic. Had we been faced with the need to distribute antiviral drugs to multiple health care and other venues, to a large percentage of our population, over a prolonged period of time, we would have been severely challenged to do so in a secure, accountable, consistent, and equitable manner. Given decreasing public health resources, I do not foresee an improvement in our capacity to do this anytime in the near future.

Early during the pandemic, the main challenges centered on ramping up response efforts, such as determining uses and target groups for antivirals, ascertaining information about antiviral availability in the commercial market, finding temperature-appropriate storage, and managing confusion about the use of public versus private stockpile antivirals. All challenges were cited less frequently during the later time period, with the exception of relabeling antivirals, which was mentioned twice as frequently during the later time period.

For those LHDs experiencing each challenge, the issues most likely to be reported as "very challenging" were staffing and personnel issues, changing antiviral guidance and multiple sources of information, and administrative hurdles (these "very challenging" issues are marked with an asterisk in Figure 6-1). An example of the type of administrative hurdles faced by LHDs was illustrated by one respondent,

> We [the LHD] were advised [by the county] . . . that the county would need to consider rapid purchase of antivirals for protection of essential county workers and possibly health care workers. We were asked to develop a special agreement to have local pharmacies make the purchase investment and guarantee them employee utilization and billing of insurance. At the start of the pandemic, this additional administrative task to avoid a sizeable county expenditure in antivirals for ongoing prophylaxis was an added task for our small health department.

Feedback from Community Partners

LHDs reported receiving negative feedback from community partners regarding a number of issues related to antivirals (Table 6-4). The most frequently mentioned issues centered on confusion around appropriate uses and target groups for antivirals, especially publicly purchased antivirals.

Private clinicians and hospital/healthcare facilities were the most frequently cited sources of negative feedback, reported by 30% and 16% of LHDs, respectively. LHDs that received negative feedback from these entities commonly also reported negative feedback in the following areas: confusion regarding clinical guidance for antiviral use, dissatisfaction regarding which patients should receive publicly purchased antivirals, and confusion regarding the use of the public versus private sources of antivirals. Medium-size health departments (those serving populations between 50,000 persons and 499,999 persons) were more likely to report hearing negative feedback regarding antiviral availability.

Only five LHDs reported difficulties or concerns in providing antivirals to specific populations. The populations noted by respondents included homeless/transient populations, undocumented persons, and pregnant women. One respondent described how reimbursement issues in Medi-Cal (California's state Medicaid insurance program for the poor and underserved) made it difficult to reach pregnant women early during the pandemic:

> [w]e had issues in the beginning with Medi-Cal patients namely pregnant women that did not get access to the stockpiled antivirals because Medi-Cal took so long to change their formulary and a communication (or other) issue related to getting the women to a location with the antivirals existed. This was remedied when Medi-Cal changed their formulary.

TABLE 6-4 Negative Feedback Received by LHDs from Community Partners (n = 44)

FEEDBACK	N	LHDs (%)
Confusion regarding clinical guidance for antiviral use	18	41
Confusion regarding the use of public- versus private-stockpile antivirals	11	25
Dissatisfaction regarding which patients should receive antivirals from public stockpile	11	25
Antiviral availability	10	23*
Administrative challenges associated with antivirals	10	23
Burdensome paperwork associated with tracking antiviral use	4	9
Difficulty determining whether local stockpiles had been depleted	3	7
Reported misuse of publicly purchased antivirals	2	5
Antiviral storage or security	1	2

*Statistically significant difference with respect to population size served by LHDs (Fisher's exact test, $p < .05$).
LHD, local health department.

LHDs also noted positive experiences working with the state health departments, including the following: "The antiviral acquisition, allocation, distribution, and dispensing was probably the smoothest [part of the] response during the H1N1 campaign. State did a great job getting them out to the LHDs as well as retrieving them."

Discussion

This chapter demonstrates how qualitative and quantitative methods were paired to assess LHD experiences managing antiviral drugs during the 2009 H1N1 pandemic. In social science research, mixed methods are often used as a mechanism for building on the inherent strengths of qualitative and quantitative approaches, and for attempting to reduce biases therein (Greene and Caracelli, 1997; Greene et al., 1989; Sosulski and Lawrence, 2008). By first engaging a multidisciplinary focus group of pandemic planners, we were able to capture the rich and contextual experiences of our public health preparedness informants.

This focus group narrative was then used, in conjunction with other data sources (literature reviews, prepandemic planning with the PIVA Advisory Group, experiences of study personnel, and pilot testing with practice-based and academic-based experts) to inform the development of a Web-based survey. Several key areas were added to the survey based exclusively on the focus group discussion, including the issue of administrative hurdles (contracting, purchasing that had to go out to bid, public posting, preferred vendors), the importance of capturing challenges early during the pandemic period versus later, and the problems posed by requiring dispensing sites to prove they had depleted commercial sources of antiviral drugs before they could receive publicly purchased antivirals.

Although many of the issues described by the PIVA Advisory Group were reflected broadly in the results of the Web-based survey, others appeared to affect only a fraction of LHDs. For example, during the focus group, the issue of requiring dispensing sites to prove they had depleted commercial sources of antiviral drugs appeared to be a universal issue. However, our findings indicate this issue was relevant only for about a one-fourth of health departments in our sample. This finding points to another strength of the mixed-methods approach. Because we used a representative sample of LHDs in California, our quantitative data provide research consumers with a better understanding of the relative frequency of antiviral management practices and challenges.

Last, although most questions on the Web-based survey had designated response options, there were several open-ended responses that allowed respondents either to elaborate on a previous response or to provide additional information. These quotes, which are presented in the Results section, help to provide a level of detail and context that could not otherwise be ascertained from the quantitative responses.

A major finding of this research is that, although the number of publicly purchased antivirals dispensed was limited in most communities (fewer than 10% of LHDs reported that more than 250 courses were dispensed in their jurisdiction), LHDs nevertheless devoted considerable resources to this effort and were required to draw on their previous experiences and knowledge to carry out this part of their H1N1 response. LHDs coordinated successfully with the state health department to receive antivirals from the SNS, made decisions regarding when and where these antivirals would be dispensed in their community, determined which groups would be eligible for these antivirals, allocated and distributed antivirals to dispensing sites for the purpose of reaching target groups, developed systems for verifying eligibility for antivirals and tracking antiviral use, and provided guidance to the clinical community.

This study also documents specific challenges presented by the 2009 H1N1 pandemic that were faced—and overcome—by LHDs. Our research corroborates and complements a recent qualitative investigation on this topic conducted by National Association of County and City Health Officials (NACCHO) researchers (National Association of County and City Health Officials, 2010b). Using different methods, both studies found that LHDs had difficulty reconciling multiple sources and versions of antiviral guidance from state and federal agencies, and that this was a major challenge at the local level. This was not only the most commonly reported difficulty in our respondents, but also was one of the most likely to be characterized as "very challenging." NACCHO researchers aptly describe two potential contributors to confusion at the local level that appear to be supported by our findings. First, federal antiviral guidance during the H1N1 response focused primarily on clinical recommendations for antiviral use and did not address directly how public stockpiles should be used. Second, clinical antiviral guidance changed during the course of the pandemic, originally focusing on postexposure prophylaxis, and later on early treatment (National Association of County and City Health Officials, 2010b).

Since the article by Hunter et al. (2012) was published, NACCHO released a research brief based on a second qualitative study, which recommends that pharmaceutical distributors and pharmacies be used for the distribution and dispensing of federal SNS supplies of antiviral drugs during a pandemic emergency (National Association of County and City Health Officials, 2012). If LHDs in California are representative of other states' experiences, this would represent a major shift in current practice. We found that only half of medium and large LHDs used commercial pharmacies for dispensing, and several health departments specifically cited difficulties using pharmacies to dispense publicly purchased antivirals.

This research also demonstrates that the recommended uses and recipients of publicly purchased antivirals during the H1N1 response differed from what LHDs had anticipated in their prepandemic plans, and that this resulted in additional difficulties. During the 2009 H1N1 pandemic, antivirals were generally available through normal wholesale and retail markets. As a result, the state health department recommended that LHDs use publicly purchased drugs for the treatment of uninsured or underinsured persons and for communities experiencing shortages (California Department of Public Health, 2009a; Centers for Disease Control and Prevention, 2011b). For many health departments, this represented a significant shift in their prepandemic antiviral implementation strategy, which had focused on the use of publicly purchased antivirals for treatment of ill persons after retail supplies had been depleted and had emphasized the role of antivirals in protecting healthcare workers and other first responders (Centers for Disease Control and Prevention, 2011b). As a consequence, LHDs revised their plans to support these new strategies, although implementing and communicating these strategies caused a strain on some local health departments and community partners.

Another outcome with particular relevance to public health planning is the effect of staffing and personnel shortages on the public health antiviral response. Of the 19 agencies that cited staffing issues as a challenge during their antiviral response, nearly half found this to be "very challenging." These findings are consistent with the documented workforce reductions in local public health since 2008 (National Association of County and City Health Officials, 2010b). As noted by one participant, current public health resources are insufficient for local health agencies to deliver antiviral services confidently in a "secure, accountable, consistent, and equitable manner" during a pandemic with a larger scope or greater severity. These concerns should be taken into account in the future development of antiviral and medical countermeasure plans and policies.

Public health systems researchers have noted that variations in the availability of community resources and community preferences will influence how public health services will be delivered (Mays et al., 2010). In this study we observed great variability in the approaches used by LHD to manage publicly purchased antiviral drugs. A similar phenomenon was seen in the LHDs' vaccination efforts (see Chapter 10).

It is expected that some of this variability is attributable to differences in the circumstances faced by LHDs (e.g., influenza illness incidence, community demographics, availability of antivirals in the retail market), whereas other variation is the result of differences in disease control and prevention strategies. It is beyond the scope of this study to evaluate the effectiveness of different approaches; however, the findings may inform preparedness conversations regarding which variations in practice are seen as beneficial and adaptive, and which areas might benefit from more standardization. State and local health departments, in California and elsewhere, can study these variations in practice and select models and promising practices to be included in their response planning.

Limitations

There are several limitations to this study. First, we chose to permit only one response per LHD and allowed anyone within the LHD to respond. Thus, we received responses from SNS coordinators, health officers and other LHD personnel. It is possible that SNS coordinators and other health department staff, especially health officers, experienced the 2009 H1N1 influenza pandemic differently given their different roles. To account for this, we gave LHDs the flexibility of choosing the person who was most familiar with their antiviral response. Given that 98% of respondents stated they knew "a lot" about their agency's antiviral response activities, we consider their perspectives to be a valid representation of the LHDs' experience.

A second limitation is the number of LHDs represented in the study. Although this sample includes health departments that represent nearly three-fourths of the 40 million residents in California, our unit of analysis is the health department, resulting in a small absolute number of cases. Furthermore, the communities served by these LHDs differ dramatically with respect to organizational and demographic factors. For example, the smallest health department represents 1,200 individuals and the largest serves more than eight million. Because of these differences, we present some of our results stratified by the size of the population served by the LHD. However, when the data are divided by population size (or any other community characteristics of interest), the number of health departments represented in each stratum is very small, requiring caution when drawing strong conclusions about any of the observed differences. This challenge has been noted by other studies of public health systems, particularly when the local health department is the unit of analysis (Thiede et al., 2012).

Last, because this research focused on LHDs in California, it is possible the findings are unique to this state. However, given the concurrence of our research findings with previous qualitative work with a wider geographic scope (National Association of County and City Health Officials, 2010b), we believe these results are applicable more broadly beyond California. To improve our understanding of the role of LHDs in the management of antivirals, this work should be replicated in a state with a different organizational, political, or authority structure in place, which might be expected to contribute to different experiences at the local level (e.g., a large state with a centralized public health authority) (Lister, 2005). Additional studies from other nations that also used publicly purchased antivirals during the H1N1 influenza response, particularly those with different policies on antiviral drug use, would cast important light on this issue.

Acknowledgments

This chapter was based on a research article developed with funding support awarded to Cal PREPARE, University of California at Berkeley Center for Infectious Diseases and Emergency Readiness, under cooperative agreements with the U.S. CDC (grant no. 5P01TP000295, Preparedness and Emergency Response Research Center). Its contents are solely the responsibility of the authors and do not necessarily represent the official views of the CDC or other partner organizations. The authors acknowledge all those individuals who participated in this research, especially the LHD representatives, the members of the PIVA Advisory Group. They also acknowledge the following individuals for reviewing survey materials and providing editorial support: Dr. Deborah Miller, Dr. Harvey Kayman, Mark Hunter, Donata Nilsen, Adam Crawley, and Jane Yang. Last, they thank Dr. Gwendolyn Hammer, Lisa Goldberg, and the California Department of Public Health for establishing the PIVA Advisory Group and developing the related decision-making methodology.

References

California Department of Health Services. (2006). Pandemic influenza preparedness and response plan. Available online at http://www.cdph.ca.gov/programs/immunize/Documents/pandemic.pdf

California Department of Public Health. (2009a). California Department of Public Health interim guidance on antiviral distribution and dispensing of state and federal antiviral medications.

California Department of Public Health. (2009b). Interim guidance: prioritizing populations for pandemic influenza vaccine in California.

California Emergency Management Agency. (2009). Mutual aid and administrative regions. Accessed March 3, 2013, at www.oes.ca.gov/WebPage/oeswebsite.nsf/PDF/Cal%20E.M.A.%20Mutual%20Aid%20Regions/$file/emaMutaid.pdf.

Centers for Disease Control and Prevention. (2008). Influenza pandemic operation plan: annex F community interventions.

Centers for Disease Control and Prevention. (2009). Interim guidance on antiviral recommendations for patients with confirmed or suspected novel influenza A (H1N1) (swine flu) virus infection and close contacts.

Centers for Disease Control and Prevention. (2010). The 2009 H1N1 pandemic: summary highlights, April 2009–April 2010. Accessed March 3, 2013, at www.cdc.gov/h1n1flu/cdcresponse.htm.

Centers for Disease Control and Prevention. (2011a). Public health preparedness capabilities: national standards for state and local planning. Available online at http://www.cdc.gov/phpr/capabilities/

Centers for Disease Control and Prevention. (2011b). Updated interim recommendations for the use of antiviral medications in the treatment and prevention of influenza for the 2009–2010 season. Accessed March 3, 2013, at www.cdc.gov/h1n1flu/recommendations.htm.

Greene, J., Caracelli, V. (1997). Advances in mixed-method evaluation: the challenges and benefits of integrating diverse paradigms. *New Directions for Evaluation.*

Greene, J. C., Caracelli, V. J., Graham, W. F. (1989). Toward a conceptual framework for mixed-method evaluation designs. *Educational Evaluation and Policy Analysis, 11*, 255–274.

Hunter, J. C., Goldberg, L., Hammer, G. (2009). *Pandemic influenza vaccine and antiviral advisory group antiviral recommendations report.* For the California Department of Public Health, Immunization Branch. Richmond, CA.

Hunter, J. C., Rodríguez, D. C., Aragón, T. J. (2012). Public health management of antiviral drugs during the 2009 H1N1 influenza pandemic: a survey of local health departments in California. *BMC Public Health, 12*, 82.
Lister, S. A. (2005). *An overview of the United States public health system in the context of emergency preparedness.* Washington, DC: Library of Congress, Congressional Research Service.
Mays, G. P., Scutchfield, F. D., Bhandari, M. W., Smith, S. A. (2010). Understanding the organization of public health delivery systems: an empirical typology. *Milbank Quarterly, 88*, 81–111.
National Association of County and City Health Officials. (2008). National profile of local health departments. Available online at http://nacchoprofilestudy.org/wp-content/uploads/2014/01/NACCHO_2008_ProfileReport_post-to-website-2.pdf
National Association of County and City Health Officials. (2010a). Local health department job losses and program cuts: overview of survey findings from January/February 2010 survey.
National Association of County and City Health Officials. (2010b). Public health use and distribution of antivirals. NACCHO think tank meeting report.
National Association of County and City Health Officials. (2012). Issue brief: local perspectives on managing antiviral medication during the 2009 H1N1 pandemic.
Sosulski, M. R., Lawrence, C. (2008). Mixing methods for full-strength results: two welfare studies. *Journal of Mixed Methods Research, 2*, 121–148.
Thiede, H., Duchin, J. S., Hartfield, K., Fleming, D. W. (2012). Variability in practices for investigation, prevention, and control of communicable diseases among Washington state's local health jurisdictions. *Journal of Public Health Management and Practice, 18*, 623–630.
U.S. Census Bureau. (2000). Census 2000 data for California. Accessed March 3, 2013, at www.census.gov/census2000/states/ca.html.
U.S. Department of Health and Human Services. (2008). Guidance on antiviral drug use during an influenza pandemic.
U.S. Department of Health and Human Services. (2009a). Determination that a public health emergency exists. Accessed March 3, 2013, at www.flu.gov/professional/federal/h1n1emergency042609.html.
U.S. Department of Health and Human Services. (2009b). Local pandemic influenza preparedness: vaccine and antiviral drug distribution and dispensing.
U.S. Government Working Group. (2009). Assessment of states' operating plans to combat pandemic influenza. Available online at http://www.flu.gov/planning-preparedness/states/state_assessment.pdf

CHAPTER 7

The H1N1 Response from the Perspective of State and Territorial Immunization Program Managers

Managing the Vaccination Campaign

ALLISON T. CHAMBERLAIN, MELISSA A. HIGDON, KATHERINE SEIB, AND ELLEN A. S. WHITNEY

Introduction

One of the major aspects of the public health response to the 2009 H1N1 pandemic was a national influenza vaccination campaign. Although the purchase and distribution of vaccine was a federal responsibility, organizing and implementing population-wide immunization campaigns was delegated primarily to state and local health departments, which required state-level immunization programs to activate plans to expand their vaccine management and distribution capabilities (Rambhia et al., 2010).

The Centers for Disease Control and Prevention (CDC) Advisory Committee on Immunization Practices (ACIP) met July 29, 2009, to develop the guidance for the mass vaccination campaign, and ultimately recommended a target group for priority vaccination that included an estimated 159 million Americans, of whom 62 million were designated to be the highest priority should vaccine supplies be inadequate to immunize all. Recommendations were based on available clinical and epidemiologic data, and input from the general public. ACIP assumed that approximately 120 million doses of vaccine would be available by mid October and that individuals would require two doses of vaccine to be fully immunized (Schnirring, 2009). As data from clinical trials became available in the fall, the CDC ultimately recommended that a single dose would be sufficient to protect people 10 years and older. Children younger than 10 years would require two doses (Centers for Disease Control and Prevention,

2009a). ACIP recommended that vaccination efforts focus on five initial target groups:

1. Pregnant women
2. People who lived with or cared for infants younger than six months
3. Healthcare and emergency medical services personnel
4. Infants six months and older through young adults aged 24 years
5. Adults 25 through 64 years who were at greater risk for complications because of chronic health disorders or compromised immune systems (Centers for Disease Control and Prevention, 2009a).

The CDC worked with McKesson, a logistics company, to ensure distribution of vaccine to state and local health departments through its centralized distribution network, which would fill orders placed by these departments. McKesson had prior experience with centralized vaccine distribution from its involvement with CDC vaccination programs, including the Vaccines for Children program (McKesson Corp, 2009). Initially, health departments were informed they could expect to receive shipments of vaccine in advance of the fall epidemic wave, but various technical issues delayed vaccine manufacture (Schnirring, 2009).

Despite federal organization of vaccine ordering and distribution, decisions regarding how to implement the vaccine programs were made at the state and local levels. Vaccine began to arrive in local communities in mid October, as the influenza epidemic was reaching its peak. Additional waves of disease were expected to continue throughout the winter influenza season, so public health entities moved forward with mass vaccination campaigns. ACIP's recommendations on vaccine priority groups were nonbinding, leaving health departments with the flexibility to adapt the guidance to local conditions. The mass vaccination campaign started October 2009 (Schnirring, 2009), with most localities focusing on limited, vulnerable populations. Because only 23.2 million doses had shipped by October 30, 2009, regional health officials had to make decisions quickly on how to refine priority groups further into "subpriority" groups—taking account both risk and demand—and how to communicate these decisions to vaccine providers and to the public. Vaccine providers were challenged with determining whether to turn away individuals who sought vaccine but did not fall into priority or subpriority groups.

Determining how to disseminate H1N1 influenza vaccine rapidly to thousands of new and existing vaccine providers and to the public was a major challenge for state and local health departments as a result of changing estimates of vaccine availability, uncertainties in distribution, and changing prioritization strategies. To expedite vaccine delivery, many state-level immunization programs worked closely and in novel ways with their state-level emergency preparedness programs. Under the National Incident Management System, the federal government encourages all levels of government, including state health departments, to use incident command systems (ICS) and emergency operations centers (EOCs) to help manage response activities and personnel efficiently and consistently, and such systems were used to manage this unique mass vaccination campaign. Ultimately, the vaccination campaign was expanded as more vaccine became available and continued into spring 2010.

Previous studies and after-action reports from other incidents have highlighted the benefits of using ICS and EOCs to help organize personnel, responsibilities, and resources (Adams et al., 2010; Mignone and Davidson, 2003; Porter et al., 2011). Understanding how immunization programs collaborated with emergency preparedness programs and how they used ICS and EOCs during the H1N1 vaccination campaign can inform future preparedness and response initiatives. Similarly, learning how immunization information systems (IISs; also know as *vaccine registries*) helped immunization programs manage H1N1 vaccine inventory and track vaccine administration will be key to improving the usefulness of these systems during future vaccine-related events. Capturing lessons learned to enhance systems becomes especially important in light of substantial cuts and changes to federal and state budgets, including the expiration of the American Recovery and Reinvestment Act funds to immunization programs, the Affordable Care Act, and potential reorganization of the CDC's immunization grant program (Association of Immunization Managers, 2011; Centers for Disease Control and Prevention, 2009b; U.S. Department of Health and Human Services, 2011). In an effort to explore how state-level immunization and emergency preparedness programs worked together, and how IISs assisted the relationships and systems implemented during the H1N1 vaccination campaign, a survey was conducted of city, state, and territorial immunization program managers (IPMs) in July 2010.

Methods

An electronic survey was sent to approximately 64 IPMs representing the city, state, and territory grantee jurisdictions supported by the CDC's National Center for Immunization and Respiratory Diseases (Centers for Disease Control and Prevention, 2012). These CDC grantee jurisdictions include the 50 states, American Samoa, Guam, the Republic of Marshall Islands, Micronesia, the northern Marianas Islands, Palau, Puerto Rico, the Virgin Islands, Chicago, the District of Columbia, Houston, New York City, Philadelphia, and San Antonio. This survey was conducted in collaboration with the Association of Immunization Managers (AIM), a national professional organization that represents IPMs from all 64 grantee jurisdictions. The survey was open between June 30, 2010, and July 28, 2010. It was distributed initially by e-mail; follow-up with nonrespondents began two weeks after initial survey dissemination, and included reminders posted in AIM weekly reports to IPMs and follow-up phone calls to nonrespondents.

The 35-question survey asked IPMs about their health department's management structure during the H1N1 vaccination campaign, including whether the department had used an ICS, the role of their incident commander, and whether they opened an EOC. The survey also ascertained perceptions of the helpfulness of existing pandemic influenza plans. In addition, questions about cooperation between the immunization and emergency preparedness programs examined the extent of collaboration before the pandemic, and the delineation of tasks between the two programs during the H1N1 vaccination campaign. Using a 5-point scale with values of "very effective," "effective," "neither effective nor ineffective," "ineffective," or "very ineffective," with an additional "not applicable" response option, respondents were asked to describe their perceptions of the effectiveness of the emergency preparedness staff in regard to specific activities related to facilitating their state's overall mass vaccination campaign, supplementing immunization staff, and developing risk communication materials for the public and vaccine providers. IPMs were asked about successes and challenges in working with emergency preparedness programs. Free-text responses to these qualitative questions were analyzed for themes by two individuals using a code book developed a priori.

This survey has several limitations. Although surveys of state directors of emergency preparedness have been conducted separately (Kun et al., 2013), the focus and specific questions were different than those reported here. Results from this survey have been shared and discussed with directors of emergency preparedness, and obtaining their responses to similar questions would be particularly useful to comprehensive planning for future public health emergencies. Furthermore, respondent self-report may be biased as a result of both staff turnover and an inability to recall events precisely from the prior year. Another limitation is that the beliefs of IPMs regarding collaborations with emergency preparedness programs, use of ICS/EOCs, characteristics of IIS reporting requirements, and other issues were not compared against outcome measures such as immunization coverage in their respective jurisdictions.

Results

Eighty-four percent of the city, state, and territorial IPMs or individuals responsible for the immunization program responded to the survey. These individuals represented 46 states, six U.S. cities and two U.S. territories. Respondents to this survey represented programs covering approximately 93% of the estimated 2010 U.S. population (Mackun and Wilson, 2011).

Use of ICS, EOCs, and Pandemic Influenza Plans

Survey results found that nearly 76% IPMs indicated that their health department used an ICS to manage the H1N1 vaccination campaign. Of those, more than one-third said their incident commander was the state public health officer and nearly one-third said the public health preparedness coordinator was the incident commander. Almost 50% of IPMs indicated their health department opened an EOC to manage the influenza vaccine campaign. Of these, half opened an in-person EOC, approximately 40% opened both an in-person and virtual EOC (i.e., a Web-based EOC), and less than 5% opened a virtual EOC only. Nearly 60% found their existing pandemic plan helpful, specifically citing the plan's role in providing an established framework for response and forging collaborations among stakeholder partners as particularly helpful.

Collaborations with Emergency Preparedness Programs

Forty percent of responding IPMs shared the programmatic lead for the 2009 to 2010 H1N1 influenza vaccination campaign with their emergency preparedness program. Of the remaining managers, 28% indicated their immunization program was the programmatic lead, 28% indicated the emergency preparedness program was the lead, and only 4% indicated other leadership arrangements. When stratified by programmatic lead, there were no meaningful differences regarding which program performed the majority of the work related to specific H1N1 mass vaccination activities, except for the activity of establishing point-of-distribution (POD) centers.

Of the IPMs who indicated the immunization program was the programmatic lead for the H1N1 influenza vaccination campaign, responses varied regarding which entity performed the majority of the work related to establishing PODs: 33% indicated that regional or local health departments performed the majority of the POD-related work, 29% indicated that the immunization program performed the majority of the work, another 30% indicated that the work was shared jointly between the immunization program and the emergency preparedness program, and the remainder indicated that POD establishment was the responsibility of the emergency preparedness program. In contrast, nearly half the IPMs from jurisdictions whose emergency preparedness program was the lead for the vaccination campaign indicated that POD establishment was the responsibility of the emergency preparedness program, whereas half the IPMs from jurisdictions whose immunization and emergency preparedness programs shared programmatic leadership of the campaign indicated that establishing PODs was also a joint effort between the immunization and emergency preparedness programs.

Seventy percent of IPMs indicated their immunization program staff coordinated with their emergency preparedness program staff within the previous two years to conduct an actual and/or simulated mass vaccination. The majority of IPMs perceived their emergency preparedness staff to be effective in facilitating their state's overall H1N1 influenza vaccination response and in supplementing immunization program staff. However, those managers who had coordinated with their emergency preparedness program on actual and/or simulated mass vaccination events in the two years before the H1N1 influenza vaccination campaign were more likely to perceive their emergency preparedness staff as effective in specific H1N1-related activities than those who had not coordinated with their emergency preparedness program. These activities included allocating scarce vaccine inventory to providers, facilitating decisions about who should receive scarce vaccine among subpriority groups, developing risk communications materials for providers about the H1N1 influenza vaccine, and developing risk communications materials for the public about H1N1 influenza vaccine.

The top three successes cited by IPMs in regard to working with their emergency preparedness programs during the H1N1 influenza campaign were (1) resource sharing, (2) logistics, and (3) social capital. Social capital describes comments that implied a beneficial understanding of a particular role, establishment of good working relationships, or positive collaboration between groups developed before the H1N1 vaccination campaign or during the campaign event. The top three challenges cited were (1) cultural differences between the programs, (2) resource allocation, and (3) leadership conflict or ambiguity. Communication was the theme indicated most commonly as both a success and a challenge.

Emergency Management Systems

During the 2009 to 2010 H1N1 vaccination campaign, state-level immunization programs used a variety of strategies to expand their programmatic and technological capacity to distribute H1N1 influenza vaccine in an efficient and timely manner. More than 75% of IPMs indicated their health department activated an ICS, nearly 50% indicated their health department opened an EOC to manage the vaccine campaign, and 40% indicated having shared the role of programmatic lead for the campaign with their state-level emergency preparedness program.

IPMs' perception of the helpfulness of their department's emergency preparedness staff was also perceived to be higher if they had collaborated previously with the emergency preparedness program for simulation or other emergency preparedness activities. More than half of the IPMs working in jurisdictions with IISs required providers to enter data into their system, and more than one-third of managers indicated using their IIS as a way to push important communications out to providers. Each of these strategies used during the H1N1 vaccination campaign illustrates the value of collaborating with emergency preparedness program partners. In addition, IPMs' responses demonstrate the importance of an IIS in the management of vaccine-related public health emergencies.

The extent to which ICS/EOC structures were used for this vaccination campaign was substantial, which was encouraging given that these management structures were largely foreign to public health agencies before the 2003 adoption of the National Incident Management System, which uses an ICS for emergency response (Homeland Security Presidential Directive 5, 2003).

Because the hierarchical nature of the ICS is not used typically to manage state and local health departments, implementation of the relatively unfamiliar ICS was initially met with some reticence by public health agencies (Sergienko, 2006).

Results from this survey suggest that although some IPMs indicated resistance and frustration with the culture of an ICS, more felt that using an ICS helped them work effectively and efficiently with collaborators, especially their emergency preparedness partners. In addition, use of existing pandemic influenza plans was substantial; many IPMs attested to the value of these plans for providing a structured basis for planning and operations, and for enacting previously established partnerships with entities such as hospitals and federally qualified health centers that proved integral to the coordination of the campaign. In addition to the roles the ICSs/EOCs and pandemic influenza preparedness plans played in managing the H1N1 vaccination campaign, shared programmatic leadership and degree of prior collaboration among immunization and emergency preparedness programs also had an impact on IPMs' perceptions of their emergency preparedness counterparts during the campaign.

Maintenance of Collaborations among Immunization Programs and Emergency Preparedness Programs

Despite having very different programmatic histories in state health departments, findings from this survey suggest collaborations between state immunization programs and emergency preparedness programs may be beneficial into the future. Immunization programs have existed for nearly 50 years, with funding having been provided historically by the Vaccination Assistance Act (Section 317 of the Public Health Service Act) and the Vaccines for Children program, a federally funded entitlement program that provides childhood vaccines free to children who might otherwise be unable to afford vaccines (Hinman et al., 2004; Rein et al., 2006). Public health emergency preparedness programs were created primarily after the enactment of the Public Health Security and Bioterrorism Preparedness and Response Act of 2002, and they receive the majority of their funding through grants from the CDC and the Health Resources Services Administration (Buehler and Holtgrave, 2007). This survey found that, among jurisdictions in which the responsibility of campaign management was shared between the immunization program and the emergency preparedness program, the majority of the work needed to establish PODs was also shared. Because both programs operate largely on discretionary funding that varies from year to year, and has either remained constant or declined in recent years, it may be mutually beneficial for these programs to share resources and personnel.

IPMs' perception of the helpfulness of their emergency preparedness colleagues was also affected by their degree of prior collaboration with the emergency preparedness program. Although results suggest that IPMs' perceptions of their emergency preparedness programs' general helpfulness in facilitating their jurisdiction's mass vaccination response was not significantly associated with exercise collaborations in the previous two years, perceptions of the emergency preparedness program's helpfulness on more specific, targeted activities associated were significantly with prior collaborations. Taken together, these findings underscore the importance of interprogram pre-event planning, and highlight benefits to structuring exercises and responding to actual events in ways that familiarize staff from each program with the specific needs and nuances of the other.

Use of Immunization Information Systems

Of the 51 respondents who indicated their jurisdiction has an IIS, the majority indicated that provider registration in their IIS was a precondition for receipt of H1N1 influenza vaccine. Similarly, more than half indicated that data entry into their IIS was mandatory for H1N1 influenza vaccine providers. Forty-four percent and 51% indicated providers were "compliant" or "somewhat compliant," respectively, with entering data into their IIS. Compared with IPMs from jurisdictions that did not mandate that providers enter data into their IIS, managers from jurisdictions that did mandate IIS data entry were more likely to rate their IIS as valuable for facilitating registration of nontraditional vaccine providers such as obstetricians and pharmacists, and for tracking recalled influenza vaccine. This association could mean either jurisdictions that mandated data entry subsequently found the IIS to be useful, or that program managers who believed a priori that the IIS would be a useful management tool were more likely to mandate data reporting.

IPMs rated the IIS as a valuable tool for supporting H1N1 influenza vaccination clinics, facilitating reminder/recall for children needing a second dose of vaccine, and tracking vaccine coverage rates. Fifty-seven percent of IPMs who indicated their IIS has the capability to "facilitate the registration of nontraditional vaccine providers" and 59% who indicated their IIS has the capability to "push communications out to providers" rated those functionalities as valuable or extremely valuable to the campaign, whereas nearly 40% of IPMs indicated their IIS did not have those functionalities. Of 35 respondents who provided comments regarding the capabilities or functionalities they "wished" their IIS had, the most frequent response was more provider participation in their IIS (26%).

Methods for streamlining and targeting communications, and determining resource allocation plans can contribute greatly to the success of programmatic collaborations. In addition to the importance of strong personnel management, the use of IIS technology was also emphasized during the H1N1 influenza vaccination campaign. Mandating provider participation in an IIS was an approach some states took to improve the ability to track vaccine, with states reporting problems tracking vaccine administration more frequently if their state did not require mandatory reporting through their state IIS (Elliott, 2010).

Lack of provider compliance with entering data into a registry system such as an IIS limits the benefits these systems can have for activities such as inventory management, reminder/recall, and strategic planning on behalf of health departments. The ability to use an IIS to push communications out to vaccine providers is especially important in an emergency situation when mass quantities of vaccine need to be distributed and monitored across a diverse population. Although many IPMs realized the value of having an IIS with these capabilities during the H1N1 vaccination campaign, more than 40% indicated their IIS could not facilitate the registration of nontraditional vaccine providers or push communications out to providers. Enabling more IISs to include these types of functionalities would benefit management of future vaccine-related emergencies. For those programs that did require providers to participate in their IIS for the H1N1 influenza vaccine campaign, it will be important to assess how this affects their willingness to participate in the system over the long term.

Moreover, with the push toward adoption of electronic medical records (EMRs) systems, it will be important to integrate IISs with EMR systems. As this transition occurs, health systems will be looking for ways to determine the most effective ways to either merge IISs with EMRs or to enable the two systems to exchange information efficiently (Stevens et al., 2013).

Implications for Policy and Practice

The 2009 to 2010 pandemic influenza H1N1 vaccination campaign holds useful lessons regarding preparation for and implementation of future mass vaccination programs. This chapter illustrates the use of an Internet-based survey of 64 city, state, and territorial IPMs. Despite some limitations, the results clearly show differences in perceptions of IPMs regarding effectiveness of a variety of measures, and point the way forward to improved collaborations and preparedness. Close collaborations among state-level immunization programs and emergency preparedness programs, and use of existing pandemic influenza plans, ICSs, and EOCs, were important in many jurisdictions across the country. Strong partnerships between staff within immunization and emergency preparedness programs are integral to preparedness against future vaccine-related emergencies. Coupling these programmatic collaborations with new approaches to the use of an IIS, such as mandatory provider participation, can assist jurisdictional responses to future vaccine-related public health threats.

Reductions to health department budgets and public health preparedness grants from the CDC are likely to result in corresponding reductions in state and local public health programs and staff. Fostering alignment of immunization and emergency preparedness programs at a national level could help diffuse the consequences of tighter budgets. In March 2012, AIM released pandemic preparedness collaboration principles to explicitly encourage state, territorial and local immunization and emergency preparedness programs to establish relationships and work together in routine and ongoing ways (Association of Immunization Managers, 2012). Overt promotion of this type of active maintenance of interprogram relationships and expanded use of an IIS cultivated during the H1N1 vaccination campaign experience are important, especially as public health budgets remain low.

During April 2010 and May 2010, the Institute of Medicine hosted a series of three workshops reflecting on the 2009 H1N1 influenza vaccination campaign (Stroud et al., 2009), the findings of which were largely similar to the findings of this study. The Institute of Medicine workshops found that the greatest challenges in vaccine distribution and administration often arose because vaccine supply and demand were poorly matched throughout the 2009 H1N1 influenza vaccination campaign, according to those at the workshops. In fall 2009, demand far outstripped supply, and in spring 2010, supply far exceeded demand. Workshop participants characterized the supply of vaccine as "trickling in" during fall 2009 (Stroud et al., 2009). Participants acknowledged that both the pharmaceutical industry and the CDC faced a number of challenges to develop, produce, and test the 2009 H1N1 vaccine in just six months, yet emphasized the importance of developing new technologies and manufacturing techniques to accelerate vaccine production. In a more virulent pandemic, six months to develop the vaccine may be too long for the vaccine to prevent the spread of disease effectively.

Given that the federal governance structure in the United States provides autonomy to the states regarding budgetary decisions, encouraging discussions of programmatic collaborations at the level of professional organization such as those endorsed by AIM (Association of Immunization Managers, 2012), might be most practical. Despite such budgetary constraints, maintaining and improving the capacity of public health to respond to health threats remains more important than ever as a result of the increasing threat of catastrophic illness or injury resulting from natural or man-made disasters (Andrus et al., 2010; Johns and Blazes, 2010). Moving from a general understanding of which aspects of collaboration worked well during the 2009 to 2010 H1N1 influenza vaccination campaign to which functionalities and policies adopted during the pandemic have actually been sustained over time will be even more informative for preparation against the next great vaccine-related emergency. Such a longitudinal evaluation of policies and practices adopted during the 2009–2010 H1N1 campaign by immunization program mangers is the focus of a Moriarty and colleagues (November 2014). Although immunization programs have been able to maintain improvements in communications between their programs and partners such as healthcare providers, specific functionalities added to IISs (e.g., identification of high-risk populations and disease risk mapping using Geographic Information Systems [GIS]) have not been maintained by many jurisdictions (Moriarty et al., 2014). Although it may not be practical to sustain all policies, capabilities, or protocols implemented during a pandemic postemergency, certain capabilities should not be lost and, in fact, can be applied to nonemergency situations. It is prudent for jurisdictions to have a sense of which activities or collaborations are important to maintain over time (or can be alternatively useful) so that response activities need not be relearned or reimplemented at the outset of the next public health emergency. This knowledge will be critical for health department staff ability to sustain and improve on the programmatic partnerships and policies most useful over time and across a variety of emergency and nonemergency events.

Acknowledgments and Disclosures

This research was conducted with funding support under a grant (no. 5P01TP000300) from the CDC to the Emory Preparedness and Emergency Response Research Center, Emory University, Atlanta, GA. The authors specifically thank all co-authors from the original manuscript presenting this data (citation at the end of the paragraph). They are grateful for collaborations with AIM and the American Immunization Registry Association on the development and distribution of this survey. They also thank the many state and territorial IPMs for their responses to this survey. The data and conclusions presented in this chapter were published previously (Chamberlain, A. T., Seib, K., Wells, K., Hannan, C., Orenstein, W. A., Whitney, E. A., Hinman, A. R., Berkelman, R. L., Omer, S. B. (2012). Perspectives of immunization program managers on 2009–10 H1N1 vaccination in the United States: a national survey. *Biosecurity and Bioterrorism, 10*(1), 142–150.

References

Adams, E. H., Scanlon, E., Callahan, J. J., Carney, M. T. (2010). Utilization of an incident command system for a public health threat: West Nile virus in Nassau County, New York, 2008. *Journal of Public Health Management and Practices, 16*(4), 309–315.

Andrus, J. K., Aguilera, X., Oliva, O., Aldighieri, S. (2010). Global health security and the international health regulations. *BMC Public Health, 10*(Suppl 1), S2.

Association of Immunization Managers. (2011). National ARRA funds for immunization. Accessed April 24, 2014, at http://c.ymcdn.com/sites/www.immunizationmanagers.org/resource/resmgr/Fact_Sheet/ARRA_Fact_Sheet_National.pdf.

Association of Immunization Managers (2012). Preparing for the next pandemic: immunization program & emergency preparedness program pandemic collaboration principles. Accessed April 24, 2014, at http://c.ymcdn.com/sites/www.immunizationmanagers.org/resource/resmgr/files/collaboration_principles.pdf.

Buehler, J., Holtgrave, D. (2007). Who gets how much: funding formulas in federal public health programs. *Journal of Public Health Management and Practice, 13*(2), 151–155.

Centers for Disease Control and Prevention. (2009a). H1N1 vaccination recommendations. Accessed April 24, 2014, at http://www.cdc.gov/h1n1flu/vaccination/acip.htm.

Centers for Disease Control and Prevention. (2009b). Recovery Act funds for Section 317 Program. Accessed April 24, 2014, at http://www.cdc.gov/vaccines/about/recovery-act-funds.htm.

Centers for Disease Control and Prevention. (2012). Grantee immunization websites. Accessed April 24, 2014, at http://www.cdc.gov/vaccines/imz-managers/awardee-imz-websites.html.

Elliott, P. I. (2010). Assessing policy barriers to effective public health response in the H1N1 influenza pandemic. Association of State and Territorial Health Officials project report.

Hinman, A. R., Orenstein, W. A., Rodewald, L. (2004). Financing immunizations in the United States. *Clinical Infectious Diseases, 38*(10),1440–1446.

Johns, M. C., Blazes, D. L. (2010). International health regulations (2005) and the U.S. Department of Defense: building core capacities on a foundation of partnership and trust. *BMC Public Health, 10*(Suppl 1), S4.

Kun, K. E., Zimmerman, J., Rose, D. A., Rubel, S. (2013). State, territorial, and local health departments' reporting of partnership strength before and after the H1N1 response. *Prehospital and Disaster Medicine, 28*(6), 580–585.

Mackun, P., Wilson, S. (2011). Population distribution and change: 2000 to 2010 (C2010BR-01). *Census Briefs*, 1–11.

McKesson Corp. (2009). CDC expands existing vaccine distribution partnership with McKesson to include H1N1 flu vaccine. News release. Accessed April 24, 2014, at http://www.mckesson.com/about-mckesson/newsroom/press-releases/2009/cdc-expands-existing-vaccine-distribution-partnership-with-mckesson-to-include-h1n1-flu-vaccine/.

Mignone, A. T., Davidson, R. (2003). Public health response actions and the use of emergency operations centers. *Prehospital and Disaster Medicine, 18*(3), 217–219.

Moriarty, L. F., Omer, S. B., Seib, K., Chamberlain, A. T., Wells, K., Whitney, E., Berkelman, R., Bednarczyk, R. A. (2014). Changes in immunization program managers' perceptions of programs' functional capabilities during and after vaccine shortages and the H1N1 influenza pandemic. *Public Health Reports, 129*(Suppl. 4), 42–48.

Porter, D., Hall, M., Hartl, B. (2011). Local health department 2009 H1N1 influenza vaccination clinics: CDC staffing model comparison and other best practices. *Journal of Public Health Management and Practice, 17*(6), 530–533.

Rambhia, K. J., Watson, M., Sell, T. K., Waldhorn, R., Toner, E. (2010). Mass vaccination for the 2009 H1N1 pandemic: approaches, challenges, and recommendations. *Biosecurity and Bioterrorism, 8*(4), 321–330.

Rein, D. B., Honeycutt, A. A., Rojas-Smith, L., Hersey, J. C. (2006). Impact of the CDC's Section 317 immunization grants program funding on childhood vaccination coverage. *American Journal of Public Health, 96*(9),1548–1553.

Schnirring, L. (2009). U.S. H1N1 vaccine delayed as cases and deaths rise. CIDRAP News. Accessed April 24, 2014, at http://www.cidrap.umn.edu/news-perspective/2009/10/us-h1n1-vaccine-delayed-cases-and-deaths-rise.

Sergienko, E. (2006). Public health and the incident command system. *American College of Emergency Physicians Newsletter*, 15.

Stevens, L. A., Palma, J. P., Pandher, K. K., Longhurst, C. A. (2013). Immunization registries in the EMR era. *Online Journal of Public Health Information*, 5(2), 211.

Stroud, C., Nadig, L., Altevogt, B. M., Institute of Medicine. (2009). *The 2009 H1N1 influenza vaccination campaign: summary of a workshop series.* Washington: National Academies Press.

U.S. Department of Health and Human Services. (2011). Justification of estimates for appropriation committees. Accessed April 24, 2014, at http://www.cdc.gov/fmo/topic/Budget%20Information/appropriations_budget_form_pdf/FY2011_ATSDR_CJ_Final.pdf.

CHAPTER 8

Implementing a National Vaccination Campaign at the State and Local Levels

Massachusetts Case Study

MICHAEL A. STOTO AND MELISSA A. HIGDON

Introduction

The Institute of Medicine (2002) has defined the public health system as the "complex network of individuals and organizations that have the potential to play critical roles in creating the conditions for health" (p. 28). For public health emergency preparedness (PHEP), this system includes not only federal, state, and local health departments, but also hospitals and healthcare providers, fire departments, schools, the media, and many other public and private organizations (Seid et al., 2006). The 2009 H1N1 pandemic required a concerted effort from the entire U.S. PHEP system, from the federal government down to local areas.

Consistent with this understanding of the public health system, to prepare for an anticipated second wave of pH1N1 during fall 2009, the Massachusetts Department of Public Health (MDPH) realized the need to seek actively the involvement and participation of local health departments and boards of health, hospitals, clinics and other healthcare providers, schools, and many other public- and private-sector public health partners across the Commonwealth.

Overall, the MDPH's response to the fall wave of pH1N1 was highly successful. The number of vaccination sites and vaccinators were increased substantially, and communications with the public and with public health partners were enhanced. Eventually, more than 3.7 million doses of vaccine were delivered, which this represents 37% of the population of the Commonwealth (60% of those 6 months to 17 years and 28% of those 18 years and older) and 51% of the initial target groups, exceeding national figures by a large margin.

Contrary to planning assumptions, however, the distribution of pandemic vaccine to local health departments was slow and unpredictable. Some providers in Massachusetts began to receive vaccine on October 6 as anticipated; but, through December, vaccine deliveries lagged behind expectations constantly, and the types and amounts of vaccine to be delivered were unpredictable. The uncertainty surrounding the timing of vaccination deliveries to Massachusetts led to a variety of challenges to the Commonwealth's response.

Building on the MDPH's pH1N1 after-action report/improvement plan, and a separate, more focused case study of the island of Martha's Vineyard (the Vineyard), this chapter focuses on lessons learned about responding to future influenza seasons, especially those characterized by a scarcity of vaccine, and a set of improvements that can be made in advance of future events—whether related to pH1N1, other types of influenza, or other disease outbreaks—to enhance public health system preparedness. Although Massachusetts is unique in many ways, this case illustrates challenges of organizing a decentralized state and local public health system response to which many communities can relate. The issues that arose are common in both urban and rural areas, and jurisdictions of all sizes.

Although, the response to pH1N1 in 2009 involved many PHEP capabilities, such as surveillance and laboratory analysis, and distribution of antivirals from the strategic national stockpile (especially during the spring outbreak), the focus of the analysis is on the state and local implementation of the national vaccination campaign in the fall. This involved efforts to allocate fairly and distribute the vaccine efficiently to local public health systems, to set priorities for its use, and to expand the capacity to administer the vaccine at the local level, and, in general, to work regionally. The public health response also required efforts to communicate between MDPH and local health departments and with their partners, and also with the public.

Methods

This chapter draws on two reports about the public health response to the 2009 H1N1 pandemic in Massachusetts. The first is the MDPH's after-action report/improvement plan for September 2009 through February 2010, which the chapter authors helped prepare. To ensure all the relevant perspectives were represented in the analysis, the MDPH contracted with Harvard School of Public Health (HSPH) to gather and analyze information from both MDPH staff and its public health partners. We began by reviewing relevant MDPH documents and communications, and Massachusetts media coverage. Between March 30, 2010, and June 8, 2010, HSPH staff conducted 29 in-person or telephone interviews. In addition, on April 29, 2010, the HSPH conducted focus groups with three groups of MDPH officials. Last, "facilitated look-back" meetings were conducted in Amherst on April 12, 2010; in Boston on May 7, 2010; and in Brockton on May 18, 2010. A facilitated look-back is an established method for examining public health system emergency response capabilities and for conducting a candid systems-level analysis. Through the use of a neutral facilitator and a no-fault approach, dimensions of decisions were probed and nuances in past decision making were explored in detail in discussions with public health leaders and key staff, in addition to a variety of community stakeholders involved with the response. A brief chronology of the events that occurred in response to pH1N1 was then reviewed. The facilitator guided the discussion and asked probing questions surrounding key issues about what happened at various points in the chronology that was presented, key decisions that were made by various stakeholders, how decisions were perceived and acted on by others, and how lessons learned were elicited (Aledort et al., 2006).

To fill in the details in this state-level analysis and to explore more fully state–local interactions, we draw on a detailed case study about the public health system response on the Vineyard (Higdon and Stoto, 2013a). This case study is based on a review of local newspapers and interviews with key stakeholders. First, we reviewed the two local newspapers—the *Martha's Vineyard Gazette* and the *Martha's Vineyard Times*——between May 2009 and December 2009. We also reviewed the *Boston Globe* for pH1N1-related material involving Massachusetts, Cape Cod, or the Vineyard. We also interviewed key stakeholders on the Vineyard in May 2010 and June 2011. The majority of the island's local health agents were interviewed in a group, including the health agents from the towns of Tisbury, Edgartown, and Chilmark. We also interviewed the chief executive officer, the chief nurse executive, the lead pharmacist, and the employee health and infectious disease nurse from Martha's Vineyard Hospital (MVH). Last, the island's school superintendent was interviewed, because the schools had a large role in the island's vaccination program.

Results

The Massachusetts Public Health System's Response to pH1N1

Massachusetts, a state of 6.5 million people (U.S. Census Bureau, 2010) and 7,800 square miles (Hayden, 2006), has 351 cities and towns, each with its own local health department and board of health. Local autonomy is deeply ingrained in Massachusetts culture. The state's decentralized public health system features local responsibility among autonomous local health boards, in addition to MDPH (Massachusetts Department of Public Health, 2000; Paulding, 2005; Salinsky, 2002; Wasserman et al., 2006). A few municipal departments such as the Boston Public Health Commission (BPHC) are large, with dozens of employees and a sizable dedicated budget. However, most local health departments are severely limited in personnel and resources, frequently represented by a part-time health director with few or no staff. Unlike many other states, local health departments in Massachusetts in general do not have clinical facilities, but rather rely on relationships with community health centers, visiting nurse associations, and other healthcare providers to administer vaccines and provide other personal healthcare services.

In 2003, after the Centers for Disease Control and Prevention's (CDC) increased dramatically funding provided to the states to enhance capacity for communicable disease emergency preparedness and response, the MDPH launched a statewide effort to establish seven public health preparedness regions, 15 subregions (plus the city of Boston), each led by a coalition (Figure 8-1). The primary rationale was to distribute federal funds more efficiently; after subtracting dedicated expenditures to enhance capacity primarily at the MDPH State Laboratory Institute and Bureau of Communicable Disease Control, simply dividing the available funds among the 351 cities and towns on a per capita basis would have created financial allocations amounting to only several thousand (or even several hundred) dollars for some communities—not enough to make a difference.

According to Koh and colleagues (2008), although the primary impetus of regionalization was to serve as a vehicle for distributing preparedness funds, this strategy had many other potential advantages. Regionalization served as a foundation for sharing resources, coordinating planning, conducting training, and strengthening the public health infrastructure on a larger scale, and after regions were established, public health officials reported better collaboration among communities and across agencies, increased public health response capacity, and improved resource sharing that led to stronger social networks and new personal connections among professionals. Regionalization also enhanced the visibility of public health as an active partner in emergency response.

2009 H1N1 in Massachusetts

Production of the pH1N1 vaccine had started nationally in May, shortly after the pH1N1 virus was identified, and deliveries were expected by late September or early October. To maximize production capacity, a number of different manufacturers produced different formulations and doses of vaccines, most of which were indicated for some population groups and not for others. In July, the CDC identified priority groups for the vaccine and, as the summer progressed, the CDC encouraged state health departments to develop plans for administering vaccine at the local level in their states (Centers for Disease Control and Prevention, 2009a, 2009b).

The first Massachusetts cases of pH1N1 were seen in early May 2009 in Boston, shortly after the pandemic emerged in Mexico, California, and New York City in April (Centers for Disease Control and Prevention, 2009a). Because children seemed to be particularly at risk for infection, these and subsequent cases triggered a wave of school closings in Massachusetts and throughout the United States. The MDPH began preparing for a large-scale immunization campaign, and other public health activities, in summer 2009. In late August, the MDPH expanded its vaccine distribution program and also alerted local health departments at that time to prepare mass

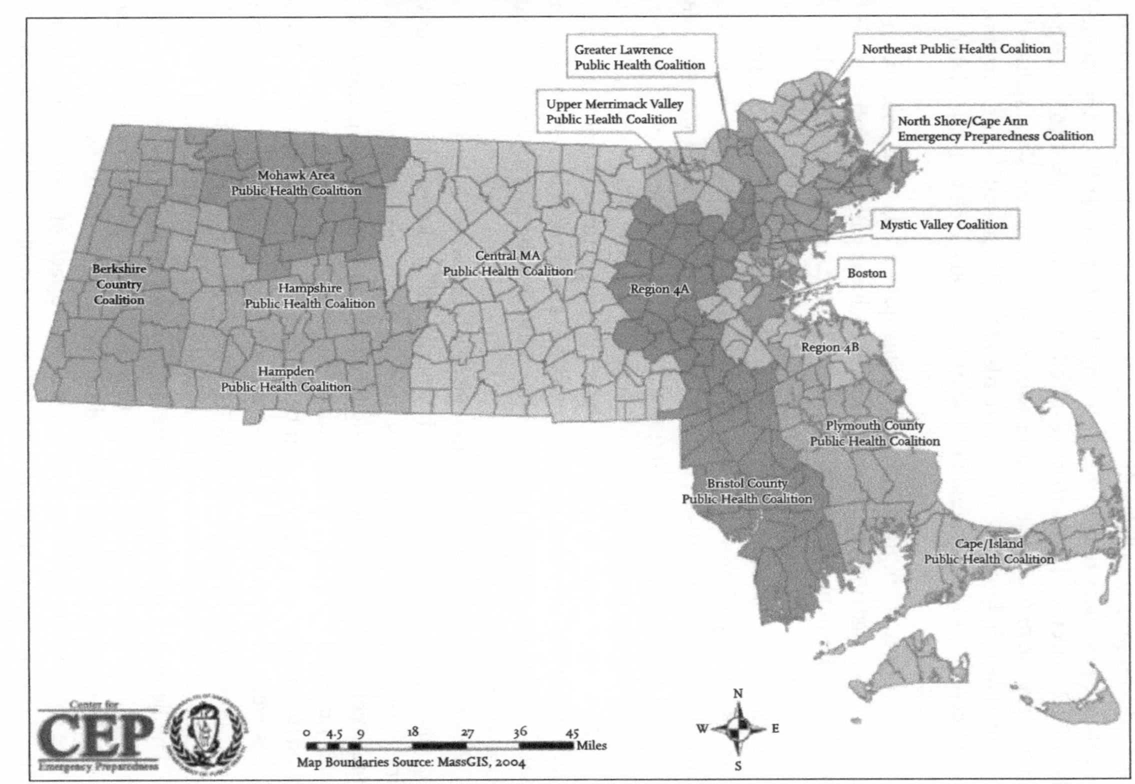

FIGURE 8-1 Massachusetts Department of Public Health (MDPH) emergency preparedness regional coalitions.

dispensing plans. And, of course, a public communication strategy was developed and launched.

Vaccination Allocation and Distribution

Anticipating a need for many more registered vaccination sites than Massachusetts had in previous years, the MDPH built on its existing Vaccine for Children program for pediatric vaccines, and urged hospitals and other healthcare providers not already in the system to register to be able to receive the pH1N1 vaccine. This action resulted in approximately 1,500 new registered sites, bringing the total to 4,500. Newly registered sites included city and town health departments and boards of health, hospitals and community health centers, and individual healthcare providers such as pediatricians and obstetricians.

However, in attempting to register sites quickly, the state lab, which was in charge of distributing vaccine, may not have gathered sufficient information on the population intended to be served, or on any plans that local health departments had made with healthcare providers in their jurisdictions. Thinking this would simplify matters, some sites registered as the representative of a group of providers but did not indicate they were doing so. Thus, when the vaccine was in short supply in October, the MDPH was not able to distinguish between sites serving many patients and sites serving few, so all sites received the minimum lot size regardless of the number of individuals they intended to serve. In addition, the MDPH sometimes did not know which vaccine formulations were appropriate or not appropriate for certain sites, and had to make assumptions based on the nature of the provider (e.g., pediatricians vs. obstetricians).

Policies for allocating vaccine to registered sites were set by an MDPH steering committee. Because the MDPH typically did not know which types of vaccines would be delivered until they arrived, these policies were driven by the epidemiology of the disease, striving for equity in the allocation, and were not determined by a formula or algorithm. Every day, the shipments received by the state lab were assessed for number of doses and formulation of each dose. Doses were then assigned to registered sites based on their recipient population profiles, taking into account the sites' priority group populations. The MDPH used its judgment to ensure allocation was equitable.

The benefit of this allocation method was its flexibility in response to the constantly changing situation, and therefore shipments could be tailored to meet the greatest need. The downside of tailoring the response so specifically to the composition of vaccine shipments was a lack of transparency. The lab was unable to communicate a detailed allocation plan to the public because they did not know how the allocation would look until the vaccine shipment arrived. Another weakness of the allocation process was that its reliance on the facility's capacity and constituent reporting made allocation susceptible to intentional or unintentional misinformation. Disparities in facilities' reporting of the populations they served and their vaccination capacities might also be responsible in part for the confusion that resulted.

Another complication was that it was not always understood, at the local level, whose responsibility it was to vaccinate certain populations. Were doses allocated to hospitals intended for the hospital staff or for the hospital's patients? Cities were concerned that allocations to large hospitals in their jurisdiction, which had staff and served populations from outside the city, counted against them. Although the MDPH worked closely with the state Emergency Medical Services (EMS) councils in developing a program to vaccinate the state's EMS and paramedic community, at the local level boards of health and EMS councils were sometimes not clear whether public health was supposed to vaccinate paramedics or if EMS councils were responsible for vaccinating their own personnel. In some jurisdictions, it was not clear whether local public health agencies, hospitals, or community health centers had the responsibility for vaccinating vulnerable populations.

Expansion of Vaccination Administration Capacity

During the 2009 H1N1 pandemic, local public health agencies made a wide variety of arrangements with schools (including colleges and universities), healthcare providers (hospitals, community health centers, long-term care facilities), shopping malls, and many other sites for vaccine administration. In addition, a regulation was passed to allow for paramedics, pharmacists, medical students, and dentists to administer vaccines. To ensure there would be enough vaccinators to meet the potential surge in people getting the vaccine, the MDPH held two kinds of trainings—one type for nontraditional vaccinators unaccustomed to vaccination, such as dentists, and a refresher course for school nurses. More than 550 school nurses attended training, as did more than 700 other nontraditional vaccinators. This regulation and the training were intended to include both traditional and nontraditional vaccinators and were successful in this regard. This was made possible by federal liability protection for pH1N1, which also covered volunteers, such as Medical Reserve Corps members.

Increasing the number and variety of vaccination sites made it more convenient for people and thus helped to make vaccine more accessible, especially for populations that historically are not vaccinated. Many of these venues knew their populations and were therefore able to target their vaccination efforts toward the highest priority groups. In addition, these venues often had their own messaging systems, which they could use to reach vulnerable populations.

Most cities and towns in Massachusetts participated in school-based vaccination programs, serving students in those schools and sometimes others in the community. In many cases, this was the first time in many years that schools had worked with public health. Drawing on MDPH planning and response frameworks prepared before the pH1N1 outbreak, several successful school vaccine clinic models were identified. School-based clinics seemed to work well on the weekends, after school, and during school hours. Some towns vaccinated school children in their town on a "per-grade system" (vaccinate all kindergarten students in the town before moving on to first-grade students, and so on) and others vaccinated school children on a "per-school system" (vaccinate the entire eligible student population in one school before moving on to a second school, for example). For a school-based flu clinic to be successful, an appropriate number of staff (both clerical and clinical) had to be present to run it. Working out the logistics of the clinic ahead of time, as opposed to relying on the schools to come up with the clinic logistics, was also important. In the end, pH1N1 presented an opportunity to forge relationships between local public health personnel and school superintendents, which is significant because schools are fairly autonomous institutions.

The primary challenge with school-based clinics was the consent process, and this was the main reason that Boston chose not to use this approach. Children would throw out their consent forms, and parents seemed not to care. Some schools solved this by holding school-based clinics in the evening or on the weekend, at which time other family members could also be vaccinated if indicated.

Throughout the Commonwealth, community health centers, large group practices, and other healthcare providers proved to be effective public health partners in administering vaccinations. A number of cities and towns worked closely with community health centers as vaccination sites. For instance, the BPHC signed memoranda of agreement with a number of Boston community healthcare centers to be the sites for almost all their vaccine clinics. Healthcare centers held numerous small vaccine clinics to minimize crowd size, deal with limited vaccine more efficiently, conserve BPHC finances, and circumvent cultural competency concerns. By having many small clinics, the BPHC avoided large groups of panicked people. This strategy helped with security concerns, and the BPHC were also able to make targeted thrusts into vulnerable populations during the initial stages of vaccine scarcity. Only one member from the BPHC staff needed to be present at these clinics to collect data, so the BPHC was able to conserve its resources. Last, the healthcare centers were trusted by the communities they served and had an appropriate translation and language infrastructure in place.

In another example, Harvard Vanguard, a large group practice in eastern Massachusetts, set up weekend clinics so they would not overwhelm pediatricians and other providers. Depending on which vaccine formulations were available at a given time, they would use information in their records to call appropriate patients and set up appointments for them in 15-minute time slots. This process could be done automatically with existing electronic medical records, and because of this preregistration and staff who knew what to expect, this course of action was all done efficiently.

Vaccination Priorities

In July, the CDC's Advisory Committee on Immunization Practices had identified the following priority groups for the vaccine: pregnant women, children six months through 24 years, caregivers of children younger than six months, and high-risk/chronically ill individuals (Centers for Disease Control and Prevention, 2009b). In the face of limited vaccine availability in the fall, however, the MDPH refined the CDC's guidance relative to vaccination priority groups, focusing attention on healthcare workers, pregnant women, and children. Experience implementing this policy at the local level, however, was mixed. Many felt it was essential to ensure the limited supply of vaccine was getting to the most vulnerable populations. Others, however, found the state guidance to be confusing because it seemed to contradict CDC guidelines. These recommendations were also problematic when, in some cases, local boards of health decided to ignore them. One large jurisdiction, for instance, started vaccinating the second tier long before anyone else, which was seen as unfair to communities without enough vaccine to do so.

Another challenge involved healthcare workers and emergency responders. The MDPH required institutions to offer vaccine to all healthcare workers, which apparently led to an increased vaccination rate among healthcare workers. But, the definition of "healthcare workers" varied, and the only mechanism for tailoring priority groups to local conditions was to ask the MDPH to evaluate each case individually. Some felt this led to inconsistent results because the level of flexibility afforded depended on the specific MDPH representative who was contacted. In addition, police and fire department personnel believed all first responders should receive the same access to vaccine as EMS personnel and other healthcare providers. This contrasted with the expectations of the emergency responders, who for years had been told they and their families would be given priority.

Communication with Public Health Partners

The MDPH communicated with local public health agencies, healthcare providers, and other public health partners primarily through weekly conference calls that were transcribed and made available to those who could not listen in. Staff from MDPHs participated as appropriate, depending on the topics being discussed. In addition, a weekly situation report was prepared and widely distributed. There were also occasional conference calls on special topics such as obstetric issues, daily e-mails about vaccine allocation, and many informal communications between MDPH staff and public health partners by individual telephone calls and through e-mail. The MDPH also conducted weekly conference calls with the health officers from the New England states, New York, and New Jersey.

Although communication was challenging as a result of the rapidly changing facts, the MDPH managed communications well and its efforts were appreciated by public health partners. The material in the weekly conference calls was seen as relevant and it communicated a consensus message from MDPH, which was seen as invaluable. Because the information was aimed at multiple kinds of public health partners, the conference calls were able to give a big-picture view to the people listening in. They also helped with community building within and among organizations, and it was helpful for the people listening in to realize they were not alone.

Prior relationships that had been developed with the support of MDPH preparedness planning efforts also seem to have been helpful in sharing information. For instance, meetings of the Council of Boston Teaching Hospitals allowed hospitals in Boston to meet and exchange information. The conference calls seem to have been especially helpful for the providers who did not have extensive contacts with drug suppliers or the MDPH, and would therefore have difficulty obtaining the information shared on the calls. Some of the preparedness coalitions in the western part of the state held regular conference calls immediately after the MDPH weekly call to discuss what was said and to coordinate local efforts.

Communication with individual providers proved to be more difficult. A major challenge was that the only way for the MDPH to obtain a list of providers was from the Board of Registration in Medicine, which had a turnaround time of one to two weeks. In addition, the point of contact listed in the vaccine site registration information was not always a clinician, making communication about medical and public health issues difficult.

Other communication problems emerged during pH1N1. For instance, some suggested there was little communication between school nurses and community pediatricians or among pediatricians as a group. Another problem was the volume of information being disseminated. Multiple e-mails were being sent by the CDC, the MDPH, and other agencies every day. Sometimes these messages were identical; sometimes they were slightly different. The MDPH webpage, some felt, also had too much information, making it difficult to find what was more important or current.

Communication with the Public

Communication with the public about the pH1N1 vaccine was viewed as an important piece of the pH1N1 response, and the MDPH used a variety of cutting-edge communication modalities, such as an interactive website that included video posts and a blog, social media such as Twitter, and hotlines to communicate with the public. Preplanning for this type of communication began during the spring and carried over into the fall/winter response. This communication required designing culturally sensitive educational materials for (1) clinicians regarding the benefits of administering vaccine and (2) specific populations about the benefits of receiving it. The MDPH also developed and widely distributed a *Flu Care at Home* booklet that clearly explained how to take care of oneself or a loved one at home. Materials were created in multiple languages and targeted to populations known to be resistant to vaccines. The blog allowed for daily updates and interaction with the public, and because people could respond, monitoring it helped the MDPH learn which populations were most nervous about the vaccine and what their concerns were. Reviewing comments posted by the public allowed the MDPH to respond to their concerns. Local health officials appreciated the use of social media as appropriate for reaching certain populations, but noted that different forms of social media are used by different populations and different socioeconomic groups.

The MDPH also worked extensively with radio, television, and newspapers to provide information to the public. In addition to working with Boston media, a number of strategies were used for communities that do not receive Boston newsfeeds. In particular, the MDPH worked with New Hampshire and Albany, New York, media outlets. The MDPH also worked to ensure that Springfield, in the western part of the state, would be able to pick up Boston feeds, and the Public Health commissioner did interviews for western Massachusetts media. Health officials in western Massachusetts, however, suggested the MDPH identify a communication specialist for western Massachusetts who understands the needs of the community, including the vulnerable populations.

Despite these efforts, it was observed that individuals who were well connected and had an existing relationship with a provider were more likely to get vaccinated. This result suggests the importance of working with healthcare providers and locating vaccine clinics at community health centers. On the other hand, those who spoke a language other than English and did not have trust in the healthcare system, the government, and so on, were less likely to accept vaccination. In addition, those with low socioeconomic status have a mistrust of government and are too concerned with day-to-day matters to worry about vaccination. Experience in 2009 suggests the importance of working with churches and schools to overcome these barriers. As noted earlier, different groups use different social media, so this should be considered in planning emergency communication. It was recommended that, before the next large-scale emergency, public health agencies identify and build relationships with nongovernmental organizations such as churches and schools that can serve as trusted channels of communication with different population groups.

Martha's Vineyard Public Health System's Response to 2009 H1N1

To analyze the local public health response in more detail, and to illustrate aspects of state–local dynamics, this next portion of our analysis focuses on the response related to the Vineyard, a 90-square mile island in Massachusetts with a year-round population of approximately 16,000. The island is composed of six towns that, together with the town of Gosnold (population 75) on a separate group of islands, make up the entirety of Duke's County, Massachusetts (Figure 8-2). Although the Vineyard has a reputation based on its wealthy summer visitors, the year-round population is comprised of mostly agricultural and service workers, with relatively low income and education in comparison with the rest of the state. A substantial number of the year-round residents are Brazilian and speak Portuguese as their primary language, and there is also a Native American community on the island known as the Wampanoag tribe of

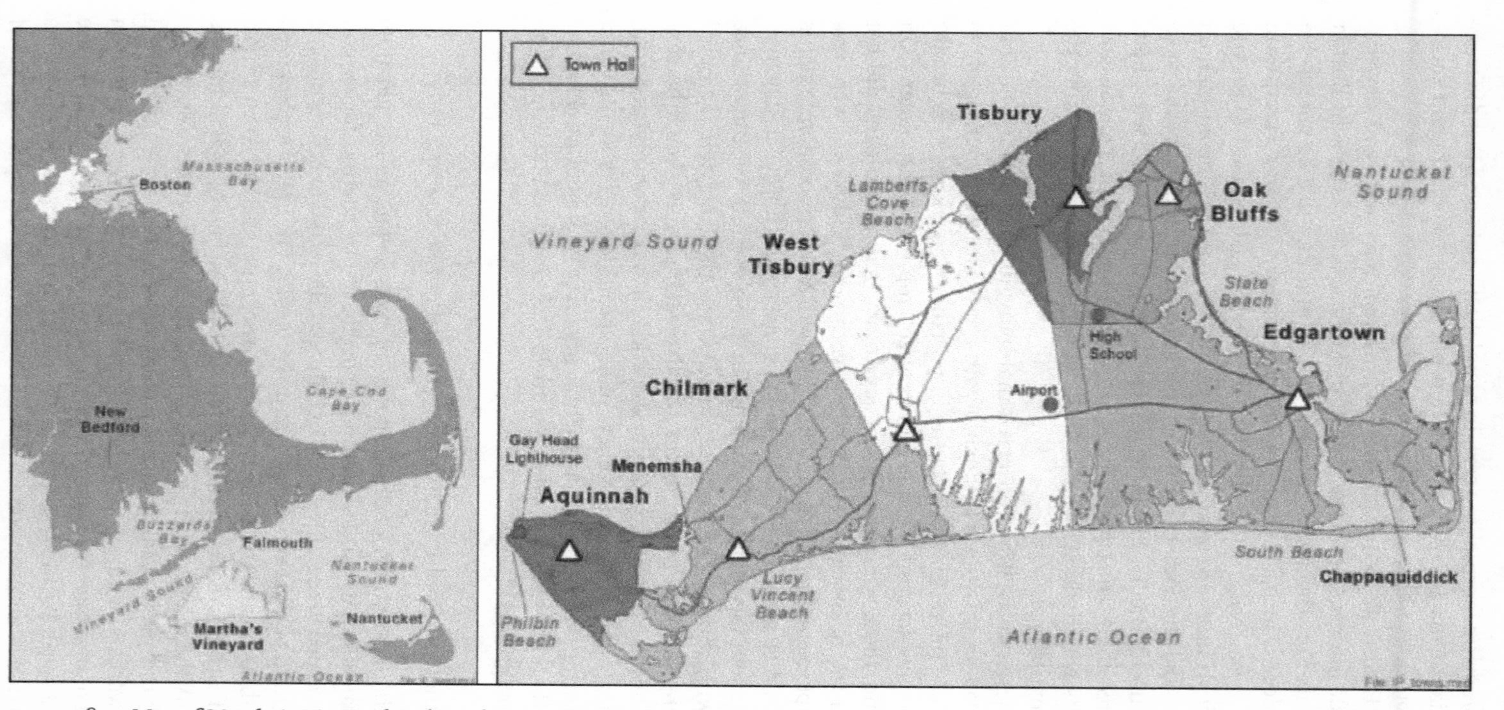

FIGURE 8-2 Map of Martha's Vineyard and southeastern Massachusetts.

Map of Martha's Vineyard. Accessed July 2011 at http://www.hihostels.com/dba/hostels-HI---Martha-s-Vineyard-060011.ends.htm and MDPH Preparedness Regions Coalitions. As it appeared in: Koh, H. K., Elqura, L. J., Judge, C. M., & Stoto, M. A. (2008). Regionalization of local public health systems in the era of preparedness. Annual Review of Public Health, 29, 205–218.

Gay Head, located predominately in Aquinnah, the island's smallest and most rural town.

The local public health system on the island is comprised of both formal and informal structures. Unlike in many other parts of the United States, Massachusetts counties have no role in public health or most administrative matters—meaning, the six town boards of health have the primary responsibility for public health matters. The largest towns on the Vineyard have a full-time health agent and up to two other staff members; the smallest towns have less than one full-time equivalent worker.

The 19-bed MVH, which is affiliated with Massachusetts General Hospital in Boston, is the only hospital on the island. Housing several hospital-owned physician practices (including the only obstetrics practice on the island), one independent practice (Vineyard Pediatrics), and the Windemere nursing home, MVH is a major part of the island's public health system. There is also a small federally qualified health center on the island, which is not officially affiliated with MVH, but also is supervised by an MVH physician. The Vineyard Nursing Association (VNA) also plays a role in the local public health system, contracting individually with each town, with the exception of Aquinnah, for standard public health nursing services including immunizations and epidemiology. In addition, the Vineyard Affordable Access Program provides access to health care for low-income island residents and is overseen by the Duke's County Health Council, which consists of representatives from MVH and the schools, the town health agents, and consumers.

The Wampanoag Health Service, which provides programs and services to members of the federally recognized Wampanoag tribe is another part is the island's public health system. The service's contract health program provides assistance to tribal members with purchasing comprehensive health services such as inpatient and outpatient care, hospital medical office visits, pharmaceutical services, and mental health counseling through members' personal healthcare providers. In 2009, Ron MacLaren managed the tribe's health affairs.

The Martha's Vineyard Regional High School (MVRHS) serves the entire island, together with one charter school that includes grades K–12. Five elementary schools exist on the island, ranging in size and composition. Tisbury, Edgartown, Chilmark, and Oak Bluffs each have one school and a regional elementary school in West Tisbury for children from West Tisbury, Aquinnah, and Chilmark that choose not to attend the small Chilmark elementary school. Each school had a limited amount of funds allocated for consultation with a physician. Anticipating the second wave of pH1N1 in fall 2009, the school superintendent, Dr. James Weiss, appointed Dr. Michael Goldfein from Vineyard Pediatrics as the school system physician on a consulting basis.

Emergency preparedness efforts on the Vineyard have been both formal and informal. In 2002, the MDPH established seven regions and 15 subregions to coordinate emergency preparedness efforts. The Cape and the Islands Emergency Preparedness Coalition, part of region 5, encompasses Barnstable

County (Cape Cod), the Vineyard, and Nantucket (Figure 8-1). In addition to the six town health departments, MVH was represented in the coalition's hospital preparedness efforts mainly through Carol Bardwell, Chief Nurse Executive. The Coalition has been the primary vehicle for the island's health departments and the hospital to access federal public health and hospital preparedness funds.

In addition, around 2005, the six towns and the Wampanoag Health Service formed the informal Martha's Vineyard Public Health Coalition (MVPHC) to strengthen communication among the six towns on MV and the Wampanoag tribe. In addition to regular meetings, the MVPHC's major activity has been to organize an annual islandwide seasonal influenza vaccine clinic, usually on Veterans Day (November 11). In addition to providing a needed preventive service, the Coalition has used these clinics to test and drill approaches to mass dispensing that would be useful in an emergency. MVH, VNA, and town emergency management agencies are brought onboard the MVPHC's activities as needed. For example, town police departments were asked to develop a traffic plan for islandwide flu clinics.

The Vineyard's public health system is characterized by the many informal connections that one finds on a small island. For instance, in addition to participating in the Cape and Islands Emergency Preparedness Coalition efforts, MVH Chief Nurse Executive Carol Bardwell is also a member of the island's Medical Reserve Corps board, as are representatives of each of the six towns.

The Public Health Response

In early August, a 26-year-old Vineyard man of Brazilian descent developed severe flulike symptoms and was treated by medical team members at MVH, who initiated a webcast medical discussion with physicians at their affiliate, Massachusetts General Hospital. pH1N1 was confirmed and the patient's conditioned worsened; he was transferred to Massachusetts General Hospital, where he ultimately died on August 14.

In September, in response to MDPH recommendations, Vineyard health agents collaborated with the VNA to register as one entity for five of the six towns on the island, and the Wampanoag Health Service registered for the tribe and the town of Aquinnah, where most tribal members live. MVH registered for its staff and physician offices owned by the hospital. Vineyard Pediatrics, an independent physician practice colocated at the hospital, was registered separately as part of the preexisting childhood immunization system to receive vaccine.

In addition, the town health agents and the VNA chose a single islandwide vaccination clinic at the regional high school, where previous seasonal flu clinics had been held, to administer both pH1N1 and seasonal vaccine. Given the urgency of the situation and the understanding that vaccine would be available, the clinic was planned for September 26 rather than November 11, as in previous years. As the planned date for the islandwide clinic neared, however, vaccine production delays were announced, and the clinic was postponed first until October 24 and eventually until November 11, when only seasonal vaccine was administered.

In the last week of October, students at MVRHS started to exhibit flulike symptoms. According to the *Vineyard Gazette,* for example, on Wednesday, October 28, 2009, more than 100 of the 800 total MVRHS students were out sick (Seccombe, 2009). Because the MDPH did not recommend laboratory testing or require case reporting, these cases were presumed to be pH1N1 and the students were sent home. Absenteeism increased throughout that week and the next, and health officials assumed this reflected students with influenza or students kept home by their parents out of concern they would be infected. According to the *Vineyard Gazette,* the worst day for student absences was Friday, October 30, 2009, when approximately 140 MVRHS students were absent from school (Seccombe, 2009).

The 2009 H1N1 vaccine started arriving on the island in late October, but only in small batches. Faced with a very different vaccine availability situation than expected, the MVPHC switched tactics. In a series of meetings in October with the school superintendent and the school system physician, a school-based approach was adopted. School officials did not think parents would bring their children to a mass vaccination clinic on a Saturday; they chose to vaccinate students at their own school when it was in session. Because the school did not have enough staff to vaccinate every student in a day, the MVPHC assembled "shooter teams" consisting of health officials and EMS staff from every town on the island and from the VNA that would go from school to school. Every Vineyard school has a full-time nurse, and because they know the children well, the school nurses were assigned the administrative paperwork and follow-up work with the students' parents as necessary. The smaller schools—the Chilmark School and the Public Charter School—were done first, beginning November 9, when 100-dose batches of vaccine first arrived. The larger schools were done later, when more vaccine became available.

MVH, meanwhile, had used its first doses of vaccine during a hospitalwide flu clinic on October 29, at which 209 hospital and Windemere nursing home staff were vaccinated. Rather than waste vaccine in multidose vials that had been opened, MVH also vaccinated emergency medical technicians and paramedics at this time. Having observed a fatal case at close range in August, the hospital chief executive officer, Mr. Tim Walsh, wanted to be sure the vaccine was used as soon as it became available. Because he assumed (incorrectly, as it turns out) the towns were waiting to assemble enough vaccine to hold the islandwide clinic, MVH also took on the responsibility of vaccinating the pregnant women on the island (because the only obstetrics practice on the island was based at the hospital) and preschool children. On Saturday, October 31, 2009, MVH brought on Portuguese translators to assist with the large population of Brazilian residents on the island and hosted a flu clinic for pregnant women. On the same day, MVH held a separate clinic at which 206 preschool-age children were vaccinated.

Despite the concerted efforts of the towns and schools, the hospital and its providers, and the tribe, there were a number of problems that emerged as more vaccine became available in November. MVH, for instance, originally assumed that because it housed the island's only obstetrics practice, all pregnant women were covered in the hospital's October 31 clinic. Town health officials pointed out that some women received their prenatal care off island or were not covered at all. Vineyard Pediatrics, which had registered to receive vaccine separate from the hospital and the towns, committed to vaccinating its own patients. Confusion arose, however, about whether this should include the patients of Dr. Melanie Miller, who works at Vineyard Pediatrics but is a hospital employee. Although these problems were resolved quickly, they created confusion and frustration.

Lessons Learned

Overall, there were notable successes in how the Vineyard handled the 2009 H1N1 pandemic, especially with regard to mass dispensing. The decision to share personnel and resources across towns to constitute shooter teams was essential in vaccinating school children in a timely manner. Moreover, the decision to vaccinate the children attending smaller schools first, and the children at larger schools as vaccine became available, was easy to explain to the general public and was well accepted. It also represents an adroitly flexible response to uncertainty about when vaccine would arrive.

Perhaps the most important achievement was the way the towns, the hospital, the tribe, the schools, and others came together as a public health system and shared personnel and other resources across towns to protect the health of those on the island. MVH, for instance, stepped up to vaccinate not only its employees but also pregnant women and preschool children on the island. The traditional fierce independence of the Vineyard towns, as one of those involved put it, with their own schools and health agents, makes this even more remarkable.

One important lesson from this experience relates to communication within the public health system: Do not assume that informal communication channels are either accurate or complete. For instance, despite best intentions across the board, however, there were a number of missed cues. MVH apparently believed that MVPHC was still planning a single islandwide pH1N1 clinic even after the focus had switched to the school-based plan. And as mentioned earlier, for instance, the hospital assumed that its obstetrics practice covered all pregnant women on the island. In addition, the complicated arrangement between Vineyard Pediatrics (owned by Dr. Goldfein but located at the hospital) and MVH (which employs Dr. Miller, who works with Vineyard Pediatrics) caused trouble when Vineyard Pediatrics received its own supply of vaccine. Parents were confused about whether their children should be immunized at school, at the hospital's preschool clinic, or by Vineyard Pediatrics (and whether it mattered whether they were Dr. Goldfein's or Dr. Miller's patient). Some officials and parents apparently assumed the effort to vaccinate children through Vineyard Pediatrics was coordinated with hospital, given Vineyard Pediatrics' location on hospital property, but the effort was separate and uncoordinated.

Many of these problems were the result of incomplete knowledge of the scope of the outbreak and who had received vaccine supplies, and the assumptions made about what others were planning to do with the vaccine they had. Despite the best efforts of the MVPHC and its informal connections to the hospital and many community health partners, communication and coordination within the local public health system located on the Vineyard did not always run smoothly. Throughout the fall, some of those involved felt that the hospital maintained a level of independence from the MVPHC. Town health agents, the VNA, the Wampanoag tribe, the schools, and public safety officers were generally represented at Coalition meetings, but a hospital representative was present less consistently. Some health agents and school representatives felt there was a one-way relationship with the hospital and the Coalition. For instance, Coalition members were frustrated when the hospital would ask the Coalition for information about the location and number of pH1N1 cases with which they came in contact, but would not provide information from their records to the Coalition. The hospital sometimes cited the Health Insurance Portability and Accountability Act Privacy Rule as a barrier to discussing the number and locations of cases of pH1N1 confirmed. One Coalition member thought the hospital was standoffish in general. In the future, it was suggested the Coalition should seek to include both MVH and Vineyard Pediatrics formally in their planning and response efforts. More generally, this experience highlights the need to build trust within the public health system.

In addition, this experience reflects MDPH's inability to recognize ad hoc regional public health systems formally, even if they were natural collaborations of existing relationships amongst colleagues at different organizations, such as the case on the Vineyard. For instance, Vineyard officials could have coordinated their efforts better if they knew how much and what kinds of vaccine were coming to the island. Although Ron MacLaren, Director, Wampanoag Health Service, became known as the voice of the Vineyard, the state health department was not able to report on the amount of vaccine that had been delivered to the island. Rather, the MDPH vaccine distribution system produced reports for the formally designated emergency preparedness regions only, such as the Cape and the Coalition.

Communication between the state and the Vineyard was complicated further by the nature of the vaccination registration process. Faced with an urgent need to increase the number of potential vaccinators rapidly, the MDPH chose to adapt an existing registration system designed for the federal Vaccines for Children program. The resulting ad hoc system did not account adequately for the diversity of the sites to which the vaccine was being distributed. Dealing with approximately 4,500 registered sites, it was difficult for the MDPH to know that the VNA had contracted to vaccinate children in the Vineyard schools rather than the elders that are typically served by visiting nursing associations. In addition, given that the hospital and Vineyard Pediatrics were also registered, it also may not have been clear that the VNA was responsible for all the island's school children because most Massachusetts towns registered individually. This became an issue when vaccine was in short supply and available in batches of 100. If the five towns had registered separately, they might have received one batch each, whereas the VNA received only one. It is ironic that the Coalition's effort to simplify the process by having the VNA register for the towns may have resulted in fewer doses being available.

Thus, another lesson from this experience is that more clarity is needed about the purpose of the registration process, and the implications for the amount of vaccine supplied to each registered site. Moreover, in the future, more detailed demographic information on the population served by the registered site should be collected from the point of registration.

Implications for Policy and Practice

To prepare for an anticipated second wave of the 2009 H1N1 pandemic during fall 2009, the MDPH began preparing for a large-scale immunization campaign, and other public health activities, in summer 2009. Responding effectively to this event required the involvement and participation of local health departments and boards of health, hospitals, clinics and other health-care providers, schools, and many other public- and private-sector public health partners across the Commonwealth. The number of vaccination sites and vaccinators were increased substantially, and communications with the public and with public health partners were enhanced. Eventually, more than 3.7 million doses of vaccine were delivered, immunizing 37% of the population and 51% of the initial target groups, exceeding national figures by a large margin. Contrary to planning assumptions, however, the distribution of pandemic vaccine to local health departments was slow and unpredictable, leading to a variety of challenges in a decentralized public health system.

Managing under Uncertainty

Before 2009, state and local public health systems throughout the Commonwealth had spent many years preparing for mass dispensing of vaccines or other countermeasures in public health emergencies. Consistent with such planning, and based on federal and state assurances in the summer and early fall that vaccine would be produced and delivered in large amounts starting in early October, the MDPH adopted a mass-dispensing approach to the 2009 H1N1 pandemic vaccination effort by increasing markedly the number of registered vaccination sites and trained vaccinators (Massachusetts Department of Health and Human Services, 2011a, 2011b). The number of registered vaccination sites was expanded, and record-keeping methods were developed to be streamlined as possible, as would be needed if vaccine was arriving in large amounts as expected. The reality, of course, is that vaccine did not arrive nearly as quickly or in as large numbers as had been promised, and demand waned after the perception developed that the crisis has passed. The simple registration database that had been developed, however, created difficulties in allocating vaccines to registered sites and tracking which populations were vaccinated. The ad hoc allocation process and tracking methods also made it difficult for local public health partners and other registered vaccinators to know when vaccine would arrive so they could plan and advertise clinics.

Because some future public health emergencies may be more like 2009 H1N1 pandemic acute events on which many planning assumptions are based, plans should be developed for situations that emerge over extended periods of time and are characterized by uncertainty. For instance, the Vineyard's decision to pool resources to constitute shooter teams and to vaccinate the children attending smaller schools first was easy to explain and well accepted by the public, and thus was an efficient, fair, and flexible response to uncertainty about when vaccine would arrive.

Although decision making under uncertainty is never easy, consultation with experts in logistics and supply chain management can help to plan for uncertainty. Management databases and tracking systems, for instance, might be developed in advance to improve the management of future responses.

Allowing for More Local Involvement in Decision Making and Program Management

In a decentralized public health system such as that in Massachusetts, local involvement in decision making and program management is essential. Many local health agencies, for instance, collaborated with hospitals and other providers in their jurisdictions and with schools to pool vaccine allocations and to ensure that it got to the population most in need. In addition, many towns collaborated with their neighbors in a variety of configurations throughout the state. These collaborations allowed small communities, for instance, to set up regional vaccine clinics and share personnel. Local involvement also included activities to coordinate activities more generally. In some areas, for instance, health agencies held conference calls immediately after the weekly statewide calls organized by the MDPH to be sure they understood what had been said, and to translate the recommendations into local actions.

There were, however, a number of challenges in this regard. As the Martha's Vineyard case demonstrates, for instance, limitations in the state's vaccine registration system meant that no one either at the MDPH or on the island had the information needed to coordinate local efforts to share vaccines or to ensure the available vaccine was going where it was needed most. This result is because the registration system did not include complete information on the population served by each registered site, nor did it provide any information on the number and types of vaccine that had been delivered to the Vineyard. The MDPH allowed for coalitions to register as a group for vaccination allocation, but many did not know this was allowed and that there was a form for this purpose.

Similarly, the BPHC collaborated with community health centers, which have existing relationships with vulnerable populations, as the primary venue for vaccine administration. To manage this, the BPHC developed a Web-based clinic staffing and scheduling calendar, from which information was uploaded automatically to a BPHC website where the public could view clinic scheduling information. Interfacing this with the MDPH's clinic scheduling calendar, which was developed later in the 2009 H1N1 pandemic, proved to be a challenge and required a lot of staff effort to translate information from one system to another.

Balancing Clear and Precise Policies with Flexible Implementation

In many ways, the 2009 H1N1 pandemic in Massachusetts illustrates the need for clear and precise policies. When the vaccine was in short supply, for instance, clear definitions of priority groups and tiers was essential to ensure the available supply went to those most in need. In some instances, clear priorities articulated by the CDC and the MDPH helped local health departments fend off political pressure to vaccinate local politicians and their families. On the other hand, lack of clarity about the definition of "healthcare worker" or the intended uses of vaccine allocated to hospitals caused problems. Some local officials were unsure, for instance, whether vaccine allocated to hospitals were for healthcare workers or patients, and whether it could be used for workers and/or patients who lived in other towns. The MDPH had no way to enforce its priorities, and inconsistencies at the local level led to perceptions of inequity.

At the same time, diversity in local public health structures throughout the Commonwealth, and differences between public and private vaccinators virtually require that policies be implemented flexibly, reflecting the local context and resources available. For instance, priorities were relatively easy to enforce in healthcare systems that alerted individual members of their need for vaccination and scheduled an appointment. On the other hand, in public and school-based clinics, some felt that turning away family members who did not meet the strict definitions of the priority groups would be counterproductive. Should opened batches of vaccine left over at the end of a school clinic be used for the EMS workers who helped with the clinic, even if they are not in the MDPH's first tier?

Some local health departments or large healthcare providers developed local policies based on their own analysis of the situation, others sought permission from the MDPH to alter policies to local needs, and others still did not feel they could deviate from state policies at all. When permission was sought, some reported the answer seemed to depend on which individual was asked.

Increasing the Transparency and Clarity of Communications

The allocation of vaccine to communities and registered vaccination sites during the pandemic was not determined by a formula or algorithm. Rather, the MDPH assessed the number of doses and formulation of each dose in the shipments received, and assigned doses to registered vaccination sites based on recipient population profiles based not only on which facilities had high percentages of constituents in priority groups, but also how many of the constituents could receive a particular vaccine formulation. In this way, the MDPH used its judgment to ensure allocation followed the epidemiology and was equitable. The benefit of this allocation method was its flexibility to respond to the constantly changing situation, tailoring shipments to meet the greatest need.

The downside of this approach was a lack of transparency. Sites compared the amounts of vaccine they received with the amounts received by neighboring providers and did not always understand why a particular site received more vaccine than they did, which resulted in confusion and, sometimes, resentment. The allocation process was addressed during the MDPH's weekly conference calls and in its blog, but only in generalities in order not to appear inconsistent. MDPH staff answered questions about allocation every day, and eventually local public health agencies were provided with a spreadsheet each week that tracked the allocation of vaccine to each provider in their jurisdiction. Although there was clearly a benefit in tailoring the response to the epidemiology and specific composition of daily vaccine shipments, the cost was a lack of transparency—and trust.

Beyond the issues of the vaccine allocation process, the case also illustrates the importance of not assuming that informal communication channels are either accurate or complete, potentially compromising situational awareness, which includes awareness of what one's partners are doing. For instance, the MVH believed that the MVPHC was still planning a single, islandwide pH1N1 clinic even after the focus had switched to a school-based plan. In addition, parents were confused about whether their children should be immunized at school, at the hospital's preschool clinic, or by Vineyard Pediatrics, and whether it mattered which doctor's patient they were.

Building Strong Partnerships

The pH1N1 experience provides many examples of how trusting relationships can enhance—and their absence impede—an effective public health emergency response. The PHEP "system" required to respond effectively includes the MDPH, local public health, school nurses, hospitals, educational institutions, EMS, long-term care providers, community health centers, community centers, colleges, and universities. For this system to work effectively, relationships must be facilitated between governmental agencies and nongovernmental agencies within a community and statewide.

Efforts to build relationships between public health and the schools, which started with including a school representative on the MDPH steering committee, were particularly successful in 2009. In many instances, pH1N1 was the first time school nurses had worked with local public health authorities. Some school nurses had been concerned about administering shots because they felt it might hurt their relationship with students, but in the end nurses were "heroes."

Trusting relationships are also central to the effectiveness of regional activities, as mentioned earlier in the discussion of "local" involvement in decision making and program management. For instance, the Vineyard experience illustrates the importance of encouraging and enhancing relationships among all the organizations connected with health, including school nurses, hospitals, and EMS. The Vineyard's approach to pooling resources in the form of vaccine and shooter teams that moved from the small to the larger schools as vaccine came available would not have been possible without everyone involved trusting that this was the most appropriate way to ensure the most populations were best protected.

Implications for Measuring and Assessing PHEP

What was said earlier about flexibility has implications for measuring and assessing PHEP. In particular, this case study demonstrates how the most effective way to implement a given capability—mass administration of a medical countermeasure (specifically, the pH1N1 vaccine)—depends on the local context. For instance, because children made up a large proportion of the target population, most communities found school-based clinics to be an effective way to administer the vaccine. Boston, on the other hand, found that its network of community health centers with established, trusted links to the populations they serve worked well. And a large group practice used its existing electronic medical record system effectively to call and set up appointments for patients on any given weekend for whom the available vaccine was appropriate. On the Vineyard and in other rural settings, small, local health departments found it useful to collaborate and pool resources to conduct regional clinics. Flexibility and ability to adapt were more important than local health departments having capacities that met a statewide or national standard for points of distribution (PODS).

This example also demonstrates the importance of a capability-based approach to measuring PHEP. What matters is how well a PHEP system can administer a countermeasure to the target population, not whether local health departments meet national capacity standards for, say, PODS. In 2009, the national capacity standard was the pH1N1 vaccine to children and other high-risk populations, but in future emergencies it could be another countermeasure and a different population. The 2009 experience shows the local public health system in Massachusetts had this capability, including the flexibility to adapt to local context and conditions. This positive experience is probably a better measure of the state's ability to respond effectively to future emergencies than capacity-based measures focusing on PODS standards.

Acknowledgments and Disclosures

This research was conducted with funding support awarded to the Harvard School of Public Health under cooperative agreements with the U.S. CDC (grant no. 5P01TP000307-01). The authors are grateful for comments from John Brownstein, Tamar Klaiman, John Kraemer, Larissa May, Christopher Nelson, Hilary Placzek, Ellen Whitney, Ying Zhang, the staff of the CDC Public Health Surveillance Program Office, and others who commented on presentations. The authors also thank the many staff members at Georgetown University who helped to collect the data used in this analysis.

References

Aledort, J. E., Lurie, N., Ricci, K. A., Dausey, D. J., Stern, S. (2006). Facilitated look-backs: a new quality improvement tool for management of routine annual and pandemic influenza. RAND. Accessed January 12, 2013, at http://www.rand.org/pubs/technical_reports/TR320.html.

Centers for Disease Control and Prevention (CDC). (2009a). H1N1 meeting the challenge: A new virus. Accessed on July 11, 2011 at http://www.flu.gov/timeline#event2

Centers for Disease Control and Prevention (CDC). (2009b). Vaccine against 2009 H1N1 Influenza Virus. Accessed on July 11, 2011 at http://www.cdc.gov/h1n1flu/vaccination/public/vaccination_qa_pub.htm#recommendations.

Hayden, E. W. (2006). Defragmenting public health. *The Boston Globe*, November 16, A19.Accessed May 19, 2010.

Higdon, M. A., Stoto, M. A. (2013a). Martha's Vineyard public health system responds to 2009 H1N1. *International Journal of Public Health*, 5(4), 356–371.

Higdon, M. A., Stoto, M. A. (2013b). The Martha's Vineyard public health system responds to 2009 H1N1. In: Weisfuse, I., Landesman, L., editors. *Preparing public health to respond to disaster: case studies.* Burlington, MA: Jones & Bartlett Learning, pp. 345–358.

Institute of Medicine (IOM). (2002). *The future of the public's health in the 21st century.* Washington, DC: National Academies Press.

Koh, H. K., Elqura, L. J., Judge, C. M., Stoto, M. A. (2008). Regionalization of local public health systems in the era of preparedness. *Annual Review of Public Health*, *29*, 205–218.

Massachusetts Department of Health and Human Services. (2011a). H1N1 (swine) flu. Accessed August 5, 2011, at http://www.mass.gov/?pageID=eohhs2onlineservices&L=7&L0=Home&L1=Provider&L2=Guidelines+and+Resources&L3=Guidelines+for+Services+%26+Planning&L4=Diseases+and+Conditions&L5=Influenza&L6=H1N1+%28Swine%29+Flu&f=H1N1+%28Swine%29+Flu_more&sid=Eeohhs2.

Massachusetts Department of Health and Human Services. (2011b). Guidelines for the vaccination of employees of licensed clinics, dialysis centers, hospitals and long term care facilities against seasonal influenza and pandemic influenza

H1N1. Accessed August 5, 2011, at http://www.mass.gov/Eeohhs2/docs/dph/quality/hcq_circular_letters/dhcq_0908521_attachment.pdf.

Massachusetts Department of Public Health. (2000). Census 2000 dataset. Mass CHIP v3.0 r319. Boston, MA: Massachusetts Department of Public Health.

Paulding, T. (2005). *Organizational structure for public health in Massachusetts.* Boston, MA: Massachusetts Public Health Association.

Salinsky, E. (2002). *Public health emergency preparedness: fundamentals of the "system."* Washington, DC: National Health Policy Forum, George Washington University.

Seid, M., Lotstein, D., Williams, V. L., Nelson, C., Lurie, N., Ricci, K. A., Diamant, A., Wasserman, J., Stern, S. (2006). Quality improvement: implications for public health preparedness. RAND. Accessed January 11, 2013, at http://www.rand.org/pubs/technical_reports/TR316.html.

Seccombe, M. (2009). Flu Hits High School Hard; - Clinic Nov. 11. Accessed November 11, 2009 at http://mvgazette.com/news/2009/11/05/flu-hits-high-school-hard-clinic-nov-11?k=vg542c1235d4bd1.

U.S. Census Bureau. (2010). State & county quick facts: Massachusetts. Accessed January 11, 2013, http://quickfacts.census.gov/qfd/states/25000.html.

Wasserman, J., Jacobson, P., Lurie, N., Nelson, C., Ricci, K. A., Shea, M. (2006). *Organizing state and local health departments for public health preparedness.* Santa Monica, CA: RAND Center for Domestic and International Health Security.

CHAPTER 9

The Italian Response to the 2009 H1N1 Pandemic

ELENA SAVOIA, PIERLUIGI MACINI, AND MARIA PIA FANTINI

Introduction

In 2009, the global spread of pH1N1 prompted countries worldwide to intensify their efforts to protect the population's health and to minimize the impact of the pandemic on society and the economy. Despite this common goal, considerable variability in health policies were observed around the world. This chapter analyzes the Italian public health system's infrastructure and organizational characteristics, and the policies implemented during the response to the 2009 H1N1 pandemic by using data obtained through semistructured interviews and a facilitated look-back activity. Italy and the United States faced similar challenges in the response to the pandemic, including difficulties in interpreting surveillance data, the late availability of the vaccine, and barriers in communication with the public in the midst of uncertainty regarding the evolution of the outbreak and media hype. However, the two countries differed in the way they addressed specific issues, mainly as a result of substantial differences in their organizational structure. This chapter analyzes the differences between Italy and the United States in the policies and procedures implemented to allocate vaccines, in the role and responsibilities of national and local public health agencies, and in the coordination of efforts between private and public providers. This chapter also aims to provide contextual information to enable readers to understand the reasons behind specific public health decisions and, eventually, compare them with decisions undertaken in the United States. This chapter begins with a brief description of the context and characteristics of the Italian public health system, including a brief introduction to its organization, a history of major healthcare reforms, and a description of the steps undertaken during the past 10 years by national and regional governments in the development of pandemic preparedness plans. This description is followed by an analysis of the challenges, strategies, and decisions made in the response to the pandemic.

Background

National Reforms and Regional Governance

In 1978, Law 833/1978 launched a thorough reform of Italy's healthcare system aimed at instituting a national health service with tax-based financing and an expansion of public services with the goal of providing universal, free access to health care to all Italian citizens. At that time, the law was also seen as an opportunity to reduce the geographic imbalance in the distribution of healthcare services between the North and South of the country and to promote integration of services across levels and categories of care. From an organizational point of view, this reform led (1) to the creation of local health units (LHUs), inspired by the United Kingdom's model of district health authorities in terms of their functions and jurisdictional area, and (2) to the creation of regional governments with responsibility for hospital planning, management, and distribution of resources across the LHUs.

Legislative Decrees 502/1992 and 517/1993, issued in 1992, launched the "Reform of the Reform," creating measures to devolve healthcare powers and financial accountability to regional governments. The 21 regional governments became responsible for the regulation of regional healthcare markets, the performance of LHUs and hospital trusts, and appointments of their chief executive officers.

It was not until 1997 to 2000, however, with Bassanini Law 59/1997 and Visco Decree 446/1997 that regional fiscal federalism was established, marking an important breakthrough toward regional financial autonomy and accountability. Regions were transferred full responsibility for providing healthcare coverage to their residents, and the 1998 to 2000 National Health Plan began to set guidelines toward defining what a "core healthcare benefit" package should consist of. Therefore, in the past decade the Italian national health service has been decentralized and the 21 Italian regions given responsibility for organizing and delivering health services within their territory, including providing the necessary actions to contain and mitigate the impact of large-scale public health emergencies such as not-so-infrequent earthquakes or infectious disease outbreaks.

The Emilia Romagna Region

Given the complexity of the Italian public health infrastructure and differences across regions, in this chapter we focus on the experience of one particular region: the Emilia Romagna region (ERR) in northeast Italy.

This region shares certain sociodemographic similarities with the state of Massachusetts, which is the subject of a case study in Chapter 8. The ERR has a population of 4.5 million residents, of which approximately 10% were born outside the country, and is a fairly wealthy region, with an individual average annual income of €14,000 per capita. The region is comprised of numerous cities with high-density populations, and has a healthcare network consisting of 3,144 primary care physicians, 61 hospitals, and 11 public health departments. Public health officials in this region are familiar with large and small-scale emergencies, and everyone can recall the August 2, 1980, terrorist attack at the Bologna train station that caused 85 deaths and injured 200 people; several moderate earthquakes that have hit the region during the past century; and seasonal extreme temperatures (heat waves) that affect the most vulnerable elderly on a yearly basis.

The ERR distinguishes itself by its cultural approach to prevention. In this region, there has been a historical emphasis on the development of a multidisciplinary and multisectorial public health system, which aims to integrate various types of public and private providers to address common population health problems. A tangible sign of this leadership role was shown by its government in the year 2000, when ERR authorities renamed the nine "prevention departments" located across the region to "departments of public health." The regional government assigned them the task of promoting, protecting, and improving the health, well-being, and quality of life of the population they serve, with actions that go beyond the provision of healthcare and preventive services and aim to engage the whole civil society. In doing so, regional public health leaders reaffirmed their belief that a multidisciplinary and multisectorial approach is the best and most reasonable strategy to reduce the social, economic, and environmental factors associated with disease incidence, unhealthy behaviors, and, most importantly, health inequalities.

Ten Years of Pandemic Planning

Since the emergence of the avian influenza threat in 1999, the Italian Ministry of Health (MOH), in collaboration with the Instituto Superiore di Sanità, initiated the development of an influenza pandemic plan. The first document, published in 2002 and titled *Italian Multiphase Plan for a Pandemic Influenza* (Gazzetta Ufficiale n°72, 2002), was updated in 2006 in accordance with the 2005 World Health Organization (WHO) recommendations (Centro Nazionale per la Prevenzione e il Controllo delle Malattie del Ministero della Salute, 2009). The 2006 plan aimed to improve surveillance, implement prevention and disease control measures, ensure medical care, develop surge plans, develop a training plan, develop appropriate communication strategies, and monitor the efficacy and efficiency of the interventions undertaken. Thereafter, regional governments developed their own regional pandemic preparedness plans, as did the LHUs within each region. During this process, very limited preparedness funds were allocated to public health emergency preparedness efforts, leaving no LHU's personnel fully dedicated to emergency preparedness activities.

In the ERR, a committee was created to develop the regional pandemic plan which included representatives from regional and local healthcare, social, and public health services. The plan was released July 2, 2007 (Bollettino Ufficiale

TABLE 9-1 Scenario at 15 Weeks in the Pandemic

	AGE, %			
VARIABLE	0–14 Y	15–64 Y	≥65 Y	TOTAL
Attack rate	45	23	20	25
Mortality	0.1	0.25	1.2	0.44
Expected hospitalized cases	0.2	1.3	3.7	1.5

Proportion of expected cases that required a primary care visit was 50%.

SOURCE: (2006). *Italian multiphase plan for a pandemic influenza. (Centro Nazionale per la Prevenzione e il Controllo delle Malattie del Ministero della Salute, 2009)*

Della Regione Emilia-Romagna, 2007), and the interventions included in response to a pandemic were based on the WHO pandemic phases and on potential scenarios reflecting the spread and severity of the outbreak. The scenarios were developed based on two scientific studies, which were the only ones available for the Italian context. The first study assessed the impact of a potential pandemic in terms of number of cases, deaths, hospital admissions, and access to the healthcare system using temporal data derived from the 2004 to 2005 flu season (Greco et al., 2006). The second study compared the potential impact of the pandemic in the presence and absence of specific interventions (Gruppo di Lavoro EPICO, 2006). Table 9-1, from the pandemic plan, summarizes the impact in the Italian context, assuming certain attack and mortality rates.

Methods

To gather data on the strengths and challenges of the Italian public health system response to the H1N1 pandemic, we partnered with the University of Bologna and used different types of techniques, including a literature review, interviews, and a facilitated look-back meeting.

A review of the literature found that the Italian scientific community has produced several works that describe the impact of specific interventions on the detection and control of the spread of the 2009 H1N1 pandemic. We reviewed these documents and relevant governmental materials, national and local pandemic plans, and local journals and TV news scripts released between April 2009 and July 2010.

Next, our colleagues from the University of Bologna interviewed public health officials within the ERR who assumed a leadership role during the response. An interview guide developed originally to assess the Massachusetts public health system's response to the 2009 H1N1 pandemic (see Chapter 8) was translated, adapted, and tested for its face and content validity in the

Italian language. This guide was then used to conduct nine interviews with representatives from the regional public health office and local public health departments, including two health department directors, a director of primary care, two infectious disease control program directors, a pharmaceutical coordinator, and a local director of communication and marketing. The interviews focused on the topics of surveillance systems, allocation and distribution of vaccine, communication with the public, and coordination across agencies. The interviews were performed by peers, recorded, and then transcribed by a team of public health students.

Subsequently, interview transcripts were analyzed, summarized, and used by the Harvard School of Public Health research team to develop a set of questions to guide the implementation of a facilitated look-back activity, which was conducted in April 2011 in Bologna. A facilitated look-back is an established method for examining public health system emergency response capabilities and for conducting a candid systems-level analysis. Through the use of a neutral facilitator and a no-fault approach, dimensions of decisions are probed, and nuances in past decision making are explored in detail in discussions with public health leaders, key staff, and a variety of community stakeholders involved with the response (Aledort et al., 2006). This activity included the participation of eight people: the director of public health services of the ERR, the regional director of infectious disease control programs, an LHU director of communication and marketing, and five representatives from local health departments. Look-back participants were asked to comment on what went well, what did not go well, and what could be improved during the response with regard to the three main topic areas described earlier. The activity was welcomed by the participating public officials, who contributed with their knowledge and exceptional analytical skills. They described the look-back technique as a great opportunity to analyze the decision-making process sustained during the response because of its structured and focused methodology.

Results

Very little is known about the impact of the 1918 Spanish influenza in Italy, which is mainly the result of significant military censorship during World War I aimed at avoiding the impact of "bad news" on the morale of both the troops and the civil population. The extent of the censorship was such that even the main national newspaper *Corriere della Sera* reported few articles regarding the pandemic. However, it is estimated that, in Italy, the 1918 flu caused 390,000 deaths with a death rate of 10.6 per 1,000 individuals, which (after Spain) was the highest reported across Europe. In Bologna, the capital of the ERR, public officials at the time attributed about 2,000 deaths to the flu. According to the interviewees, such historical records and more recent assumptions based on the potential attack rate of H5N1 avian influenza set the scenario and mind-set for the development of the 2003 national and 2006 regional pandemic plans.

When the first case of pH1N1 in Italy was reported on May 2, 2009 (Rizzo et al., 2010) (Table 9-2), Italian public health authorities and many colleagues around the globe referred to worst-case scenarios to elaborate containment strategies. In the ERR, the first case of pH1N1 was identified in July, and response efforts were put in place based on limited and difficult-to-interpret information about the case fatality rate from Mexico and the United States. What the Italian officials repeated frequently during the interviews and the facilitated look-back activity is that, "although past experience may help to understand new phenomena, history does not necessary repeat itself." They argued that data derived from the southern hemisphere during summer 2009, showing a mild clinical spectrum and an reproductive number (R_0) estimated by the Italian epidemiologists to be approximately 1.5, should have had more influence on the decision-making process than historical data on past pandemics or the initial data derived from Mexico.

Surveillance Systems

In Italy, as in other countries, several national and regional surveillance systems are used to monitor seasonal influenza cases. The national surveillance network, InfluNET, monitors data from the "sentinel physicians" system, which consists of a national network of approximately 1,000 primary care physicians and pediatricians in the 21 regions and autonomous provinces

TABLE 9-2 Timeline of Events in the ERR

DATE	EVENT
May 2	First pH1N1 case in Italy
May 25	First imported case in ERR
June 11	WHO pandemic level
July 3	First indigenous case in ERR
August 10	Development of a vaccination plan and modalities for hospital and homecare assistance
September 24	MOU between school district and public health commissioner on the operational plan in response to the pandemic
September 29	Change in surveillance approaches
October 1	Release of priority groups for vaccine distribution
October 13	Distribution of the first 13,000 doses
October 15	School absences monitoring
October 15	Start of regional vaccine campaign
October 16	Hygiene practices campaign
November 10	Creation of a regional website
Mid November	Start of a decrease in the number of cases

ERR, Emilia Romagna region; MOU, Memorandum of Understanding; WHO, World Health Organization.

(Ajelli et al., 2011). This system collects data on the incidence of influenza-like symptoms and, not long after the pandemic influenza alert was announced in April 2009, was expanded to begin collecting data earlier in the year than usual (Rizzo et al., 2010). At the regional level, FLUNET, a surveillance system implemented by the WHO for monitoring flu-related emergency department visits and hospital admissions, was also enhanced to increase the number of emergency departments being surveyed.

In addition to these national surveillance systems, the ERR used community-based pediatric services (CBPSs) to gather further surveillance data. The CBPSs are pediatric units established within the primary care sector and are providers of pediatric public health services to the community. These services work under the leadership of the primary care units within the LHU and are part of the healthcare system. The services, which are fully integrated within the school system, include routine children immunization practices. This is an example of the multisectorial approach described earlier, in which the integration of public health, health care, and the school sector are used to address children's health. To monitor school absences, a sample of 200 schools within the ERR was identified, and a single day of the week was selected to gather data. The CBPSs were in charge of collecting the data from the schools' administration offices and communicating them to the regional public health office for further analysis. According to the facilitated look-back participants, this type of monitoring system was seen as very cost-effective and something that worked particularly well because it relied on an existing system for reporting the number of children present in the school to manage meal services. The peak of school absences was consistent with hospital data on admissions and emergency department visits, demonstrating the reliability of this new surveillance system, compared with the others, and its potential use for future outbreaks.

The Distribution and Allocation of Vaccine

The interviewees and look-back participants reported that, during a pandemic, the question of who should be vaccinated is always challenging, with ethical and operational consequences. There was wide consensus that essential workers, including healthcare workers, should be protected, and that people at risk of severe disease should be a priority. However, whether or not healthy school children and adolescents should be a target, to limit spread in the community (see Chapter 4), was debated, and Italy did not embrace this category as a priority group. The priority groups were established by the MOH and were communicated to the regional public health authorities by decree. Regional governments are required by law to execute the decree and to follow national guidelines, so local public health officials have little or no ability to modify the priority groups to accommodate local needs. By law, any variation in the priority groups has to be discussed with the MOH, and the decree modified accordingly before allocating the vaccine. The role of the MOH, in this case, is very different from the one assumed by the Department of Health and Human Services in the United States, where the Centers for Disease Control and Prevention provides guidelines on the recommended priority groups to state and local officials, who have the authority determine whether those guidelines are appropriate to meet the needs of the population they serve.

During the early phase of pH1N1 pandemic, in the fall, the priority groups identified by the MOH were limited to "essential workers" in charge of maintaining the functioning of public services. These groups—healthcare personnel, law enforcement, public transportation workers, and so on—were established originally by the National Pandemic Preparedness Plan. However, as the pandemic evolved, several regional public health officers, including those representing the ERR, expressed concerns regarding the feasibility and medical consequences of this approach. The greatest concern was for patients affected by chronic diseases who had been actively calling the health departments to request the vaccine because of their greater risk of morbidity and mortality, and because typically they were the first to be vaccinated during the influenza season. Multiple discussions between the MOH and the regional public health officers during pandemic weekly meetings led to a change in the decree which added people with chronic diseases to the priority groups. At this point in time, public health agencies were charged with the allocation and distribution of the vaccine to the local providers based on the revised priority groups.

Ultimately, when the public interest in the vaccine waned, the vaccine was recommended for a greater number of people. However, as in other European countries, it was never recommended for everyone. In Italy, unlike in the United States, vaccines are only recommended for at-risk populations which would exclude, for example, children in good health.

In the ERR, the allocation of the vaccine to the healthcare providers was supported by current information systems used by healthcare providers to record medical data, transfer prescriptions, schedule appointments, and verify that patients are assigned to the correct "insurance status." Data are accessed at the regional level and entered by primary care physicians (PCPs), pediatricians, and hospital personnel on a daily basis.

As an example, providers use the system to verify the patient is exempt from copayments when affected by a chronic disease. The existence of this system allowed public health officials at the regional level to easily calculate the number of vaccines needed by each PCP for his or her patients with chronic disease and to generate a formula to allocate the vaccine based on such data. The vaccination of children was the responsibility of the CBPS.

Italy eventually reached an overall vaccine uptake rate of 4% of the population. The ERR reached 7%, the highest rate in the country. Although it is not clear why the ERR had such a high rate, the facilitated look-back participants argued that it could be attributed to the role of the CBPS and good communication and integration among regional and local services. However, rates of 4% to 7% are low compared with the target of 40% set by the MOH.

One of the major difficulties in the distribution of vaccine and, as a consequence, the overall low population uptake, was the lack of coordination between public health organizations and PCPs. Every Italian resident is allowed to choose a PCP independently of their insurance or income status, so PCPs are an important source of information regarding population needs, and are the best source of dissemination of public health measures. However, PCPs are private providers that work under a contract with the LHU; they are not employees of the national public health system. During the pandemic preparedness phase, PCPs were identified as the main providers in charge of administering vaccine because of their potential access to the majority of the population. However, they were not included in planning discussions at the level needed to ensure their participation. When the 2009 H1N1 pandemic occurred, they denied this role and public health officials had to negotiate with the PCPs' union to determine their role in the distribution of vaccine and compensation, which delayed the development of vaccine distribution plans. This was not an issue in this particular case because of the delay in the arrival of vaccine; but it could have caused serious delays in population uptake under different circumstances, such as a more severe outbreak.

Communication and Coordination among National, Regional, and Local Offices, and the Public

In some instances, the lack of evidence to support the recommendations provided by the MOH, and inconsistency in the messages being delivered by other national agencies, made it difficult for regional and local public health officers to communicate with the public effectively. The situation became more challenging when local public health officials were asked to execute decrees with which they disagreed. For example, the time interval recommended by the MOH between the inoculation of the two influenza vaccines, seasonal and pH1N1, was not supported by scientific evidence. This fact caused organizational issues in the distribution of vaccine and difficulties in explaining to the public why they needed to make two appointments rather than one. Another source of confusion was the MOH's recommendation not to vaccinate patients with autoimmune diseases, which occurred at the same time the MOH was suggesting the vaccination of patients with type I diabetes, which is a disease with an autoimmune mechanism.

Although inconsistency of messages from the national agencies was reported as an issue by many local health officers, they also said that when communication was handled at the regional level messages were consistent and no particular issues of miscommunication between regional and local agencies were recalled. The ERR pandemic preparedness plan had established that, during day-to-day operations, staff members of LHUs and local departments of public health work autonomously from the regional office. However, in the case of a crisis such as a pandemic in phases 4 to 6 on the WHO scale, the response becomes centralized, with regional officers in charge of the decision-making process and communication to the public. During the 2009 H1N1 pandemic, such centralization was made possible by strong preexisting relationships between regional and local agencies and mutual trust among their leaders, which allowed local perspectives to be integrated in the regional decision-making process.

The purpose of centralization was to shorten the time of the response and to maintain consistency and coherence in public communication efforts. This unified approach was perceived by the look-back participants as something that went particularly well, especially in light of the fact that, in Italy, the town administrator is designated by law to be the health authority, and public health agencies are to provide technical support to the town administration and other offices. For this reason, public health decisions need a formal vehicle to be executed, which is in the hands of nonpublic health officials. In this context, relationships across agencies and personal relationships among the people leading such agencies, are necessary to execute health policies and public health orders to integrate the technical guidance of public health agencies to protect the health of the population. As one of the interviewed public health officials reported, "the strength of the relationships between agencies and their officials is what makes the decision acts undertaken to be perceived as transparent." This statement emphasizes the importance of trust between individuals and agencies during a crisis, and how such trust allows public officials to work in a confident way within the reporting and incident command system in which they are operating.

Communication with the Public

The interviewees reported that another response challenge during the 2009 H1N1 pandemic was rumor control. The way in which the pandemic vaccines were licensed was one of the main reasons of concern and low compliance with vaccine uptake among healthcare workers. The pH1N1 vaccines were licensed by the European Medicine Agency, based on a mockup vaccine procedure, on the basis of clinical data supporting the safety and effectiveness of vaccines developed using the influenza A(H5N1) strain, which had been thought would cause the next pandemic. This approach made many healthcare workers uncomfortable about the vaccine's safety, and, as a result, the vaccination rate in this group was low (15%). Moreover, PCPs ended up not recommending the vaccine to their patients.

Another concern was the fact that the vaccine being distributed in Italy contained the adjuvant MF59-squalene, which had not been approved by the U.S. Food and Drug Administration. This inconsistency between the United State and Italy reinforced preexisting concerns among healthcare workers and parents about the safety of vaccines containing the specific adjuvant. The fact that the 2009 H1N1 vaccine was recommended to risk groups that differed from those included in seasonal vaccination (e.g., children and pregnant women rather than the elderly) also added to miscommunication and mistrust. On the other hand, nonpharmaceutical measures such as hand washing and cough etiquette were welcomed by the general population, and some data support an increase in the use of such good hygiene practices (Trivellin and

Gandini, 2011). Interviewees and look-back participants also pointed out how the media played a role in generating phobia during the early phase of the pandemic, and how public opinion and mistrust during a time of great political and economic difficulties in the country may have generated additional barriers in communication.

Implications for Policy and Practice

In this chapter we described the Italian response to the H1N1 pandemic, focusing on the ERR in northern Italy. This analysis is based on a series of interviews and a facilitated look-back activity with local- and regional-level public health officials. The methods we used were the same ones used in Massachusetts, as described in Chapter 8. Because of the similarity of the methods applied, we were able to gather information to analyze the Italian response in a comparative way, focusing on the impact the Italian context, including its public health infrastructure and regulations, had on policy implications. We were also able to identify common lessons learned that seem to be independent of country-specific contextual factors.

The first lesson from both countries' experience is the challenge of managing a crisis under conditions of uncertainty. For instance, the early estimates of the severity of the pandemic (as measured by the case fatality rate) ranged between the mildest possible pandemic envisaged in preparedness planning to a level of severity requiring highly stringent interventions (Fraser et al., 2009; Garske et al., 2009; President's Council of Advisors on Science and Technology, 2009; Secretarìa de Salud, Mexico, 2009; Wilson and Baker, 2009). Another form of uncertainty was whether the severity, drug-sensitivity, or other characteristics of the infection might change as the pandemic progressed or varied across countries. With such uncertainty and the historical precedent of a mild infection turning virulent in a matter of months, public officials in both countries ended up making an investment in vaccine procurement and other prevention activities regardless of the estimated severity of the disease (Lipsitch et al., 2011).

The second lesson is the need to balance clear and precise policies with flexible implementation, taking into account the local situation. For example, the two countries prioritized vaccinations in very different ways. Limited vaccine supplies create a tradeoff between vaccinating those at greatest risk (to provide direct protection) and those most likely to transmit the infection (herd immunity). In such circumstances, the key questions that policymakers need to address are: Who is at the greatest risk and how can they be readily identified? And, on the other side, who are the transmitters? ERR public health officials, similar to their colleagues across the country, decided to embrace the "direct protection" strategy. They could do this thanks to the current health information system and network of PCPs that allowed them access to the exact number of individuals in each healthcare provider affected by chronic conditions and, therefore, who were at greater risk of severe complications or death if infected. In the United States, public health agencies, during the allocation and distribution of the vaccines, had to rely on estimates provided by the healthcare providers, which were unreliable and inaccurate. Because of differences in the legal relationship between national, regional/state, and local health authorities, the U.S. guidance on priority groups was more flexible, and local agencies embraced the herd immunity strategy because it was more convenient logistically. Thus, comparing vaccine allocation strategies in the two countries suggests that access to accurate and reliable population data can have a great impact on policy implications and overall strategy in the response to an emergency. Vaccination coverage rates achieved in ERR (7%), however, were far less than those in Massachusetts (60%). In retrospect, we know that supplies of vaccine did not arrive in time to reduce transmission significantly, which makes the herd immunity strategy likely to be less effective than the direct protection one. This is an example of how data extrapolated from a specific context does not describe the effectiveness of an intervention. Taking into account the local situation and context is important, and should lead to a flexible implementation and interpretation of the results of local policies.

A third lesson from this analysis is that clear and consistent communication across agencies is important to sustain population trust in governmental institutions and to reduce the need for rumor control. Interestingly, the difference between the use of vaccine adjuvant in Italy and the United States was the source of the greatest concern in the population, reminding us that differences in policies and communication messages are noticed by the public. Such differences, especially when highlighted by the media, can generate a safety or equity argument.

The fourth lesson is the importance of generating trusting relationships between individuals and agencies. Trust contributes to transparency. Absence of preexisting relationships or clear definition of roles and responsibilities may undermine the execution of simple public health policies. Community involvement is needed to build trust in decision making and program management so that, when a crisis hits, such relationships generate a solid foundation for a more centralized response compared with daily routine activities. Especially in Italy, where regulations are strict and are applied by decree, the preexistence of trusting relationships is extremely important to generate the possibility of the feedback necessary from the local to the regional and national levels to improve the response while the emergency is still evolving.

Acknowledgments and Disclosures

This research was conducted with funding support awarded to the Harvard School of Public Health under cooperative agreements with the U.S. Centers for Disease Control and Prevention (grant no. 5P01TP000307-01). The authors acknowledge Drs. Alba Carola Finarelli and Maria Grazia Pascucci from the Servizio Sanità Pubblica, Assessorato Politiche per la Salute, Regione Emilia Romagna, for providing their expertise in the interpretation of facts and findings. The authors thank Drs. Cristiana Crevari, Maria Cristina Molinaroli, and Giuseppe Sergi from the Azienda Unità Sanitaria Locale of Piacenza, and those students of the Alma Mater Studiorum, Università di Bologna, Master II Livello in management dei servizi sanitari per le funzioni di direzione 2010 to 2011, for conducting the interviews. Last, the authors thank Dr. Valentina Di Gregori, resident in hygiene and preventive medicine, Alma Mater Studiorum, Università di Bologna, for her assistance in the coordination of the project, and Sarah Short from the Harvard School of Public Health for editing and providing comments on the chapter.

References

Ajelli, M., Merler, S., Pugliese, A., Rizzo, C. (2011) Model predictions and evaluation of possible control strategies for the 2009 A/H1N1v influenza pandemic in Italy. *Epidemiology and Infection, 139*(1), 68–79.

Aledort, J. E., Lurie, N., Ricci, K. A., Dausey, D. J., Stern, S. (2006). Facilitated look-backs: a new quality improvement tool for management of routine annual and pandemic influenza. Accessed March 3, 2013, at http://www.rand.org/pubs/technical_reports/TR320.html.

Bollettino Unfficiale Della Regione Emilia-Romagna. (2007). Piano regionale di preparazione e risposta a una pandemia influenzale. Accessed March 3, 2013, at http://www.h1n1registry.com/Portals/0/pandemia_Emilia-Romagna_07.pdf.

Centro Nazionale per la Prevenzione e il Controllo delle Malattie del Ministero della Salute. (2009). Piano nazionale di preparazione e risposta a una pandemia influenzale. Accessed March 3, 2013, at http://www.epicentro.iss.it/focus/flu_aviaria/pianopandemico.pdf.

Fraser, C., Donnelly, C. A., Cauchemez, S. (2009). Pandemic potential of a strain of influenza A (H1N1): early findings. *Science, 324*(5934), 1557–1561.

Garske, T., Legrand, J., Donnelly, C. A. (2009). Assessing the severity of the novel influenza A/H1N1 pandemic. *British Medical Journal, 339*, b2840.

Gazzetta ufficiale n°72 del 26-03-2002. Piano italiano multifase d'emergenza per una pandemia influenzale (2002) Accessed March 3, 2013, at http://www.gazzettaufficiale.it/atto/serie_generale/caricaDettaglioAtto/originario?atto.dataPubblicazioneGazzetta=2002-03-26&atto.codiceRedazionale=02A03262&elenco30giorni=false

Greco, D., Rizzuto, E., Paramatti, D. (2006). A possible scenario of pandemic influenza in Italy. *Igiene e Sanità Pubblica, 62*, 201–214.

Gruppo di Lavoro EPICO. (2006). Scenari di diffusione e controllo di una pandemia in Italia. Rapporti ISTISAN 06/33. Accessed March 30, 2013, at www.iss.it/binary/publ/cont/06-33.1165244461.pdf.

Lipsitch, M., Finelly, L., Hefferman, R. T., Leung, G. M., Redd, S. (2011). Improving the evidence base for decision making during a pandemic: the example of 2009 influenza A/H1N1. *Biosecurity and Bioterrorism*, 9(2), 89–115.

President's Council of Advisors on Science and Technology (PCAST). (2009). *Report to the president on U.S. preparations for 2009-H1N1 influenza.* Washington, DC: Executive Office of the President.

Rizzo, C., Rota, M. C., Bella, A., Giannitelli, S., De Santis, S., Nacca, G., Pompa, M. G., Vellucci, L., Salmaso, S., Declich, S. (2010). Response to the 2009 influenza A (H1H1) pandemic in Italy. *Eurosurveillance, 15*(49), 197–744.
Secreterìa de Salud, Mexico (2009). Defunciones, Descripcion preliminar. Accessed March 3, 2013, at portal.salud.gob.mx/descargas/pdf/influenza/graficas_defunciones060509.
Trivellin, V., Gandini, V., Nespoli, L. (2011). Low adherence to influenza vaccination campaigns: is the H1N1 virus pandemic to be blamed? *Italian Journal of Pediatrics, 37*, 54.
Wilson, N., Baker, M. G. (2009). The emerging influenza pandemic: estimating the case fatality ratio. *Eurosurveillance, 14*(26), 199–255.

CHAPTER 10

Local Health Department Vaccination Success during 2009 H1N1

TAMAR KLAIMAN, KATHERINE O'CONNELL, AND MICHAEL A. STOTO

Introduction

The 2009 pH1N1 vaccination campaign was the largest such effort in U.S. history. More than 75 million Americans, or close to 25% of the population, were vaccinated against the pH1N1 virus in late 2009 and early 2010 (Roos, 2010). The federal government was responsible for procuring vaccine from manufacturers, and state health departments received vaccine on a per-capita basis and delivered it to local health departments (LHDs) for administration to the public (Vinter et al., 2009). The Centers for Disease Control and Prevention (CDC) and the Advisory Committee on Immunization Practices identified key priority groups for early vaccination during limited supply and gave guidance on reaching out to the community. LHDs, however, were responsible for administering vaccines as they deemed appropriate, especially because the vaccine supply was limited.

Public health authorities used varied methods for distributing vaccine to the public, including mass vaccination clinics, school clinics, private providers, and pharmacies. In many ways, the public health system responded well to the challenge. In less than a year, for instance, a new 2009 pH1N1 vaccine was developed, produced, and delivered to 81 million people. From another perspective, however, the response had its limitations. For example, less than half the population was vaccinated and nearly half of the 162 million 2009 pH1N1 vaccine doses produced went unused (Association of State and Territorial Health Officials, 2010; Institute of Medicine, 2010; National Association of County and City Health Officials, 2010).

Because LHDs held primary responsibility for implementing public and school-based clinics, practices varied widely. Public clinics were often modeled after existing mass dispensing plans, whereas many school-based clinics had to be designed and implemented during the response. Because the national campaign was unique in its initial urgency, limited supply of vaccine, and high public demand, LHDs could not depend on previous experience or established "best practices" to decide how to administer vaccines to the public most efficiently. The high demand for vaccine during a time of uncertainty regarding vaccine delivery timing and quantity made this task especially challenging. As a result, there were extensive local differences in vaccination processes (Institute of Medicine, 2010), which suggests there is room for improvement in the quality of the response across locations (Association of State and Territorial Health Officials, 2010).

To date, no formal evaluations of approaches for local vaccine distribution have been reported. We implemented a positive deviance approach to identify and learn from LHDs that were successful in local vaccine distribution via public and school-based clinics. We used a realist evaluation perspective to conduct in-depth analyses of top performers to discern mechanisms for successful vaccine distribution practices in specific contexts.

Methods

Traditionally, emergency response evaluations (1) focus on individual response agencies, jurisdictions, or geographic regions that document their experiences in after-action reports (AARs) and (2) create a list of lessons learned to receive federal reimbursement funds. However, AARs are rarely probing enough to learn valid lessons from one location, let alone to make comparisons across locations. This chapter illustrates an approach to taking a more in-depth look at the 2009 pH1N1 public vaccination response to understand the nuances of what made some LHDs successful and to share those lessons with others with similar contexts.

Positive Deviance Approach

The positive deviance approach is a framework for identifying and learning from top performers. This approach was first used in public health to identify interventions designed around uncommon but beneficial health behaviors that some community members already practiced, and it has been used traditionally for individual-level behavior interventions (Marsh et al., 2004). The positive deviance framework also has been used to learn about effective practices in healthcare organizations (Bradley et al., 2009), community health programs (Marsh et al., 2004), and health intervention planning (Walker et al., 2007).

The positive deviance approach typically involves four key steps: (1) identification of positive deviants—those that perform consistently beyond expectations, (2) in-depth study of these units using qualitative methods to generate hypotheses or theories about practices that lead to success, (3) hypothesis testing in a statistically representative sample, and (4) working in partnership with key stakeholders to disseminate best practices (Bradley et al., 2009). Because objective performance measures to identify positive deviants are lacking, and the 2009 pH1N1 pandemic experience cannot be replicated, this analysis focused on step 2, using a rigorous qualitative approach, realist evaluation, to learn about best practices from high-performing LHDs that can be useful in similar contexts.

Realist Evaluation

Realist evaluation is an approach grounded in realist philosophy, which asserts that both the material and the social worlds are "real" and can have observable effects, and that it is possible to work toward a closer understanding of *how* an intervention causes change. This approach assumes that, rather than universally, programs "work" under different circumstances for different people or organizations. The realist perspective posits that interventions provide catalysts that change organizations' reasoning processes, their motivations, capacities, opportunities, and the like, to promote change. The "context" in which an organization operates (its resources, staff, funding, and so on) makes a difference in the outcomes it achieves. Different contexts might enable or prevent certain "mechanisms" from being triggered. Thus, there is always an interaction between context and mechanisms that influences outcomes, represented as: Context + Mechanisms = Outcomes, or C + M = O.

Rather than simply asking *whether* a program works, realist evaluation seeks to understand *how* context and program mechanisms interact so findings can be generalized to similar situations. Program mechanisms, rather than specific interventions, trigger change (Pawson, 2002). Our C + M = O approach allowed us to learn about which contexts triggered specific mechanisms that, when combined, led to good outcomes. Positive deviance and realist evaluation offer an organized way to learn from the experience of frontline public health professionals during a challenging time. We identified LHDs deemed by their peers to have done well in one or more of the process map areas noted in Figure 10-1, rather than focusing on vaccination coverage rates alone. We used a systematic approach (the process map) to guide interviews about what happened, what (in their professional opinion) seemed to work well, and what problems arose. Last, we analyzed data qualitatively to identify combinations of C + M that led to good outcomes (O), so LHDs can learn from their peers in a way that takes into account their individual contexts.

Identifying Positive Deviants

Initially, we reviewed the National Association of County and City Health Officials (NACCHO) Model Practices Database for model health departments in the areas of emergency preparedness and/or vaccination. The Model Practices Database is an online searchable collection of innovative best

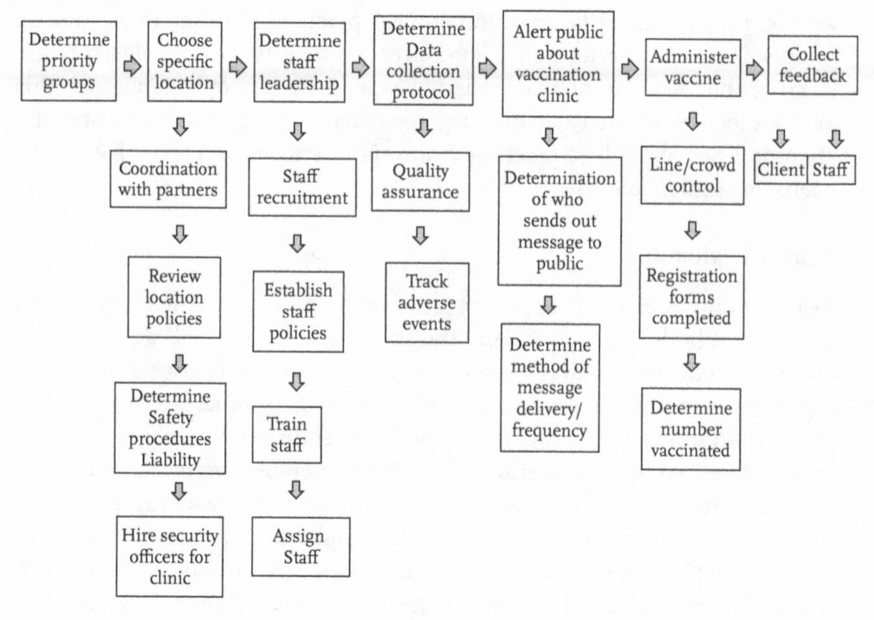

FIGURE 10-1 Public distribution. Public Health Emergency Preparedness.

practices across public health areas. Health departments self-select to share their experiences with NACCHO, and if their work is deemed to be a promising or model practice after review by NACCHO, it is entered into the online database. We searched the NACCHO database for all 2009 submissions for model or promising practices (n = 55). We included only those submissions focused on emergency preparedness, immunization, and/or infectious diseases, of which there were 18.

We reviewed a sample of state and local AARs that were compiled from practice partners through the Harvard Preparedness and Emergency Response Research Center, attendance at the NACCHO Emergency Preparedness Summit, and recommendations from LHDs. We reviewed 10 state and local AARs. We also reviewed more than 100 published reports, mass media reports, and other relevant documents (Institute of Medicine, 2010).

Working with local emergency preparedness and response public health partners, we developed an initial list of high-performing LHDs in the 2009 pH1N1 vaccination campaign (n = 35). We used a snowball sampling method in which we asked LHD staff to recommend peers who they believed performed well in the distribution of pH1N1 vaccine from the perspective of our process map. Our interest was in a purposive sample of high-performing LHDs, rather than a representative sample of all LHDs. We selected LHDs to ensure those with varying contexts (size, demographics, geography) were represented in the analysis.

Learning from Positive Deviants

After reviewing LHD vaccination processes from across the country, we created process maps to define the key activities LHDs conducted during public and school-based vaccination clinics to develop an "observational grid" that identified key activities on which to focus, and we used them as the basis for in-depth interviews of staff from positive deviant LHDs. We circulated the process maps to members of the Harvard CDC-funded Preparedness and Emergency Response Research Center Advisory Board and to principle investigators to validate the list and narrow down the most important focus areas.

We concentrated on activities conducted in public vaccination clinics and school-based clinics because they were the most common approaches, and they were the methods for vaccine distribution that were most dependent on local public health system infrastructures, unlike the use of pharmacies or private providers for vaccine distribution. Figure 10-1 notes the key areas that each LHD had to consider when setting up its public and school-based vaccination clinics.

We conducted in-depth interviews with health department officials from 20 LHDs defined as high performers based on the process maps and peer recommendations who agreed to be interviewed. We used a semistructured interview protocol in which we asked questions about each of the key process domains. The lead author (T. K.) conducted the interviews, and a research assistant (K. O.) assisted in taking notes during each of the interview calls. Notes were compiled and typed within 24 hours of each call. At the completion of all the interviews, we organized the data by process map domain areas to look for consistency and patterns that suggested C + M = O stories. Some health departments did not address specific domains, but focused on the areas in which they felt they performed best.

Thomas Jefferson University's Institutional Review Board ruled this project exempt.

Results

The 20 LHDs chosen for in-depth analysis represented a variety of geographic locations across the contiguous United States. The LHDs served populations in urban, suburban, and rural communities in Washington, Texas, California, Illinois, Pennsylvania, New York, Massachusetts, Louisiana, and Kansas. There were five LHDs in communities with less than 100,000 people, six with populations between 100,000 and 500,000, four with between 500,000 people and one million people, and five serving communities with more than one million residents. The number of employees working in LHDs during the vaccination campaign ranged from as few as two to more than 1,800 full-time employees.

Of the 20 LHDs studied, eight held both public and school vaccination clinics, five held public clinics only, and five held school clinics only. One LHD held public clinics and contracted with pharmacists to administer vaccine, whereas one LHD held public clinics and distributed vaccine to primary care providers to administer as well.

Boxes 10-1 and 10-2 note specific examples of the C + M = O stories we discovered in our interviews. For example, we discovered that small, rural LHDs depended on informal relationships with school administrators and nurses, whereas larger, more urban LHDs used more formal relationships. This is a reflection of the local community in which the school nurse may be the neighbor or fellow community group member of the local emergency planner. Personal relationships allow for less formality in partnerships,

Box 10-1 SELECT CONTEXT + MECHANISM = OUTCOMES STORIES FOR PUBLIC CLINICS

Defining Priority Groups

- Local vulnerable populations + Access to vulnerable populations (through shelters, nursing homes, etc.) = Greater vaccination rates among underserved
- Small local health department (LHD) + Large Orthodox Jewish community + Sunday clinics = Jewish attendance at clinic
- Limited English-speaking community + Materials in multiple languages = Greater immigrant vaccination rates

Communicating with the Public

- Public questions/concerns + LHD hotline + Website = Informed public
- Public questions about clinics + Social media (e.g., Facebook, Twitter) = Informed public
- LHD need to advertise + Multiple media outlets (TV, newspaper, website, radio, religious institutions) = Reaching the public
- Rural LHD + Flashing road sign borrowed from police = Public notification about clinic
- Reverse 911 system + Clinic information = Public notification about clinic

Staffing

- Small LHD + Large population + Trained Medical Reserve Corps (MRC) = clinic staff
- Large population + Trained MRC = Clinic staff
- Numerous clinics + Local health professions (schools) = Clinic staff
- Small LHD + Public health emergency response funds = Contract nursing staff for clinics
- Small LHD + Local health professions (students) + Clinic training added to school curriculum = Well-trained clinic staff

Community Partnerships

- Community venues + Existing memoranda of understanding (MOU) = Clinic location
- Large turnout expected + Relationship with large venue = Clinic location
- Many local churches + Meeting with clergy = Coordination with local partners and greater vaccination rate
- Rural community + Close relationship with venue security = Clinic security staff
- Large LHD + Formal MOU with local police = Clinic security
- Local police engagement in LHD activities + Traffic direction = Clinic safety

Flexibility

- High demand for vaccine + Large community event (e.g., county fair) = High vaccination rate
- Multiservice LHD + Weekend clinics = Minimal service interruptions
- Small LHD + Limited budget + Completed registration forms = Reimbursement from insurance companies for those vaccinated who were privately insured
- Emergency declaration + Access to additional resources = More effective vaccination campaign

Box 10-2 SELECT CONTEXT + MECHANISM = OUTCOMES STORIES FOR SCHOOL-BASED CLINICS

Defining Priority Groups

- Local vulnerable populations + Access to vulnerable populations (through shelters, nursing homes, and so on) = Greater vaccination rates among underserved
- Small local health departments (LHDs) + Large Orthodox Jewish community + Sunday clinics = Jewish attendance at clinic
- Limited English-speaking community + Materials in multiple languages = Greater immigrant vaccination rates

Communicating with the Public

- Public questions/concerns + LHD hotline + Website = Informed public
- Public questions about clinics + Social media (e.g., Facebook, Twitter) = Informed public
- LHDs need to advertise + Multiple media outlets (TV, newspaper, website, radio, religious institutions) = Reaching the public
- Rural LHD + Flashing road sign borrowed from police = Public notification about clinic
- Reverse 911 system + Clinic information = Public notification about clinic

Staffing

- Small LHD + Large population + Trained Medical Reserve Corps (MRC) = Clinic staff
- Large population + Trained MRC = Clinic staff
- Numerous clinics + Local health professions (schools) = Clinic staff
- Small LHD + Public health emergency response funds = Contract nursing staff for clinics
- Small LHD + Local health professions (students) + Clinic training added to school curriculum = Well-trained clinic staff

Community Partnerships

- Community venues + Existing memoranda of understanding (MOU) = Clinic location
- Large turnout expected + Relationship with large venue = Clinic location
- Many local churches + Meeting with clergy = Coordination with local partners and greater vaccination rate
- Rural community + Close relationship with venue security = Clinic security staff
- Large LHD + Formal MOU with local police = Clinic security
- Local police engagement in LHD activities + Traffic direction = Clinic safety

Flexibility

- High demand for vaccine + Large community event (e.g., county fair) = High vaccination rate
- Multiservice LHD + Weekend clinics = Minimal service interruptions
- Small LHD + Limited budget + Completed registration forms = Reimbursement from insurance companies for those vaccinated who were privately insured
- Emergency declaration + Access to additional resources = More effective vaccination campaign

whereas formal relationships may solidify partnerships that would not exist otherwise. In rural communities, a neighbor may also be the local police chief who has a child in the same school. Large, urban LHDs may require formal memoranda of understanding because organizational staff do not know each other.

Public Clinics

Defining Priority Groups

Given the uncertainty of vaccine supplies, all the LHDs we interviewed felt one of the keys to success was defining the priority groups clearly before implementing public clinics. Some LHDs interpreted the CDC priority group recommendations strictly, which made no distinctions among large numbers of people, whereas others decided to address the community members they felt were most vulnerable. Success in reaching priority groups required access to vulnerable populations, which depended on strong, previously established partnerships with community organizations. Approximately half the successful LHDs held separate clinics for particularly vulnerable populations, such as individuals with cognitive or physical disabilities, the uninsured, the homeless, and senior citizens. These special clinics were usually held at municipal buildings or buildings that were familiar to the population (e.g., shelters, long-term care facilities, senior centers).

Communicating with the Public

Most of the LHDs we interviewed established a call center early during the pandemic to give information to the public about pH1N1 and vaccinations. Smaller LHDs depended on volunteers to staff the call centers; larger LHDs sometimes used staff and volunteers. Larger LHDs with more financial resources were able to have longer call center hours than smaller LHDs. A number of LHDs used social media sites such as Facebook and Twitter to disseminate information to the public. As evidenced by the number of people who attended vaccination clinics, particularly during the early days of the pandemic, the majority of LHDs felt their dissemination efforts were quite effective.

Staffing

Successful LHDs had various ways of ensuring sufficient numbers of trained staff for public clinics. All 20 LHDs used the Incident Command System, an all-hazards emergency management approach used to organize leadership roles during a response to define leadership positions in the public clinics. All but one LHD was located in an area where a state of emergency had been declared, and most interviewees felt the state and federal resources activated by the emergency declaration made it easier to function and complete the necessary tasks.

Three of the LHDs collaborated with nursing and pharmacy schools in the area, and used the students as volunteers to administer the immunizations as an educational activity. In one community that used volunteer students from professional schools as vaccinators, the LHD was able to incorporate just-in-time training into the students' curriculum before the clinic opened.

Some larger LHDs used public health emergency response (PHER) funds to hire temporary staff for data entry and quality assurance. Hired staff reviewed completed forms, followed up whenever possible with individuals who had missing data, and double-checked data being entered into electronic systems. Smaller LHDs depended on volunteers or LHD staff to do the same, but this was challenging given the many different tasks that required completion during the vaccination response effort.

Smaller LHDs and those serving a large population often depended on contract nurses, paid for by federal H1N1 PHER funds, to supplement volunteers or when volunteers were unavailable. LHDs also used PHER funds to pay for staff overtime. Each of the eight LHDs that used public vaccination clinics only to administer vaccine reported they would not have been able to afford the overtime or been able to hire contract nurses without these funds.

One large LHD with a sophisticated information technology system assigned clinic volunteers and staff based on clinic distance and areas of interest/expertise. To reduce LHD service interruptions, one jurisdiction held public clinics on weekends only. Although this strategy allowed the community easier access to vaccine, it did create a stressful situation for LHD employees, who had to work overtime.

Community Partnerships

Community partners were vital in lending support to LHDs in areas such as safety and line control, vaccine administration, space donation, and help to set up and take down the clinics. LHDs that had existing relationships with community partners had fewer challenges getting stakeholders to agree on priorities, and had more streamlined clinic planning processes. In the majority of the communities we interviewed, partners included schools and law enforcement, and local emergency medical technicians. LHDs leveraged their relationships with other local public agencies for clinic locations, security, and administrative support.

For example, one small, rural LHD worked with a local large employer to hold clinics at the centrally located business office. Employees and their families received vaccine, and onsite security oversaw clinic safety. Another community held its annual fall community fair during the time frame of the HINI vaccination campaign and reached a large number of residents in a short amount of time. One LHD in a rural community worked with local law enforcement to set up flashing road signs on the busiest streets in its town to notify residents about the location and time of the vaccination clinics.

Flexibility

The LHD staff we interviewed felt that flexibility in decision making, staffing, and clinic implementation early during the vaccination campaign helped them to be successful. LHDs used situational awareness to build from existing plans, but altered them as needed. LHDs had to implement new staff training, recruit new staff and volunteers, and establish new policies while they were responding to an emergency. The LHDs we interviewed maintained flexibility throughout the response as information and resources changed.

School-Based Clinics

Relationship with Local School Authorities

Initially, LHDs had to choose the schools where they would hold clinics for local children. Some chose to hold clinics at all schools in a local district;

others chose key, centrally located schools. Many of the successful LHDs that we interviewed had previously established relationships with the school districts in their jurisdiction, making the vaccination location decision clear. Some LHDs previously held mass vaccination drills or seasonal flu clinics in local schools, so the clinic setup and implementation had already been practiced. Most successful LHDs had worked with school officials during the emergency preparedness planning process. Small, rural LHDs often had fewer locations to visit, but sometimes had more children to vaccinate in each location. Small, rural LHDs also had more informal relationships with school officials whereas large, urban LHDs often had formalized agreements with school officials for clinic implementation.

School nurses served a vital role in the relationship between LHDs and local schools. The school nurses helped with the planning and organization of the clinics, and acted as liaisons between the LHDs and the schools. In some locations, school nurses were employees of the LHD, which solidified the relationship between the schools and the LHD. In other locations, the LHD had to work closely with nonemployee school nurses to coordinate the clinics, and some had to convince school nurses initially that school-based vaccination would be an effective and feasible way to reach children.

Most LHDs held regular conference calls with school nurses and administrators once or twice per week, especially during the early days of the pandemic response, when LHDs did not know when they would receive vaccine. Global buy-in of the school system, intensive planning, constant communication, and trusting relationships between health department staff and the school districts were vital to the success of the school vaccination campaign.

LHDs had to plan carefully when timing school-based vaccination clinics. Most school districts we interviewed allowed the LHD to hold clinics during the day, while school was in session, to vaccinate as many children as possible. LHDs typically visited each public school in the district—elementary through high school and preschools. Some LHDs, particularly those in smaller communities, also offered vaccinations to private and parochial schools. Some schools were uncomfortable holding vaccination clinics during the day because of class disruptions or because school administrators wanted parents to be present. When that was the case, clinics were held after school or in the evening so parents could be present. The placement and timing of the clinic was dependent primarily on what the school district felt was the least disruptive to classroom activities.

Communicating Effectively with Parents

LHDs had to work closely with schools to decide whether parents would be required to attend vaccination clinics. As noted earlier, some schools decided to hold clinics outside normal school hours to ensure parental participation. Regardless of parental attendance, all children in school-based clinics had to submit permission slips to receive the vaccine. Most LHDs depended on schools to distribute and collect permission slips. Smaller schools in which the school nurse knew most of the children and parents seemed to have more returned slips than those schools in which the nurse did not know most of the children.

Schools used a variety of mechanisms for distributing forms and communicating with parents about vaccinations. Schools that had active listservs used those to reach out to parents. Other schools used the school's website, whereas some sent paper slips home with children. Some large school districts used an automated phone system to notify parents about the clinics. LHDs found that using media outlets such as newspaper, radio, and local television stations, and sending notes out to parents also proved to be an effective way to communicate. Schools that reached out directly to parents received more feedback than those who sent slips home with children without following up with another form of communication.

Ensuring Clinic Logistics

LHDs that held clinics during the school day used primarily LHD staff to run the clinics. Medical Reserve Corps and other volunteers often worked other jobs during the day, and many could not attend daytime clinics. Medical Reserve Corps volunteers were used in the after-hours clinics, and some were able to help with the in-school clinics as well. Because of security concerns, however, only volunteers who had submitted to background checks were allowed in many of the schools. Most LHDs we interviewed did not have the staff available to conduct background checks on new volunteers in addition to planning for the clinics and training existing staff.

Training was challenging in school-based clinics. LHDs, for instance, had to educate first responders and teachers about vaccination priority groups, and often had to explain why children were receiving vaccine first. Some successful LHDs held just-in-time training to ensure all staff and volunteers received the same training. This was a challenge in large LHDs that held multiple, school-based vaccination clinics. In such situations, debriefing sessions at the end of each week helped vaccinators fine-tune their processes based on feedback from others, implementing an informal plan–do–study–act cycle.

For the most part, school nurses were responsible for data collection and management. Students handed in vaccine registration forms to their schools, and school nurses collected and aggregated the data. School nurses were also responsible for ensuring each child who received vaccine had a permission slip. School nurses submitted data from the forms to the LHD or to the state vaccine tracking system directly. In larger communities where the LHD had the capacity to do so, LHD staff or volunteers entered data into the state tracking system. One particular LHD in a midsize community color-coded the forms to keep track of them. This system reduced confusion when entering the data into the state system, and it also helped to prevent medication errors from occurring, because data regarding how many shots students received was entered and searchable.

School nurses reviewed each form to make sure information was correct before the child received vaccine. In some instances, the nurse had to call a parent or guardian to verify information on the form. Some LHDs were able to use electronic databases to store the information, and they did not need to store the forms physically. However, the majority of LHDs that participated in school-based clinics, regardless of population size, kept a physical copy of the form. Many LHDs do not have the financial resources to invest in scanning systems or other databases to house this information. Entering the data manually is very time intensive, and many LHDs had to hire extra staff to complete this process. It took one LHD nine months to enter all the children's forms. Because it took so long for most LHDs to enter the information about those vaccinated, they resorted to counting the forms to determine how many children were vaccinated at each clinic, thus undermining the value of the system for providing real-time tracking information.

Some children had to receive two doses of the vaccine, and many LHDs and schools found it challenging to track whether students had received their second dose. Some LHDs with enough staff and vaccine went back to schools a second time and provided the second dose to students, whereas others sent information to parents about where children could receive a second dose, and put the onus on them to ensure their child was immunized.

LHD staff worked with school administrators to set up clinics in a way that ensured rapid flow, accurate data collection and quality controls, and calm children. In most clinics, qualified LHD staff and nurses vaccinated the children, and many broke into teams with two vaccinators per team. At larger schools, the school nurses also vaccinated children, especially if the LHD was relatively small or understaffed. One LHD was able to vaccinate a school district by visiting each of their 21 buildings in a matter of three and a half weeks. Vaccination in other locations sometimes took longer because of scheduling concerns, regardless of whether parents would be in attendance and whether the clinic would be held during school hours or after school.

Teachers aided in controlling the flow of the students, and most schools opted to bring classes to the clinic one at a time to reduce possible issues. Two schools gave snacks to the children after they received the vaccine as a way to keep them calm. Schools that separated the vaccinators from the entrance of the vaccination room experienced success at keeping children calm who were waiting in line. Children who saw others being vaccinated tended to have more anxiety about receiving a vaccine.

Limitations

This study has a number of limitations. Given its retrospective nature, our interviews depended on the memories of interviewees, which may be inaccurate. However, retrospective analysis does allow for consideration of why things went particularly well (or poorly). Because this project focused on successful activities, the retrospective interviews likely yielded more information than interviews would have if they were conducted during the response.

In addition, although the 2009 pH1N1 pandemic will not be repeated in exactly the same way and LHDs differ, we cannot test our hypotheses in a statistically representative sample (step 3 of the positive deviance methodology). Rather, the realist evaluation perspective has helped to identify what may work in particular contexts in the future.

Our project focus was on identifying and learning from positive deviants, rather than comparing their experience with the LHDs that did poorly. This approach is innovative because it focuses on learning from those who did well, rather than learning what *not* to do. In addition, defining LHDs that did poorly is a challenge, because peers are unlikely to tell researchers who did not do well. LHDs that did poorly are also less likely to share their experience than those that did well.

The experience of successful LHDs outlined here can assist others in implementing successful public vaccination clinics in the future. This work can be integrated into future vaccine distribution policies currently being debated. The lessons learned can be applied to both large and small immunization clinics because the mechanisms for success can be scaled to the appropriate circumstances. Our findings show that context triggers specific mechanisms that lead to good outcomes. Often, these activities required minimal financial commitment from LHDs and augmented regular LHD activities by increasing community buy-in and partnerships, thereby making a more resilient community. We focused on successful LHDs, but all the staff we interviewed felt strongly that they wanted to share the lessons they learned throughout the 2009 pH1N1 vaccination campaign process to improve responses in the future.

Implications for Policy and Practice

The U.S. public health system allows for great local autonomy in practice with oversight from state and federal authorities. The benefits of local control are that context can be considered when planning public health interventions, and based on our findings we know that local context makes a difference in how interventions are designed and how they work. Rather than a one-size-fits-all approach, LHDs can reach their constituents as they see fit. However, the challenge with such a system is that there is a limited evidence base for what works, when it works, and how it works. We know that school-based vaccination leads to greater vaccination rates in children (Bednarczyk et al., 2013; Cawley et al., 2010; King et al., 2005; Kwong et al., 2010; Piedra, 2013) and that the 2009 pH1N1 school vaccination campaign delivered vaccines at lower cost per dose than public clinics (Kansagra et al., 2012), but there is a limited evidence base of effective, replicable practices for distributing vaccine in schools, especially during emergencies. Lessons learned from a large LHD in a major city may not apply to a rural community. Our research shows how context and mechanisms interact, leading to better (or worse) outcomes. The key is understanding what works, when, and for whom.

In this context, our positive deviance/realist evaluation approach allowed us to learn from successful LHDs during the public and school-based vaccination processes in response to the 2009 H1N1 pandemic. There is great variation in the size, structure, and function of LHDs, and in the practices they used to administer pandemic vaccine. The goal of this project was to understand how LHD context triggered specific mechanisms that led to good outcomes so similar LHDs can learn from peers. As noted in Box 10-1 and Box 10-2, LHDs addressed the challenges they faced creatively, given their specific circumstances.

Conclusion

Local health departments faced many challenges during the pH1N1 response, not least of which was getting vaccine to the public on a very large scale. Many LHDs were successful in reaching the public by building on their existing strengths, and capitalizing on plans and partnerships that were already in place. School-based clinics were especially successful in communities with school nurses and administrators who had an existing relationship with the LHD. There is evidence that parents will consent to school-based vaccination (Brown et al., 2014; Herbert et al., 2013; Middleman and Tung, 2010; Middleman et al., 2012), making it an ideal mechanism for getting vaccine to children in future public health emergencies. Learning from exemplary LHDs can help all public health systems in the future.

Acknowledgments and Disclosures

This research was conducted with funding support awarded to the Harvard School of Public Health under cooperative agreements with the U.S. CDC (grant no. 5P01TP000307-01). The authors are grateful for comments from John Brownstein, Melissa Higdon, John Kraemer, Larissa May, Christopher Nelson, Hilary Placzek, Ellen Whitney, Ying Zhang, the staff of the CDC Public Health Surveillance Program Office, and others who commented on presentations. They also thank the many staff members at Georgetown University who helped to collect the data used in this analysis.

References

Association of State and Territorial Health Officials. (2010). Assessing policy barriers to effective public health response in the 2009 H1N1 influenza pandemic. Accessed April 2, 2012, at http://www.astho.org/Display/AssetDisplay.aspx?id=4933.

Baty, S. A., Aurimar, A., Odish, M., Cadwell, B. L., Schumacher, M., & Sunenshine, R. H. (2013). Factors associated with receipt of 2009 pandemic influenza A (H1N1) monovalent and seasonal influenza vaccination among school-aged children: Maricopa County, Arizona, 2009–2010 influenza season. *Journal of Public Health Management and Practice, 19*(5), 436–443.

Bednarczyk, R., Duvall, S., Meldrum, M., Flynn, M., Santilli, L., Easton, D., Birkhead, G. (2013). Evaluating the most effective distribution strategies to assure administration of pandemic H1N1 influenza vaccine to New York state children and adolescents: evaluation using the New York state immunization information system. *Journal of Public Health Management and Practice, 16*(6), 589–597.

Bradley, E. H., Crurry, L. A., Ramanadhan, S., Rowe, L., Nembhard, I. M., & Krumholz, H. M. (2009). Research in action: Using positive deviance to improve quality of health care. *Implementation Science, 4*, 25.

Brown, D. S., Arnold, S. E., Asay, G., Lorick, S. A., Cho, B. H., Basurto-Davila, R., & Messonnier, M. L. (2014). Parent attitudes about school-located influenza vaccination clinics. *Vaccine, 32*(9), 1043–1048.

Cawley, J., Hull, H. F., Rousculp, M. D. (2010). Strategies for implementing school-located influenza vaccination of children: a systematic literature review. *Journal of School Health, 80*(4), 167–175.

Herbert, N. S., Gargano, L. M., Painter, J. E., Sales, J. M., Morfaw, C., Murray, D., Hughes, J. M. (2013). Understanding reasons for participating in a school-based influenza vaccination program and decision-making dynamics among adolescents and parents. *Health Education Research, 28*(4), 663–672.

Institute of Medicine. (2010). The 2009 H1N1 influenza vaccination campaign: summary of a workshop series. Accessed March 11, 2012, at http://iom.edu/Reports/2010/The-2009-H1N1-Influenza-Vaccination-Campaign.aspx.

Kansagra, S. M., McGinty, M. D., Morgenthau, B. M., Marquez, M. L., Roselli-Fraschilla, A., Zucker, J. R., Farley, T. A. (2012). Cost comparison of 2 mass vaccination campaigns against influenza A H1N1 in New York City. *American Journal of Public Health, 102*(7), 1378–1383.

King, J. C., Cummings, G. E., Stoddard, J., Readmond, B. X., Magder, L. S., Stong, M. (2005). A pilot study of the effectiveness of a school-based influenza vaccination program. *Pediatrics, 116*(6), e868–e873.

Kwong, J. C., Ge, H., Rosella, L. C., Guan, J., Maaten, S., Moran, K., Guttman, A. (2010). School-based influenza vaccine delivery, vaccination rates, and healthcare use in the context of a universal influenza immunization program: an ecological study. *Vaccine, 28*(15), 2722–2729.

Marsh, D. R., Schroeder, D. G., Dearden, K. A., Sternin, J., & Sternin, M. (2004). The power of positive deviance. *British Medical Journal, 329*(7475), 1177–1179.

Middleman, A. B., Short, M. B., & Doak, J. S. (2012). School-located influenza immunization programs: factors important to parents and students. *Vaccine, 30*(33), 4993–4999.

Middleman, A. B., & Tung, J. S. (2010). Urban middle school parent perspectives: the vaccines they are willing to have their children receive using school-based immunization programs. *Journal of Adolescent Health, 47*, 249–253.

National Association of County and City Health Officials. (2010). NACCHO H1N1 policy workshop report. Accessed April 3, 2012, at http://www.naccho.org/topics/H1N1/upload/NACCHO-WORKSHOP-REPORT-IN-TEMPLATE-with-chart.pdf.

Pawson, R. (2002). Evidence-based policy: in search of a method. *Evaluation, 8*(2), 157–181.

Piedra, P. O. (2013). Why vaccinate school-aged children against influenza? *Contemporary Pediatrics*. Available online at http://contemporarypediatrics.modernmedicine.com/contemporary-pediatrics/RC/why-vaccinate-school-aged-children-against-influenza?page=full

Roos, R. (2010). US H1N1 vaccine uptake estimated at 75 million. CIDRAP. Accessed March 7, 2012, at http://www.cidrap.umn.edu/cidrap/content/influenza/swineflu/news/feb0410nvac.html.

Vinter, S., Levi, J., & Segal, L. M. (2009). Ready or not? Protecting the public's health from diseases, disasters, and bioterrorism. Accessed December 8, 2011, at http://healthyamericans.org/reports/bioterror09/pdf/TFAHReadyorNot200906.pdf.

Walker, L. O., Sterling, B. S., Hoke, M. M., & Dearden, K. A. (2007). Applying the concept of positive deviance to public health data: a tool for reducing health disparities. *Public Health Nursing, 24*(6), 571–576.

CHAPTER 11 | Public Communication during the 2009 H1N1 Pandemic

ELENA SAVOIA, LEESA LIN, AND
KASISOMAYAJULA VISWANATH

Introduction

During a crisis, federal, state, and local public health agencies typically engage in a variety of communication efforts to inform the public, encourage the adoption of preventive behaviors, and limit the adverse impacts of specific events. These efforts to communicate with the public to provide guidance about preparing for, responding to, and recovering from emergencies is a critical component in public health emergency preparedness (PHEP) and response (Centers for Disease Control and Prevention, 2011; Wingate et al., 2007). Moreover, the strength of a society's response to a public health emergency depends on meeting the needs of all segments of the population, especially those who are most vulnerable and subject to a disproportionate share of adversity. Failing to address the great diversity of special health and medical concerns, language and cultural barriers, and other life circumstances can decrease the effectiveness of the public health response to specific threats, including reducing the benefits of timely interventions. Salient, if not central, to these factors is the phenomenon of communication inequalities, differences among individuals and social groups in accessing and using health information, and the consequential impact on knowledge and behaviors (Taylor-Clark et al., 2010; Viswanath, 2006). Yet, individuals and groups may not be able to access and use some of the resources offered to them, including information on health and specific threats, because of the existing inequalities manifesting along many fault lines, including class, race, place, ethnicity, and physical and mental disability, among others (Viswanath and Ackerson, 2011).

This chapter is a case study of the 2009 H1N1 pandemic that illustrates the complexities that public health authorities experience in conveying information using public communication during pandemics. We describe how we approached an assessment of the impact of public communication around pH1N1 on the U.S.

population during the pandemic. Although the adverse impact of the pandemic was not as severe as initially expected, it provided an opportunity to test the role of public communication in community preparedness. We begin by describing the different methods we used to study the population's reactions to information exposure and to present findings from narrative literature reviews, content analysis, focus groups, and surveys. We move on (1) to discuss how each method contributed to painting an overall picture of the generation and reception of information on the pandemic and its effect on the population's compliance with vaccination and social distancing measures, and (2) to provide an overall assessment of how public health communication worked during the pandemic. Throughout the discussion we pay specific attention to vulnerable populations. We then end with implications of our findings for policy and practice. Much of the material we present in this chapter reflects analysis of current literature, results from our research projects, and discussions between communication experts and public health officials that occurred during the last five years of our work (Galarce et al., 2011; Jung et al., 2013; Lin et al., 2014; Savoia et al., 2012, 2014).

Specifically, our research during the 2009 H1N1 pandemic focused on investigating communication inequalities, defined as differences in social groups in accessing and using health information, and the consequential effects of such differences, including knowledge and behaviors (Prus, 2011; Tichenor et al., 1970; Viswanath, 2006; Viswanath and Finnegan, 1996). In this chapter we describe what we learned through the use of multiple research methods about gaps in knowledge experienced by the U.S. population during the 2009 H1N1 pandemic and how we found social determinants to be associated with such gaps. We also examine how vaccine uptake varied by sociodemographic groups, H1N1-related beliefs, and seasonal influenza immunization practices, and discuss how early vaccination, a cost-effective solution to prevent contagion that reduces morbidity and mortality, can be affected negatively by inadequately targeted public communication practices. Unlike some aspects of the public health system response to the 2009 H1N1 pandemic, we can actually measure the impact of public health communication on how information was received and, by measuring vaccine uptake, determine how it was acted on. Communication and other social science research methods allow us to document the public information environment and assess its impact on knowledge, attitudes, and behaviors of people from diverse population subgroups.

Background

Communication and Pandemics

Public health systems around the world have relied on pandemic influenza planning to protect their countries against the potentially devastating impact of a pandemic, and public communication has been recognized as a critical component in such planning efforts. Outbreaks caused by unknown or newly discovered microorganisms generate a tremendous amount of uncertainty, and often fear, among the public, influencing actions and inaction. For this reason, the World Health Organization (WHO) has issued outbreak communication guidelines indicating that communication expertise is as important as epidemiologic and laboratory expertise in infectious disease control practices (World Health Organization, 2005). More specifically, communication during pandemics is crucial because it has the potential to reduce uncertainty, limit fear and panic, and facilitate action to stop the spread of the infection. Analyses of previous crises such as the 2003 to 2004 severe acute respiratory syndrome outbreak and Hurricane Katrina underline the importance of public communication in the response to large-scale emergencies, and emphasize the value of trustworthy, transparent, and responsive communication methods to reduce the adverse impact of such events (Arguin et al., 2004; Brug et al., 2004; Guion et al., 2007). However, public communication can be effective in preparing communities to act in times of crisis only when the various segments of the population are exposed promptly to the messages, understand them, and have the capacity to take action on the information given to them to protect themselves and their families (Viswanath, 2006).

From the earliest days of the pH1N1 outbreak in spring 2009, the Centers for Disease Control and Prevention (CDC) acknowledged that public communication would be challenged by the uncertainty of the unfolding circumstances of a potential pandemic (Maher, 2010). Because it is impossible to keep outbreaks hidden, the WHO recommends early official announcement to minimize rumors and misinformation (World Health Organization, 2005). Early engagement and communication are critical in the advent of social media, when information moves faster across different groups and when official information may be contested. As a consequence, during the pH1N1 pandemic, federal, state, and local public health agencies throughout the United States engaged quickly in a variety of public communication efforts to inform the population, encourage the adoption of preventive behaviors, and limit the spread of the disease. Familiar messages that mirrored advice for reducing contagion from common colds and flu were given, including basic hygiene measures (e.g., handwashing, coughing etiquette) and ways to contain the spread of infection (e.g., staying at home with flulike symptoms, deferring nonessential travel, keeping children at home during school closures) (Ringel et al., 2009).

In spring 2009, however, policy recommendations and communication messages had to be developed in the absence of complete and accurate data on the magnitude and severity of the outbreak. Consequently, information was often communicated under conditions of uncertainty, as is typical of most public health emergencies and disasters, and with very limited knowledge of how people will react and respond to public messaging. In some circumstances, this situation led to ambiguity about the purpose of the communication itself. Instead of using the tools and principles of risk communication to create public understanding of the risks posed by the pandemic, experts and policymakers frequently used another form of communication—*persuasion,*—which is intended not so much to create understanding but to persuade the public to take certain actions (Abraham, 2010). The reality that this information was directed at social groups known to vary widely in their capacity to follow specific public health advice, because of broad disparities in underlying health and socioeconomic status, communication abilities, and health literacy (Hutchins et al., 2009; Viswanath, 2006), complicated this situation.

Social determinants such as social class, neighborhood conditions, social capital, and race/ethnicity are associated strongly with health outcomes and inequalities in communication, including knowledge gap (Viswanath, 2006; Berkman and Kawachi 2000). Research also shows that the consequences of disasters and emergencies are experienced disproportionately by members of lower social classes, racial/ethnic minorities, and underserved groups whose media use patterns differ from those of higher socioeconomic status groups. In fact, several studies have demonstrated profound inequalities in communication between low and high socioeconomic status groups, including inequalities in the communication of risk (Viswanath, 2006). Moreover, knowledge alone is not enough to get people to act during a crisis, even when information about a probable hazard is available and communicated promptly to the public. For example, Mexican Americans often have delayed responses to natural emergencies because of the time they spend in trying to communicate with their extended families (Perry, 1979). Hearing impairment has left the elderly more vulnerable to information processing, causing difficulty in understanding evacuation orders during emergencies (Fernandez, 2002), and individuals with low literacy levels have been challenged in the interpretation of written messages (Tierney et al., 2001).

Methods

Assessing Communication Outcomes

An examination of the role of communication requires a multiprong approach that includes an assessment of both the information environment and the audience exposure to, reaction to, engagement with, and effects of pandemic-related messages. During the 2009 H1N1 pandemic, we used narrative literature reviews, content analysis, focus groups, and surveys to paint an overall picture of the generation and reception of information about pH1N1 (the pandemic virus), as well as how individuals' knowledge was related to vaccination and social distancing measures, and to assess how public communication worked during the pandemic. We began by performing a systematic review of the literature and combined the results of this review with qualitative data derived from a series of focus groups to develop and validate the use of the structural influence model of communication in PHEP (Figure 11-1). The model examines the relationship between social determinants, communication processes, and PHEP outcomes, and is based on the premise that

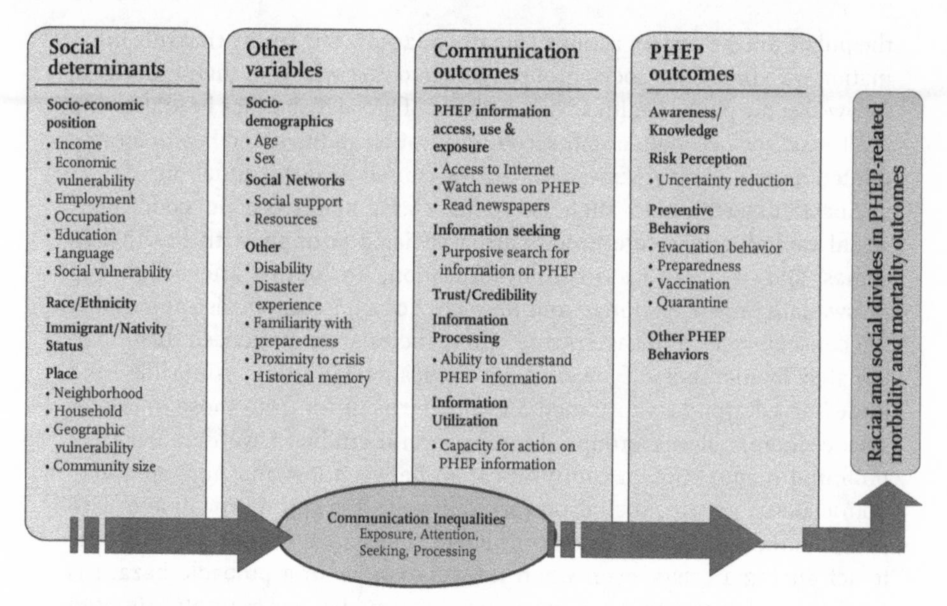

FIGURE 11-1 Structural influence model of communication in public health emergency preparedness (PHEP).

control of information is power and that whoever has the capacity to generate, access, use, and distribute information enjoys social power and the advantages that accrue from it (Tichenor et al., 1970).

To assess people's knowledge and experience about pH1N1, we conducted five focus groups between April 2009 and June 2009. The goal was to develop a better understanding of PHEP communication issues important to our target audience and to investigate the sources of information on PHEP communications among groups of different ethnic, racial, and socioeconomic position, and from urban and rural areas. This strategy helped us in determining not only what people thought about the pandemic, but also why they thought in a particular manner. This open conversation between the moderators and respondents in a group setting allowed for extensive probing, follow-up questions, and observation of emotional reactions. As with any qualitative research, the conclusions from our focus groups cannot be generalized, but the information obtained was used to develop a survey instrument to explore more systematically the themes that emerged from this initial qualitative approach. The 46 participants ranged from 26 to 72 years old and their educational level ranged from fourth grade to bachelor's degree, with the majority from underserved population groups and of low socioeconomic status. Participants were recruited mainly through newspaper advertisements and flyers. Of the five focus groups, one was conducted in Spanish. The topic of the focus groups included broad categories of questions concerning information sources, knowledge, and attitude about pH1N1; additional information desired in the event of a future outbreak;

preferred communication channels to receive such information; and general personal preparedness in the event of a public health emergency.

We subsequently developed and fielded a national survey designed to investigate information sources, knowledge, and attitudes in the U.S. population about pH1N1 itself and pH1N1 vaccine beliefs and uptake. Survey questions were based on the same structural influence model of communication in PHEP discussed previously. The survey was fielded in March 2010, in English and Spanish, using a strategy developed by the research firm Knowledge Networks, that includes both landline and cell phone-only households to obtain nationally representative samples administered online. After survey data were gathered, we used quantitative techniques to develop measures of a population's knowledge about pH1N1 in terms of symptoms and modalities of contagion, vaccine uptake, and attitude toward the vaccine. We then applied multivariate statistical techniques to study the associations between demographics, socioeconomic factors, beliefs and vaccine uptake, and knowledge about pH1N1 with the goal of determining what segments of the population were less likely to receive vaccine and less likely to be knowledgeable about how to limit the contagion (Galarce et al., 2011; Savoia et al., 2012).

Literature Review

We identified and analyzed 118 empirical studies in eight major communication, social sciences, and health and medical databases examining public communication issues during the 2009 H1N1 pandemic. Among them, 78% were population-based studies and 22% were articles that used information environment analyses techniques—a systematic analysis of news content on pH1N1 on different information channels. The pH1N1 pandemic offered a unique opportunity for researchers to assess the impact of communication efforts in response to an influenza outbreak of uncertain evolution, leading to a robust research program in the field of communications in public health emergency preparedness and risk communication. This trend was best demonstrated by the surge of empirical studies focusing on public communication during the 2009 H1N1 pandemic from 2009 to early 2012 (n = 118). These studies have outnumbered the total amount of articles investigating the same issues in all disasters from 2001 to 2011 (n = 44) (Savoia et al., 2013).

While reviewing these studies, we found that most population-based studies (82%) assessed the association between specific population characteristics (i.e., sociodemographic and interpersonal and psychosocial factors) and pH1N1-related communication and/or preparedness outcomes. Communication outcomes studied empirically during this pandemic included information source and exposure (50% of the papers analyzed), trust and credibility (32%), information use (12%), and information-seeking behaviors (11%). These communication behaviors were often identified and examined as important mediating factors of a population's preparedness outcomes. The most frequently researched preparedness outcomes were preventive behaviors such as hygiene and social distancing practices (in 70% of the studies), risk perceptions (70%), levels of knowledge and awareness about the pandemic (53%), and emotional responses such as fear and worry (47%).

Our review shows that older age, household income, level of education, and home ownership were associated positively with greater knowledge about pH1N1. Being worried about the disease was identified as an important predictor of compliance with recommended preventive behaviors, and was associated with the volume of media attention and media reporting number of pH1N1 cases (Ferrante et al., 2011; Keramarou et al., 2011; Liao et al., 2010; Olowokure et al., 2012; Pfefferbaum et al., 2012; Prati et al., 2011; Rubin et al., 2010a; Rubin et al., 2010b, 2010c, 2010d) Evidence also linked pH1N1-related knowledge to people's attitudes, which were measured by preexisting beliefs about pandemic influenza, such as social stigma and discrimination against one or more particular social subgroups, trust in the government's handling of the emergency, and/or fairness of treatment of all social groups (Boyd et al., 2012; Hilyard et al., 2010; Kumar et al., 2012; Liao et al., 2010; Y. Lin et al., 2011; Myers & Goodwin, 2011; Paek et al., 2010). Furthermore, knowledge and attitudes about pH1N1 have been proved to affect people's adoption of preventive measures (Balkhy et al., 2010; Cowling et al., 2010; Jhummon-Mahadnac et al., 2012; Jung et al., 2013; Lin et al., 2014; Wong & Sam, 2010, 2011a, 2011b; Zairina et al., 2011; Gaygisiz et al., 2012; Lin et al., 2011; Mak and Lai, 2012; Prati et al., 2011; Rubin et al., 2010a, 2010c; Kamate et al., 2009). Trust and credibility are also essential elements in all risk communication strategies and affect people's choice of information sources and attitudes toward the message received significantly (Gray & Ropeik, 2002; Reynolds, 2010; Liao et al., 2010; Prati et al., 2011; Quinn et al., 2013). People perceived their social networks—including friends, family, and physicians; communities (e.g., workplace, church); and health agencies—as trustworthy sources of information (Ferrante et al., 2011; Frew et al., 2012; Gray et al., 2012; Jhummon-Mahadnac et al., 2012; Jung et al., 2013; Quinn et al., 2013).

In fact, factors identified previously to be associated positively with knowledge and attitudes also affected pH1N1 vaccination behaviors significantly. Older age, social capital, worry, media exposure, information-seeking behaviors, and perceived severity and susceptibility to infection have a positive association with vaccine uptake (Eastwood et al., 2010; Ferrante et al., 2011; Frew et al., 2012; Jung et al., 2013; Kumar et al., 2012; (Mandeville et al., 2014); Prati et al., 2011; Rubin et al., 2010a, 2010b, 2010c; Setbon et al., 2011; Soto Mas et al., 2011). Trust in public officials, having a doctor recommending the vaccine, and a history of acceptance of the seasonal flu vaccine have been reported to increase acceptance of vaccination (Eastwood et al., 2010; Frew et al., 2012; Galarce et al., 2011; Griffiths et al., 2011; Kim et al., 2012; Lau et al., 2010; Maurer & Harris, 2011; Maurer et al., 2010; Plough et al., 2011; Ramsey & Marczinski, 2011; Rubin et al., 2010b, 2010c; Setbon et al., 2011; Walter et al., 2012; Wong and Sam, 2010b). Perceiving the vaccination as safe and effective was shown to be associated positively with vaccine uptake, whereas being concerned about potential side effects was associated negatively with such behavior. (Galarce et al., 2011; Kim et al., 2012; Li et al., 2012; Maurer et al., 2010; Plough et al., 2011a; Ramsey and Marczinski, 2011; Soto Mas et al., 2011). Our review confirms the existence of differences across various segments of the population on information exposure during the 2009 H1N1 pandemic, and their reactions and behaviors.

Results

Focus Groups Findings

Findings from the focus groups show there was a wide array of outlets where people were exposed to messages about pH1N1; the gamut of information sources included television, radio, Internet, newspapers, schools, healthcare professionals, hospitals, work, and grocery stores. Among the different sources, local television news was reported as the primary source of flu information, followed by local newspapers. However, although most participants first heard about the 2009 H1N1 pandemic outbreak from the television, they did not rate it as a highly trusted source. A majority of focus group participants did not seek out information actively regarding pH1N1, but of those who did, the Internet was used to get more information. The most trusted source for pH1N1 information was healthcare professionals, including doctors and nurses, as a participant reported and many others echoed: "It seems like a medical physician would have the updates on everything. Your doctor. Yeah. That's who you'd talk to. Definitely."

Despite some inaccuracies cited by some participants, most knew of the origin, transmission, precautions, symptoms, and treatments of pH1N1. This speaks well of the information communicated to citizens during the outbreak. There was a desire to know more specific information, such as what age groups were most at risk, because participants could only recall that the virus affected the young and the old. Focus group participants reported a willingness to comply with desirable behavior changes suggested by the media, such as frequent hand-washing, and were specifically interested in knowing more about how to protect themselves and others from a future outbreak. They also reported perceived low risk of contracting the infection. The focus group data are limited in that the research team could not assess adequately an individual participant's flu risk to determine whether his or her perceptions of risk were appropriate. Many participants discussed "information overload" and voiced concern over "media hype," as a participant reported: "I did not feel a need to actively look. I felt like I was being kind of bombarded with it."

Some participants cited a desire for one source of information and did not want to sift through all the available information. Participants also wanted clear action steps to take to care for someone who may be sick, and highlighted the importance of recognizing the line between sensationalism and reporting facts. They also cited the difficulty of following specific advice according to personal circumstances, as a participant stated: "One prepares oneself according to one's ability, because there are times that you don't have money to prepare yourself for an eventuality. You grab and buy things most necessary." A new channel of communications emerged from the discussions when participants were asked specifically about what and how they would like future information delivered to them; most reported they would like to receive information via mail (Viswanath et al., 2009).

There were urban and rural differences in information sources, with more rural residents citing a reliance on radio for communication. There were ethnic differences in information sources, with many Hispanic participants citing a reliance on ethnic media such as newspapers and television channels, as a participant described: "Yes, because that is the news from here and what is close to us. And that is what one is interested in knowing." Ethnic differences were also found in general attitudes toward emergency preparedness, with Hispanic participants voicing a fatalistic attitude in that they felt there was little they could do to prepare themselves in case of an emergency and, if a situation was to occur, they would rely on God's help.

Knowledge of pH1N1

Public health messages are often subject to differences in interpretation that can vary considerably according to individual perception of the risk and trust in the government, and according to different abilities to understand and interpret data and information—especially in the context of uncertainty. Forty-four percent of the people we surveyed answered a series of questions correctly about how the virus is transmitted from person to person, and 69% of them identified signs and symptoms of pH1N1 infection correctly. Although these data show that a sizable portion of the U.S. population had good knowledge about pH1N1, when we looked at differences in knowledge among the various segments of the population, we found substantial inequalities.

The survey results showed how socioeconomic position, and level of education in particular, was associated strongly with knowledge about pH1N1. Our research suggests that more education can prepare people for receiving and processing more complex information, even under conditions in which elements of uncertainty or changes over time complicate the message and the nuances of interpreting it. Such findings are consistent with the structural influence model presented earlier, which posits a relationship between socioeconomic position, communication, and health—with formal education standing out as a strong predictor of how much and what people know about health-related issues. The association between level of education and knowledge about pH1N1 suggests that even 10 months into the pandemic, when people were surveyed, messages about how you may get infected and what symptoms you may present if infected did not reach the less educated.

We also found that another socioeconomic position factor—home ownership—was related to knowledge about pH1N1. In the literature, home ownership has been shown to be an important predictor of good health. Those who live in rented living spaces have more symptoms and long-term illness, and they report poorer general and mental health than owner–occupiers (Dalsttra et al., 2006; Hiscock et al., 2003; Lim et al., 2010; Macintyre et al., 2003; Viswanath et al., 1990). At a time when homelessness is a national crisis, finding an association between knowledge of pH1N1 and home ownership raises concerns and brings attention to the importance of taking into consideration yet another economic indicator in communication planning efforts. Furthermore, home ownership is not only an indicator of economic status, but also of social cohesion. Owning a home anchors individuals to the community in which they live, and neighbors may serve as one potential source of information and knowledge (Viswanath et al., 1990). Moreover, better integration into the community is likely to be related to greater trust in local authorities, which in turn may affect willingness to heed the message and consequent ability to learn from the information received.

Vaccine Uptake

Early vaccination against influenza is a cost-effective solution to prevent contagion and to reduce the number of flu-related deaths (Sander et al., 2010). Nonetheless, year after year, the majority of the U.S. population fails to receive the flu vaccine (Centers for Disease Control and Prevention, 2010). The reasons for not receiving the vaccine range from socioeconomic barriers to medical, cultural, sociopolitical, and religious (Egede and Zheng, 2003; Fredrickson et al., 2004). As a consequence, vaccination uptake is not uniform across the U.S. population, but varies among different sociodemographic, political, ethnic, and cultural groups. Multiple studies have shown that ethnic/racial minorities and those of low socioeconomic status display lower seasonal influenza vaccination rates across all age groups (Bryant et al., 2006; Ostbye et al., 2003). Based on such premises, we were interested in investigating how barriers and objections to pH1N1 vaccination vary and affect vaccine uptake across different population subgroups, and we did so through the use of the survey mentioned earlier.

Our results show that pH1N1 vaccine uptake is associated with socioeconomic position and demographic factors, pH1N1-related beliefs, and seasonal vaccination uptake. Fewer than half the people with a high school degree perceived the vaccine as safe, whereas two-thirds of those with a bachelor's degree or higher did. Blacks were the ethnic/racial group least likely to report believing the pH1N1 vaccine was safe, and blacks with less than a bachelor's degree were the least likely to have received vaccine. Blacks were also more likely to have tried and failed to find vaccine. Similarly, those who had received the seasonal flu vaccine that same year were 21 times more likely to get the pH1N1 vaccine than those who had not (Galarce et al., 2011; Maurer et al., 2009). The same level of low trust was true for participants living in urban areas. These results demonstrate how measuring and analyzing belief variations across population subgroups contribute to the understanding of how perceptions associated with vaccination may influence behaviors, suggesting implications for risk communications practices.

Implications for Policy and Practice

These results suggest that public health officials take into account differences in population subgroups as they develop public communication strategies, lest they exacerbate the inequalities that already exist among the groups. Rapid surveys may be very useful to test the messages and assess their impact on the population, and to provide public health officials with a better understanding of the population they serve. Such surveys can also help officials capitalize on and adjust for existing cultural differences, and ultimately shape better communication capabilities for complex emergency situations.

Our research suggests that in areas where home ownership is limited, public health officials may want to design more creative public communication strategies. These might include developing messages that rebuild a feeling of trust in the government, and selecting nongovernmental channels of communication, such as community-based organizations, community leaders, or family networks, to ensure the diffusion of their messages among all social groups. Also, given the significant role of education, channels such as local television watched by people with less formal schooling could be an important platform to deliver messages. Similarly, communication efforts to increase vaccination rates or other preventive practices may be most effective when targeted to those who think they will get the vaccine but have not tried yet, or to those who are still unsure. On the other hand, campaigns targeted to those determined not to get the vaccine might require a different approach aimed at changing their perceptions about disease susceptibility and vaccine safety. To improve vaccination rates during seasonal influenza or other types of outbreaks, we need to improve our understanding of the multilevel nature of the barriers to vaccination. The first set of barriers has been reported extensively and refers to beliefs regarding pH1N1 vaccine safety and virus-related risk perceptions. A second set of barriers refers to vaccine access but it is not limited to physical and structural impediments; instead, it extends to social factors such as education and race/ethnicity, which are likely to interact with psychosocial barriers.

Lastly trust in public officials and journalists is a critical component for effective public communications. Our work clearly points toward the necessity to develop strategic public health communication efforts that call for communication campaigns toward audiences segmented by social class, race/ethnicity, and beliefs—often what advertisers call "psychodemographics."

Acknowledgments and Disclosures

This research was conducted with funding support awarded to the Harvard School of Public Health under cooperative agreements with the U.S. CDC (grant no. 5P01TP000307-05). The views expressed in the chapter are those of the authors and not of the CDC.

References

Abraham, T. (2010). The price of poor pandemic communication. *British Medical Journal, 340*, c2952.

Arguin, P. M., Navin, A. W., Stelle, S. F., Weld, L. H., & Kozarsky, P. E. (2004). Health communication during SARS. *Emerging Infectious Diseases, 10*(2), 377–380.

Balkhy, H. H., Abolfotouh, M. A., Al-Hathlool, R. H., & Al-Jumah, M. A. (2010). Awareness, attitudes, and practices related to the swine influenza pandemic among the Saudi public. *BMC Infectious Diseases, 10*.

Berkman, L. F., Kawachi, I. (2000). Social cohesion, social capital, and health. In: L.F. Berkman, L. F., & I. Kawachi, I., (editors). *Social Epidemiology* (pp. 174–190). New York: Oxford University Press.

Boyd, C. A., Gazmararian, J. A., & Thompson, W. W. (2012). Knowledge, attitudes, and behaviors of low-income women considered high priority for receiving the novel influenza A (H1N1) vaccine. *Maternal and Child Health Journal*. doi: 10.1007/s10995-012-1063-2.

Brug, J., Aro, A. R., Oenema, A., de Zwart, O., Richardus, J. H., Bishop, G. D. (2004). SARS risk perception, knowledge, precautions, and information sources, the Netherlands. *Emerging Infectious Diseases, 10*(8), 1486–1489.

Bryant, W. K., Ompad, D. C., Sisco, S., Blaney, S., Glidden, K., Phillips, E. (2006). Determinants of influenza vaccination in hard-to-reach urban populations. *Preventive Medicine, 43*(1), 60–70.

Centers for Disease Control and Prevention (CDC). (2010). Immunization coverage in the U.S. Accessed January 2, 2013, at http://www.cdc.gov/vaccines/stats-surv/imz-coverage.htm.

Centers for Disease Control and Prevention (CDC). (2011). Public health preparedness capabilities: national standards for state and local planning: centers for disease control and prevention (CDC), Department of Health and Human Services. Accessed January, 2, 2013, at http://www.cdc.gov/phpr/capabilities/dslr_capabilities_july.pdf.

Cowling, B. J., Ng, D. M., Ip, D. K., Liao, Q., Lam, W. W., Wu, J. T., . . . Fielding, R. (2010). Community psychological and behavioral responses through the first wave of the 2009 influenza A(H1N1) pandemic in Hong Kong. *Journal on Infectious Disease, 202*(6), 867–876. doi: 10.1086/655811

Dalsttra, J. A., Kunst, A. E., Mackenbach, J. P. (2006). A comparative appraisal of the relationship of education, income and housing tenure with less than good health among the elderly in Europe. *Social Science & Medicine, 62*, 2046–2060.

Eastwood, K., Durrheim, D. N., Jones, A., & Butler, M. (2010). Acceptance of pandemic (H1N1) 2009 influenza vaccination by the Australian public. *Medical Journal of Australia, 192*(1), 33–36.

Egede, L. E., & Zheng, (2003). Racial/ethnic differences in adult vaccination among individuals with diabetes. *American Journal of Public Health, 93*(2), 324–329.

Fernandez, L. S., Byard, D., Lin, C. c., Benson, S., & Barbera, J. A. (2002). Frail elderly as disaster victims: Emergency management strategies. *Prehospital Disaster Medicine*, 17(2), 67–74.

Ferrante, G., Baldissera, S., Moghadam, P. F., Carrozzi, G., Trinito, M. O., & Salmaso, S. (2011). Surveillance of perceptions, knowledge, attitudes and behaviors of the Italian adult population (18-69 years) during the 2009-2010 A/H1N1 influenza pandemic. *European Journal of Epidemiology, 26*(3), 211–219. doi: 10.1007/s10654-011-9576-3

Fredrickson, D. D., Davis, T. C., Arnould, C. L., Kennen, E. M., Hurniston, S. G., Cross, J. T. (2004). Childhood immunization refusal: provider and parent perceptions. *Family Medicine, 36*(6), 431–439.

Frew, P. M., Painter, J. E., Hixson, B., Kulb, C., Moore, K., del Rio, C., . . . Omer, S. B. (2012). Factors mediating seasonal and influenza A (H1N1) vaccine acceptance among ethnically diverse populations in the urban south. *Vaccine, 30*(28), 4200–4208. doi: 10.1016/j.vaccine.2012.04.053

Galarce, E. M., Minsky, S., Viswanath, K. (2011). Socioeconomic status, demographics, belief and A(H1N1) vaccine uptake in the United States. *Vaccine, 29*(32), 5284–5289.

Gaygisiz, U., Gaygisiz, E., Ozkan, T., Lajunen, T. (2012). Individual differences in behavioral reactions to H1N1 during a later stage of the epidemic. *Journal of Infection and Public Health*, 5(1), 9–21.

Gray, G. M., & Ropeik, D. P. (2002). Dealing with the dangers of fear: the role of risk communication. *Health Affairs (Millwood), 21*(6), 106–116.

Griffiths, S. M., Wong, A. H., Kim, J. H., Yung, T. K. C., & Lau, J. T. F. (2011). Authors response to Influence of country of study on student responsiveness to the H1N1 pandemic. *Public Health*, 125(10), 739–740.

Guion, D. T., Scammon, D. L., Borders, A. L. (2007). Weathering the storm: a social marketing perspective on disaster preparedness and response with lessons from Hurricane Katrina. *American Marketing Association, 26*(1), 20–32.

Hilyard, K. M., Freimuth, V. S., Musa, D., Kumar, S., & Quinn, S. C. (2010). The vagaries of public support for government actions in case of a pandemic. *Health Affairs (Millwood)*, 29(12), 2294–2301. doi: 10.1377/hlthaff.2010.0474

Hiscock, R., Macintyre, S., Kearns, A. (2003). Residents and residence: factors predicting the health disadvantage of social renters compared to owner–occupiers. *Journal of Social Issues*, 59, 527–546.

Hutchins, S. S., Fiscella, K., Levine, R. S., Ompad, D. C., McDonald, M. (2009). Protection of racial/ethnic minority populations during an influenza pandemic. *American Journal of Public Health*, 99(2), 261–270.

Jhummon-Mahadnac, N. D., Knott, J., & Marshall, C. (2012). A cross-sectional study of pandemic influenza health literacy and the effect of a public health campaign. *BMC Research Notes*, 5, 377. doi: 10.1186/1756-0500-5-377

Jung, M., Lin, L., & Viswanath, K. (2013). Associations between health communication behaviors, neighborhood social capital, vaccine knowledge, and parents' H1N1 vaccination of their children. *Vaccine, 31*(42), 4860–4866. doi: 10.1016/j.vaccine.2013.07.068

Kamate, S. K., Agrawal, A., Chaudhary, H., Singh, K., Mishra, P., & Asawa, K. (2009). Public knowledge, attitude and behavioural changes in an Indian population during the Influenza A (H1N1) outbreak. *Journal of Infection in Developing Countries, 4*(1), 7.

Kamate, S. K., Agrawal, A., Chaudhary, H., Singh, K., Mishra, P., Asawa, K. (2010). Public knowledge, attitude and behavioural changes in an Indian population during the influenza A (H1N1) outbreak. *Journal of Infection in Developing Countries, 4*(1), 7–14.

Keramarou, M., Cottrell, S., Evans, M. R., Moore, C., Stiff, R. E., Elliott, C., . . . Salmon, R. L. (2011). Two waves of pandemic influenza A(H1N1) 2009 in Wales--the possible impact of media coverage on consultation rates, April-December 2009. *EuroSurveillance, 16*(3).

Kim, S., Pinkerton, T., & Ganesh, N. (2012). Assessment of H1N1 questions and answers posted on the Web. *American Journal of Infection Control, 40*(3), 211–217. doi: 10.1016/j.ajic.2011.03.028

Kumar, S., Quinn, S. C., Kim, K. H., Musa, D., Hilyard, K. M., & Freimuth, V. S. (2012). The social ecological model as a framework for determinants of 2009 H1N1 influenza vaccine uptake in the United States. *Health Education & Behavior, 39*(2), 229–243. doi: 10.1177/1090198111415105

Lau, J. T., Yeung, N. C., Choi, K. C., Cheng, M. Y., Tsui, H. Y., Griffiths, S. (2010). Factors in association with acceptability of A/H1N1 vaccination during the influenza A/H1N1 pandemic phase in the Hong Kong general population. *Vaccine, 23*(29), 4632–4637.

Li, M., Chapman, G. B., Ibuka, Y., Meyers, L. A., & Galvani, A. (2012). Who got vaccinated against H1N1 pandemic influenza? A longitudinal study in four U.S. cities. *Psychology & Health, 27*(1), 101–115. doi: 10.1080/08870446.2011.554833

Liao, Q., Cowling, B., Lam, W. T., Ng, M. W., & Fielding, R. (2010). Situational awareness and health protective responses to pandemic influenza A (H1N1) in Hong Kong: a cross-sectional study. *PloS One, 5*(10), e13350. doi: 10.1371/journal.pone.0013350; 10.1371/journal.pone.0013350

Lim, S., Chung, W., Kim, H., Lee, S. (2010). The influence of housing tenure and marital status on smoking in South Korea. *Health Policy, 94*(2), 101–110.

Lin, L., Jung, M., McCloud, R. F., & Viswanath, K. (2014). Media use and communication inequalities in a public health emergency: a case study of 2009–2010 pandemic influenza A virus subtype H1N1. *Public Health Report, 129*(Sup4), 49–60.

Lin, Y., Huang, L., Nie, S., Liu, Z., Yu, H., Yan, W., & Xu, Y. (2011). Knowledge, attitudes and practices (KAP) related to the pandemic (H1N1) 2009 among Chinese general population: a telephone survey. *BMC Infectious Disease, 11*, 128. doi: 10.1186/1471-2334-11-128

Macintyre, S., Ellaway, A., Hiscock, R. (2003). What features of the home and the area might help to explain observed relationships between housing tenure and health? Evidence from the west of Scotland. *Health & Place, 9*, 207–218.

Maher, B. (2010). Crisis communicator. *Nature, 463*, 150–152.

Mak, K. K., Lai, C. M. (2012). Knowledge, risk perceptions, and preventive precautions among Hong Kong students during the 2009 influenza A (H1N1) pandemic. *American Journal of Infection Control, 40*(3), 273–275.

Maurer, J., Harris, K. M., Parker, A., Lurie, N. (2009). Does receipt of seasonal influenza vaccine predict intention to receive novel H1N1 vaccine: evidence from a nationally representative survey of U.S. adults. *Vaccine, 27*(42), 5732–5734. doi: 10.1016/j.vaccine.2009.07.080

Maurer, J., & Harris, K. M. (2011). Contact and communication with healthcare providers regarding influenza vaccination during the 2009-2010 H1N1 pandemic. *Preventive Medicine, 52*(6), 459–464. doi: 10.1016/j.ypmed.2011.03.016

Maurer, J., Uscher-Pines, L., & Harris, K. M. (2010). Perceived seriousness of seasonal and A(H1N1) influenzas, attitudes toward vaccination, and vaccine uptake among U.S. adults: does the source of information matter? *Preventive Medicine, 51*(2), 185–187. doi: 10.1016/j.ypmed.2010.05.008

Myers, L. B., & Goodwin, R. (2011). Determinants of adults' intention to vaccinate against pandemic swine flu. *BMC Public Health, 11*(1), 15. doi: 10.1186/1471-2458-11-15

Olowokure, B., Odedere, O., Elliot, A. J., Awofisayo, A., Smit, E., Fleming, A., & Osman, H. (2012). Volume of print media coverage and diagnostic testing for influenza A(H1N1)pdm09 virus during the early phase of the 2009 pandemic. *Journal of Clinical Virology: The Official Publication of the Pan American Society for Clinical Virology, 55*(1), 75. doi: 10.1016/j.jcv.2012.05.013; 10.1016/j.jcv.2012.05.013

Ostbye, T., Taylor, D. H., Lee, A. M. M., Greenberg, G., van Scoyoc, L. (2003). Racial differences in influenza vaccination among older Americans 1996–2000: longitudinal analysis of the Health and Retirement Study (HRS) and the Asset and Health Dynamics Among the Oldest Old (AHEAD) survey. *BMC Public Health, 3*, 41–141.

Paek, H. J., Hilyard, K., Freimuth, V., Barge, J. K., & Mindlin, M. (2010). Theory-based approaches to understanding public emergency preparedness: implications for effective health and risk communication. *Journal of Health Communication, 15*(4), 428–444. doi: 10.1080/10810731003753083

Perry, R. W. (1979). Evacuation decision-making in natural disasters. *Mass Emergencies, 4*, 25–38.

Pfefferbaum, B., Schonfeld, D., Flynn, B. W., Norwood, A. E., Dodgen, D., Kaul, R. E., . . . Ruzek, J. I. (2012). The H1N1 crisis: a case study of the integration of mental and behavioral health in public health crises. *Disaster Medicine and Public Health Preparedness, 6*(1), 67–71. doi: 10.1001/dmp.2012.2

Plough, A., Bristow, B., Fielding, J., Caldwell, S., & Khan, S. (2011). Pandemics and health equity: lessons learned from the H1N1 response in Los Angeles County. *Journal of Public Health Management and Practice, 17*(1), 20–27. doi: 10.1097/PHH.0b013e3181ff2ad7

Prati, G., Pietrantoni, L., & Zani, B. (2011). Compliance with recommendations for pandemic influenza H1N1 2009: the role of trust and personal beliefs. *Health Education Research, 26*(5), 761–769. doi: 10.1093/her/cyr035

Prus, S. G. (2011). Comparing social determinants of self-rated health across the United States and Canada. *Social Science & Medicine, 73*(1), 50–59.

Ramsey, M. A., & Marczinski, C. A. (2011). College students' perceptions of H1N1 flu risk and attitudes toward vaccination. *Vaccine, 29*(44), 7599. doi: 10.1016/j.vaccine.2011.07.130; 10.1016/j.vaccine.2011.07.130

Reynolds, B. J. (2010). Building trust through social media. CDC's experience during the H1N1 influenza response. *Marketing Health Services, 30*(2), 18–21.

Ringel, J. S., Trentacost, E., Lurie, N. (2009). How well did health departments communicate about risk at the start of the swine flu epidemic in 2009? *Health Affairs, 28*(4), w743–w750.

Rubin, G. J., Potts, H. W., & Michie, S. (2010a). The impact of communications about swine flu (influenza A H1N1v) on public responses to the outbreak: results from 36 national telephone surveys in the UK. *Health Technology Assessment, 14*(34), 183–266. doi: 10.3310/hta14340-03

Rubin, G. J., Potts, H. W. W., & Michie, S. (2010b). The impact of communications about swine flu (influenza A HINIv) on public responses to the outbreak: Results from 36 national telephone surveys in the UK. Study 1: The influence of the media on levels of worry in the community. *Health Technology Assessment, 14*(34), 183–266.

Rubin, G. J., Potts, H. W. W., & Michie, S. (2010c). The impact of communications about swine flu (influenza A HINIv) on public responses to the outbreak: Results from 36 national telephone surveys in the UK. Study 2: Factors predicting likely acceptance of vaccination against swine or seasonal flu. *Health Technology Assessment, 14*(34), 183–266.

Rubin, G. J., Potts, H. W. W., & Michie, S. (2010d). The impact of communications about swine flu (influenza A HINIv) on public responses to the outbreak: Results from 36 national telephone surveys in the UK. Study 3: The effects of advertising and media coverage on behavioural change during the early stages of the swine flu. *Health Technology Assessment, 14*(34), 183–266.

Sander, B., Bauch, C. T., Fisman, D., Fowler, R. A., Kwong, J. C., Maetzel, A. (2010). Is a mass immunization program for pandemic (H1N1) 2009 good value for money? Evidence from the Canadian experience. *Vaccine, 28*(38), 6210–6220.

Savoia, E., Testa, M. A., & Viswanath, K. (2012). Predictors of knowledge of H1N1 infection and transmission in the U.S. population. *BMC Public Health, 12*, 328. doi: 10.1186/1471-2458-12-328

Savoia, E., Lin, L., & Viswanath, K. (2013). Communications in public health emergency preparedness: a systematic review of the literature. *Biosecur Bioterror, 11*(3), 170–184. doi: 10.1089/bsp.2013.0038

Setbon, M., Le Pape, M. C., Lactroublon, C., Caille-Brillet, A. L., Raude, J. (2011). The public's preventive strategies in response to the pandemic influenza A/H1N1 in France: distribution and determinants. *Preventive Medicine, 52*(2), 178–181.

Soto Mas, F., Olivarez, A., Jacobson, H. E., Hsu, C. E., & Miller, J. (2011). Risk communication and college students: the 2009 H1N1 pandemic influenza. *Preventive Medicine, 52*(6), 473–474. doi: 10.1016/j.ypmed.2011.04.004

Taylor-Clark, K., Viswanath, K., Blendon, R. (2010). Communication inequalities during public health disasters: Katrina's wake. *Health Communication, 25*(3), 221–229.

Tichenor, P. J., Donohue, G. A., Olien, C. N. (1970). Mass media flow and differential growth in knowledge. *Public Opinion Quarterly, 34*(2), 159–170.

Tierney, K. L. (2001). *Facing the unexpected: disaster preparedness and response in the United States*, 4th ed. Washington, DC: Joseph Henry Press.

Viswanath, K. (2006). Public communications and its role in reducing and eliminating health disparities. In: Thompson, G. E., Mitchell, F., Williams, M. B., editors. *Examining the health disparities research plan of the National Institutes of Health: unfinished business* (pp. 215–253). Washington, DC: Institute of Medicine.

Viswanath, K., Ackerson, L. K. (2011). Race, ethnicity, language, social class, and health communication inequalities: a nationally-representative cross-sectional study. *PLoS One, 6*(1), e14550.

Viswanath, K., Finnegan, J. R. (1996). The knowledge gap hypothesis: twenty five years later. In: Burleson, B., editor. *Communication yearbook 19* (pp. 187–227). Thousand Oaks, CA: Sage Publications.

Viswanath, K., Finnegan, J. R., Rooney, B., & Potter, J. (1990). Community ties and use of newspapers and cable TV in a rural Midwestern community. *Journalism Quarterly, 67*, 899–911.

Viswanath, K., Minsky, S., Ramamurthi, D., & Kontos, E. (2009). *Communications under uncertainty: communication behaviors of diverse audiences during the A(H1N1) incidence of spring and summer 2009*. Report: Viswanath Lab. Harvard School of Public Health, and Dana-Farber Cancer Institute, Boston, MA.

Walter, D., Bohmer, M., Reiter, S., Krause, G., & Wichmann, O. (2012). Risk perception and information-seeking behaviour during the 2009/10 influenza A(H1N1) pdm09 pandemic in Germany. *Euro Surveillance: Bulletin Europeen Sur Les Maladies Transmissibles = European Communicable Disease Bulletin, 17*(13), 20131.

Wingate, M. S., Perry, E. C., Campbell, P. H., David, P., Weist, E. M. (2007). Identifying and protecting vulnerable populations in public health emergencies: addressing gaps in education and training. *Public Health Reports, 122*(3), 422–426.

Wong, L. P., & Sam, I. C. (2010). Factors influencing the uptake of 2009 H1N1 influenza vaccine in a multiethnic Asian population. *Vaccine, 28*(28), 4499. doi: 10.1016/j.vaccine.2010.04.043; 10.1016/j.vaccine.2010.04.043

Wong, L. P., & Sam, I. C. (2011a). Behavioral responses to the influenza A(H1N1) outbreak in Malaysia. *Journal of Behavioral Medicine, 34*(1), 23. doi: 10.1007/s10865-010-9283-7; 10.1007/s10865-010-9283-7

Wong, L. P., & Sam, I. C. (2011b). Knowledge and attitudes in regard to pandemic influenza A(H1N1) in a multiethnic community of Malaysia. *International Journal of Behavioral Medicine, 18*(2), 112. doi: 10.1007/s12529-010-9114-9; 10.1007/s12529-010-9114-9

Zairina, A. R., Nooriah, M. S., & Yunus, A. M. (2011). Knowledge and practices towards influenza A (H1N1) among adults in three residential areas in Tampin Negeri Sembilan: a cross sectional survey. *The Medical journal of Malaysia, 66*(3), 207.

CHAPTER 12

Obstacles to pH1N1 Vaccine Availability

The Complex Contracting Relationship between Vaccine Manufacturers, the World Health Organization, Donor and Beneficiary Governments

SAM F. HALABI

Introduction

When researchers in Mexico and the United States concluded that influenza-related hospitalizations in separate, noncontiguous areas of Mexico, southern California, and New York City uniquely affected children and young adults, they were alerted to the possibility that a new pandemic viral subtype of influenza had emerged (Cordova-Villalobos et al., 2009; see also Chapter 2). After the U.S. Centers for Disease Control and Prevention (CDC) received samples from two early H1N1 patients in mid April, 2009, researchers exposed banked blood samples taken before and after vaccinations from 2005 to the new virus (Centers for Disease Control and Prevention, 2009). Samples from children produced no antibodies whereas samples from adults vaccinated against seasonal flu showed a slight increase in antibodies against the pH1N1 virus. Because it did not appear that the seasonal vaccine would adequately protect adults against infection, the CDC recommended development of a vaccine specific to the new strain (Hancock et al., 2009). This recommendation was echoed in the World Health Organization's (WHO's) June 11, 2009, declaration of a Phase 6 pandemic. Under WHO classificatory scheme operating in 2009 (it has been revised in light of the H1N1 experience), in Phases 1 through 3 of a pandemic, influenza circulates predominantly in animals and there are few human infections. In Phase 4, there is sustained human-to-human transmission, and in Phases 5 and 6, sustained human transmission spreads to at least two WHO regions (Doshi, 2011).

The CDC's recommendation and WHO's declaration triggered a race by a small number of vaccine manufacturers to develop and then put into production a pandemic-specific vaccine because a market had instantaneously developed and some manufacturers already had in place agreements with governments that required them to shift to pandemic vaccine production (Centers for Disease Control and Prevention, 2012; World Health Organization, 2011b). Aside from the governments that had already put procurement policies and contracts in place, the vast majority of the world's governments and the populations they represented lacked access to vaccines and looked to WHO to work with firms and potential donor governments to facilitate access. The gene sequence of wild-type pandemic pH1N1 was made publicly available April 27, 2009. By May 8, 2009, samples of wild-type virus had been sent from reference laboratories to vaccine manufacturers, all of which were in Europe and the United States, because they had the necessary high-level biological containment facilities. This chapter analyzes the obstacles standing between WHO, vaccine manufacturers, and the populations who needed the vaccines they produced.

Vaccines are the first line of defense against influenza to prevent infection and to control spread of the disease because they are more effective and burden society less than nonpharmaceutical measures like masks, closing of public gathering places, and isolation of patients (Aledort et al., 2007; Carter and Plosker, 2008). The process by which a vaccine is first developed in a laboratory to its administration to a population engages the full range of governmental health agencies, community organizations, pharmaceutical firms, and international organizations that comprise the system the U.S. National Health Security Strategy sets at the core of improving public health emergency response.

Although recent pandemic influenza threats have originated in middle- or low-income countries, the capacity for pandemic influenza vaccine production is overwhelmingly concentrated in Australia, Europe, and North America (Crosse, 2008). These regions' pharmaceutical firms are in a persistent cycle of seasonal influenza vaccine production, which is based on surveillance reports detailing which influenza viruses are in circulation, how they are spreading, and how well the previous season's vaccine viruses protect against new strains. Although WHO recommends specific vaccine viruses after information is gathered from more than 100 national influenza centers in more than 100 countries, individual countries make their own decisions about licensing of vaccines subject to their own regulatory mechanisms.

When a new influenza strain emerges, the first step in vaccine response is to assess whether the seasonal influenza vaccine will produce adequate immunity to protect against the new strain. After researchers concluded the seasonal vaccine did not protect against pH1N1, pharmaceutical firms, five of which control approximately 80% of the influenza vaccine market, found themselves negotiating with WHO about conditions for donation, shipment, and distribution of vaccine. Governments with preexisting contracts sought to preserve as much of their firms' capacity—that is, firms located within the territorial borders of the procuring governments—as necessary to inoculate their populations first before giving or selling to others. As a result, manufacturers negotiated with a much larger than usual number of procurement officials, regulators, health-care providers, and vaccine distributors (Hanquet et al., 2011).

From the manufacturers' perspective, these negotiations occurred in the shadow of potentially large liabilities related to their existing contractual arrangements with governments; detailed processes for vaccine approval, distribution, and marketing; and more general exposure should quickly developed vaccines generate unexpected adverse reactions or safety problems. Indeed, WHO prequalified some vaccines in as little as one day, even when ongoing studies showed significant adverse events (World Health Organization, 2010). Manufacturers were required to seek approval as if it were an entirely new vaccine. Under typical regimes, manufacturers must modify the new virus to grow efficiently (generally in eggs) so it may be used for vaccine production. This modification also ensures the vaccine virus may be handled safely. To develop antigens and injectable antiserum to measure vaccine potency, manufacturers must coordinate with reference laboratories and regulatory agencies. Vaccines must then be tested in human trials to assess safety and effectiveness. Regulatory approval for marketing and use is dependent on laboratory-generated evidence and clinical trial outcomes. Even safe and effective vaccines generate adverse events among those inoculated, ranging from (common) soreness at the injection site to fever, discomfort, and muscle pain to (rare) anaphylaxis and oculorespiratory syndrome (World Health Organization, 2012). One of the vaccines produced specifically for pH1N1 by GlaxoSmithKline has been associated with an increased risk of narcolepsy (Centers for Disease Control and Prevention, 2013). In many jurisdictions, manufacturers bear legal responsibility for these adverse events.

Manufacturers therefore face a range of legal barriers to production, donation, and discounted sale of pandemic vaccines like the process by which vaccines may be approved and registered with national regulatory authorities, protection from and indemnification for liability, and preexisting advance market commitment agreements that affect the ability to enter into additional contracts after a pandemic has been declared. In short, the global public health response is dependent on private-sector actors who must balance private-sector and public-sector demands on their resources.

Methods

Contracts between private parties are rarely available for public scrutiny unless litigation exposes them. Similarly, agreements between private-sector actors and public authorities are kept confidential in most circumstances unless they are specifically covered by open records laws, the bidding process for them requires a high degree of transparency, or private-sector actors themselves make some or all of the agreements available. Confidentiality of agreements is particularly important when the agreement potentially affects national defense or security—circumstances that generally characterize governmental strategies for dealing with pandemics.

However, many aspects of the relationships between vaccine manufacturers, WHO, donor and beneficiary governments have been revealed through testimonies before legislative bodies, postpandemic analyses undertaken by WHO, including a comprehensive assessment of its response, and conversations and interviews with persons representing governments, firms, and WHO. These primary sources were supplemented by analyses of the 2009 pH1N1 vaccine development and distribution problem published in the academic literature to develop as comprehensive picture as possible of vaccine contracting obstacles.

This document review was also supplemented by informal interviews with decision makers, many of whom did not have time for extensive, formal interviews. The data collected from the academic literature, WHO reports, and interviews were organized according to major legal obstacles, which were then vetted with public health researchers, practitioners, governmental officials, and one representative from a vaccine manufacturer to maximize the chance that all key issues were captured and no critical concerns were excluded. Although these methods cannot tell us the frequency with which specific issues arose, they are sufficient to ensure the major contracting obstacles facing manufacturers, governments, and WHO have been identified and explored.

Other issues also affected vaccine distribution, including supply line breaks, and inconsistencies and inadequate infrastructure to distribute vaccines once the legal uncertainties just described were resolved (see, for example, Chapter 10), but are beyond the scope of this chapter. Those problems included the availability and resilience of cold chain packaging, shelf-life, and planning within both public-sector actors such as the United Nations' (UN) Office for Project Services, UNICEF, and development agencies, along with private-sector actors like global logistics firms.

Results

The Legal Framework for pH1N1 Pandemic Influenza Vaccine Distribution

Development, approval, and distribution of the 2009 pH1N1 vaccine was shaped by preexisting frameworks that had been established to address the outbreak of H5N1 avian flu in Southeast Asia (McConnell, 2010). That subtype spread quickly around the globe but did not (and has not to date) evolved to become easily transmissible to humans. The concern that H5N1 may become easily transmissible to and then between humans resulted in both divergent (if accelerated) regulatory approval processes, and a set of agreements entered into between two manufacturers—GlaxoSmithKline (GSK) and Sanofi Pasteur (Sanofi)—and the WHO donations of antivirals and prepandemic H5N1 vaccine doses. After the pN1H1 influenza strain was identified, WHO immediately began negotiations with "all known" influenza vaccine manufacturers (World Health Organization, 2011b). Those discussions were shaped by planning for H5N1 (Hanquet et al., 2011).

When the WHO declared a Phase 6 pandemic, GSK and Sanofi pledged 50 million and 60 million doses of H5N1 vaccine, respectively, although no legal agreements for donations were in place. GSK and Sanofi agreed to convert those commitments to pandemic influenza A pH1N1 vaccine and to increase the number of doses to 150 million. GSK and WHO signed an agreement for the donations on November 10, 2009, which resulted in just over 24 million doses actually donated. Sanofi announced a "flexible" donation of up to 100 million doses on June 17, 2009, but the donation agreement was not signed until December 2009. Novartis specifically eschewed donations, favoring pricing mechanisms to establish a "sustainable way" to deliver vaccine to developing countries.

Despite the small number of players, negotiations regarding all aspects of procurement were difficult and protracted, revealing a near-total lack of planning to move vaccine from the private-sector developers and manufacturers to the populations that needed them. Negotiations involved at least four manufacturers and 12 governments on the donor side, and nearly 100 governments on the beneficiary side (World Health Organization, 2011b). WHO's negotiation with GSK served as a template for agreements with CSL Australia, MedImmune, and Sanofi, which concluded in December 2009. Novartis signed an agreement in January 2010, although a 2011 WHO assessment of its response to the pandemic strongly suggests the Novartis agreement differed from the other four. Legal agreements with governments followed those with firms: the United States (December 16, 2009), Australia (December 22, 2009), France (January 15, 2010), Belgium (January 29, 2010), Switzerland (March 16, 2010), Norway (March 19, 2010), Italy (April 16, 2010), the United Kingdom (May 28, 2010), and Singapore (June 21, 2010). Some states perceived that WHO "shopped" different agreements with different legal terms to different governments—a practice that generated suspicion among the donor governments and caused further delay in finalizing terms.

The delay in placing agreements between firms, governments, and WHO was attributable to at least two causes. First, both firms and governments had entered into advance purchase agreements that constrained the ability of firms to donate or otherwise provide vaccines to WHO or governments directly. Second, vaccine manufacturers insisted on strong protections from liability should the pandemic influenza vaccine result in adverse health events in populations, and coverage for interests affected by specific title transfer arrangements.

Advance Purchase Agreements and Territorial Restraints

Long before WHO declared a pandemic, many countries, including Belgium, Canada, Finland, France, Germany, Italy, Switzerland, the Netherlands, the United States, and the United Kingdom, had already placed large orders of pH1N1 vaccine or had advanced agreements in place (Doshi and Jefferson, 2010). With advance purchase agreements (also known as *sleeping contracts*), a vaccine manufacturer agrees to supply its pandemic influenza vaccine as soon as possible after a pandemic has been declared and agrees to reserve a specified number of doses for the country or to more openly meet that country's orders first. When it commenced negotiations with manufacturers, WHO did not know about key aspects of the agreements. When asked whether they would be willing to reserve (not donate) 10% of real-time production for purchase by UN agencies, many vaccine manufacturers cited advance purchase agreements with high-income countries as a barrier. Contracting states noted the relatively inflexible terms of those agreements. A review of European Union member states' vaccine planning strategies after the pandemic highlighted the obstacles advanced purchase agreements pose:

> From the contracting country's perspective, it is clear that maximizing not only guaranteed access to vaccine, but also increased flexibility that can help to minimize costs and better calibrate orders to changing prognoses regarding the ongoing development of the pandemic. Convincing vaccine [manufacturers] to provide such flexibility is likely to pose a challenge and might well require finding ways of enhancing the negotiating power of contracting Member States. A forum for discussions among Member States of how to develop advance purchase contracts could be useful. (European Commission (2010)

Even aside from advance purchase agreements, the decision to dedicate physical infrastructure and human resources to pandemic influenza vaccine production is, from the manufacturers' view, a business decision. In a 2010 WHO report examining operational successes and failures of WHO Deployment Initiative (the umbrella term WHO used to describe its effort to procure vaccines from firms and governments, and to distribute them to needy countries), pharmaceutical firms noted that "support for WHO Deployment Initiative may have disrupted business in other areas and reduced their competitive strength" (World Health Organization, 2010, p. 9). Vaccine manufacturers, therefore, desire stockpiling agreements as a solution to business uncertainty, whereas procuring governments demand flexibility to fit the severity of the pandemic. The 2009 pH1N1 influenza pandemic has exacerbated this tension between firms and the governments wealthy enough to procure advanced vaccine production, and therefore what is left for populations in lesser developed or middle-income states. After the pH1N1 threat diminished, many more governments entered into advance purchase agreements with a wider divergence in legal terms for a larger number of doses of pandemic or prepandemic vaccine.

In addition to and accompanying advance purchase agreements, domestic law may nevertheless constrain the production and shipment environment of vaccine manufacturers. For example, GSK's facility in Sainte Foy, Quebec, must fill Canada's orders first before supplying to others, and Canada awarded its pandemic influenza vaccine contract to a Canadian company precisely because it feared foreign governments would restrict exports of vaccine doses (Fidler, 2010; Standing Senate Committee on Social Affairs, Parliament of Canada, 2010). The Australian government made it clear to the Australian manufacturer CSL that it must fulfill the government's domestic needs before exporting pH1N1 vaccine (Fidler, 2010). Despite clear acknowledgment that the 2009 outbreak originated in Mexico and leveled its most significant toll there, Mexico had "a terrifically difficult time getting access to the pandemic vaccine" as a result of the difficulties in assessing needs and distributing vaccines to target populations across the globe (Halabi, 2014, p. 148).

Regulatory Approval and Legal Liabilities

Each country's national regulatory authority responding to the pandemic imposed its own regulatory process for approving pH1N1 vaccines, authorizing their importation, and overseeing their distribution (World Health Organization, 2010). These processes ranged from one-time waivers of normal rules to detailed requirements for pediatric subgroup data, regulatory assessments capacity, quality control preparedness and capacity, and postmarketing safety surveillance and field assessment of efficacy and immunogenicity. Some regulatory agencies approved pandemic vaccines as a type of seasonal influenza vaccine, whereas others adapted an approval process in place for candidate H5N1 (avian flu) vaccines. The biochemistry of pH1N1 vaccines varied widely, with adjuvanted vaccines (an adjuvant is an inorganic or organic chemical, macromolecule, or entire cell of certain killed bacteria that enhance the immune response to an antigen) and vaccines produced using cell- rather than egg-based technology facing more significant regulatory review. In more than half the beneficiary countries, prequalification of a vaccine by WHO was not sufficient to obtain regulatory approval, and relatively few countries' national laws stated that products donated by the UN did not require national registration (World Health Organization, 2010).

These requirements, in turn, adversely affected efficacious donation and distribution. Even when a manufacturer agreed in principle to donate to WHO or other UN agencies (e.g., UNICEF), it might not agree to do so if the vaccine would be distributed in a country where that vaccine is not licensed (Crosse, 2008). Since at least 2006, industry representatives have stated that manufacturers would need advance assurance that governments would provide liability protection in order to donate vaccines. Indeed, some manufacturers will not even authorize use of the vaccine for clinical trials if not insured against legal liabilities. Because the initial urgency of the pandemic response required an unprecedented number of doses of a new vaccine to be deployed globally in a period of only a few months, vaccine manufacturers required that all purchasers or recipients (many of which were European and North American governments) indemnify them for adverse events resulting from the use of the pandemic H1N1 vaccine, with exceptions allowed for failure to follow current good manufacturing processes or other discrete specifications.

Manufacturers required access to information on country regulatory processes that was often difficult to obtain. Reallocating products after this work had begun led to additional work for manufacturers and delayed delivery to countries (World Health Organization, 2010). In one instance, a change in the delivery schedule necessitated switching to the product of a different manufacturer, which triggered a de novo review of all aspects of vaccine approval (World Health Organization, 2010). The delays caused by this legal wrangling were substantial. For countries in WHO's African region, vaccines were deployed, on average, 261 days after a country expressed interest in donated vaccine (World Health Organization, 2010). Legal issues surrounding both title and transfer between manufacturers, governments, and beneficiary countries added to the delay (World Health Organization, 2010). "For those countries that were first hit by the emerging pandemic, like those in the Southern Hemisphere, but also for some countries in the Northern Hemisphere, the vaccines clearly came too late and well after the pandemic struck" (Osterhaus et al., 2011, p. 2769).

The complexity of this contracting universe explains, in part, discrepancies in pledged versus contractually committed vaccines. Availability of supply and differing appreciation of available safety and efficacy data influenced where and under what circumstances certain vaccines could be deployed to certain countries (Luteijn et al., 2011). By the end of WHO Deployment Initiative in September 2010, 200 million doses of pandemic influenza A (pH1N1) 2009 vaccine had been pledged for donation, but only 122.5 million doses had been committed contractually. In total, 78 million doses of pandemic influenza A (pH1N1) 2009 were deployed to 77 countries.

Implications for Policy and Practice

Although vaccines are the first line of defense to prevent infection and to control spread of pandemic influenza, the capability to develop and manufacture vaccine is almost entirely under the control of a small number of large pharmaceutical firms whose ability and willingness to respond to a pandemic are fundamentally intertwined with their regulatory and contractual relationships. If a seasonal vaccine is inadequate against a new pandemic influenza strain, which occurred with pH1N1, manufacturers must modify the new virus, coordinate with reference laboratories and regulatory agencies, conduct human trials, and decide whether, and to what extent, to switch seasonal vaccine production to pandemic vaccine production. In 2009, some agreements in place between firms and governments effectively forced this choice (Hanquet et al., 2011). Vaccines must then be tested in human trials to assess safety and effectiveness. Regulatory approval for marketing and use is dependent on laboratory-generated evidence and clinical trial outcomes. Even safe and effective vaccines generate adverse events among those inoculated, and in many jurisdictions manufacturers bear legal responsibility for these adverse events (Swendiman and Jones, 2009).

Each of these aspects of the vaccine development process generated contracting obstacles when WHO and individual governments approached firms with requests for vaccine donation or purchase. Manufacturers faced differing regulatory and approval processes, uncertain protection from legal liabilities, constraints imposed by advance purchase agreements in place with mostly European and North American countries, and equally uncertain and undeveloped systems for distribution even if they could manufacture a limitless number of doses. In short, the global public health response to pandemic influenza in 2009 was dependent on private-sector actors who, under the circumstances then prevailing, demanded both legal assurances and relief from legal requirements in order to participate fully in that response. There were few effective mechanisms for dealing with that reality. An effective global strategy for the next influenza pandemic will require the identification of these contracting and regulatory obstacles, anticipation of new ones, and the creation of ex ante agreements and negotiation for that may facilitate vaccine development and distribution.

Although efforts are underway to increase vaccine manufacturing capacity in developing states, the capability remains overwhelmingly centered in large pharmaceutical firms located in Australia, Japan, Europe, and North America. There is a substantial consensus that capacity for vaccine production is tiny compared with the number of doses required in the event of the next pandemic. WHO, as well as North American and European governments, are funding programs to increase the supply of seasonal and pandemic influenza vaccines by expanding global coverage of seasonal flu vaccine, promoting new development sites (including in developing states), and enhancing research and development for novel influenza vaccines (Condon and Tapen, 2010).

WHO is optimistic the agreements put in place between donor governments and firms between November 2009 and March 2010 will provide a time-saving legal framework for production and distribution of vaccine or other medicines during the next pandemic (World Health Organization, 2010). However, there are reasons to doubt this will be the case based on systemwide response changes. For example, one of the controversial aspects of vaccine development and distribution between 2009 and 2010 was WHO's criteria for identifying a pandemic. Those criteria were based in some measure on geographic spread rather than severity. WHO has agreed to revise these criteria so that the next time it declares a pandemic, the declaration will reflect a more severe public health event on a widespread scale—a scenario likely to render existing legal agreements less applicable than WHO now hopes (Doshi, 2011).

As far as the 2009 pH1N1 experience goes, building capacity without a consistently updated framework for efficiently moving pandemic vaccine from the private sector to the public sphere may simply aggravate the legal and regulatory bottlenecks experienced between 2009 and 2010. The expansion of capacity in middle-income or developing countries enhances the contracting complexity that will likely be faced during the next pandemic. No agreements were reached with firms that are not members of the International Federation of Pharmaceutical Manufacturers Associations, which does not include the small but growing number of manufacturers in developing countries. For the most part, vaccine manufacturers and major purchasers still decide whether to suspend seasonal influenza vaccine production so that all production capacity can be used for pandemic vaccine. Manufacturers also decide whether production of pandemic vaccine can be safely scaled down or suspended in favor of seasonal vaccine. Advance agreements should exist between industry, WHO, and countries regarding these decisions or should at least create ongoing forums that keep relevant stakeholders current on a regular basis on how vaccine manufacturers' commitments affect overall capacity for production in the case of a pandemic.

Approval processes for national regulatory authorities created a major obstacle not just for initial agreements to donate, but also for logistical practicalities that favored deployment of pandemic vaccines as quickly as possible to countries that needed them as soon as possible. As with the vaccine framework developed for H1N1, regulatory harmonization has been shaped by pre-2009 preparations for emergence of a pandemic H5N1 influenza virus strain. WHO, in collaboration with health authorities from Canada, Japan, Spain, and the United States, convened three technical workshops between 2006 and 2007 to examine regulatory harmonization, but the results are shaped by detailed examination of countries with clear regulatory mandates and at least one major vaccine manufacturer. The 2009 H1N1 pandemic has not resulted in a measurable increase in agreements between national regulatory authorities or with WHO on data sharing, mutual recognition, of some or all aspects of vaccine approval.

Moreover, the difficulty lesser developed and middle-income countries experienced in obtaining pandemic H1N1 vaccine exacerbated already existing tensions over the process of developing medicines and vaccines (which frequently involves the use of flu samples obtained in developing countries) and making them available at affordable prices. In 2007, Indonesia withheld samples of influenza A (H5N1) from WHO, arguing that developing countries typically shared such samples for free only to have North American and European firms patent derivative medicines and vaccines for sale in richer states, out of reach (in financial and other terms) from developing countries. In response, WHO and the World Health Assembly adopted the Pandemic Influenza Preparedness Framework, under which member states and vaccine manufacturers have agreed on a standard material transfer agreement that regulates the terms under which countries agree to donate influenza samples, the entities authorized to receive and research them, and the corresponding sharing of resulting vaccines and other intellectual properties (Halabi, 2014). WHO is currently negotiating with six vaccine manufacturers based on the standard material transfer agreement, with one agreement concluded with GSK. These agreements provide several options to manufacturers regarding the contributions they must make in exchange for virus access. Some of these options involve pandemic vaccine donation, while others involve antiviral donations, and still others authorize licensing of intellectual property to developing country manufacturers. These agreements, especially the options manufacturers choose, must coexist with the advance purchase agreements and, presumably, liability issues outlined above. Together with the proliferation of advance purchase agreements and the unknown extent of vaccine stockpiling agreements, the commitments made by manufacturers under WHO's Pandemic Influenza Preparedness Framework may render the legal framework used in 2009 obsolete.

Vaccines are the front line in the global response to the next pandemic influenza outbreak, and thus their manufacturers—together with public health agencies—form a critical public–private partnership. The seasonal–pandemic influenza vaccine production balance; the process by which vaccines are developed, researched, and approved for use by regulatory agencies; the potential liability manufacturers face; and the contractual limitations imposed by advance purchase agreements all portend potential delays for the necessary global health response. WHO has already noted that advance agreements between itself, countries, and industries should be negotiated without regard to virus subtype for a specified period of time (e.g., three to five years) and should be regularly reviewed and renewed. Countries that receive donated vaccine, as any purchaser of the vaccine, should adhere to the same practices of releasing and indemnifying manufacturers from certain legal liabilities. Whether donated or purchased, vaccine manufacturers have emphasized that liability protection is a crucial part of their participation in the broader response to pandemic influenza (International Federation of Pharmaceutical Manufacturers and Associations, 2006). As WHO's Final Report on the functioning of the International Health Regulations in relation to the 2009 A(PH1N1) pandemic noted:

> Despite the ultimate deployment of 78 million doses of pandemic influenza vaccine to 77 countries, numerous systemic difficulties impeded the timely distribution of donated vaccines. Among the key difficulties was a variation in willingness to donate, concerns about liability, complex negotiations over legal agreements, lack of procedures to bypass national regulatory requirements and limited national and local capacities to transport, store and administer vaccines. Some beneficiary countries felt WHO did not adequately explain that liability provisions included in the beneficiary agreement were the same as the liability provisions accepted by purchasing countries. All these difficulties proved daunting in the midst of a pandemic; some could have been reduced by more

concerted preparation and advance arrangements among all interested parties. (Available online at http://apps.who.int/gb/ebwha/pdf_files/WHA64/A64_10-en.pdf?ua=1, p. 133)

Acknowledgments and Disclosures

This research was conducted after conversations with John Monahan, whose observations at the U.S. Department of State during the 2009 pandemic prompted the author's inquiry into the complex contracting environment in which pharmaceutical firms, governments, and international organizations operate. The author is grateful for comments from John Monahan, Bruce Gellin, Oscar Cabrera, Susan Kim, and Fernanda Alonso; and for research support from the O'Neill Institute for National and Global Health Law at Georgetown University. The data and conclusions have been published previously in one briefing report:

- Halabi, S. F. (2014). The uncertain future of vaccine development and deployment for influenza pandemic. O'Neill Institute for National and Global Health law briefing paper no. 8. Accessed March 19, 2014, at http://www.law.georgetown.edu/oneillinstitute/resources/documents/Briefing8Halabi.pdf.

References

Aledort, J., Lurie, N., Wasserman, J., Bozette, S. (2007). Non-pharmaceutical public health interventions for pandemic influenza: an evaluation of the evidence base. *BMC Public Health*, 7, 208–217.

Carter, N. J., Plosker, G. L. (2008). Prepandemic influenza vaccine H5N1 (split virion, inactivated, adjuvanted) [Prepandrix]: a review of its use as an active immunization against influenza A subtype H5N1 virus. *BioDrugs*, *22*(5), 279–292.

Centers for Disease Control and Prevention (CDC). (2009). Serum cross-reactive antibody response to a novel influenza A (H1N1) virus after vaccination with seasonal influenza vaccine. Accessed January 28, 2014, at http://www.cdc.gov/mmwr/preview/mmwrhtml/mm5819a1.htm.

Centers for Disease Control and Prevention (CDC). (2012). First global estimates of 2009 H1N1 pandemic mortality released by CDC-led collaboration. Accessed January 28, 2014, at http://www.cdc.gov/flu/spotlights/pandemic-global-estimates.htm.

Centers for Disease Control and Prevention (CDC). (2013). CDC statement on narcolepsy following Prepandrix influenza vaccination in Europe. Accessed January 28, 2014, at http://www.cdc.gov/vaccinesafety/Concerns/h1n1_narcolepsy_pandemrix.html.

Condon, B., Tapen, S. (2010). The effectiveness of pandemic preparations: legal lessons from the 2009 influenza epidemic. *Florida Journal of International Law*, 1, 7.

Cordova-Villalobos, J. A., Sarti, E., Arzoz-Padres, J., Manuell-Lee, G., Mendez, J. R. (2009). The influenza A(H1N1) epidemic in Mexico: lessons learned. *Health Research Policy and Systems, 7*, 21.

Crosse, M. (2008). Influenza pandemic: efforts underway to address constraints on using antivirals and vaccines to forestall a pandemic. Accessed March 9, 2014, at http://www.gao.gov/new.items/d0892.pdf.

Doshi, P. (2011). The elusive definition of pandemic influenza. *Bulletin of the World Health Organization, 89*, 532–538.

Doshi, P., Jefferson, T. (2010). Another question for GSK. *British Medical Journal, 340*, c3455.

European Commission. (2010). Assessment report on EU-wide pandemic vaccine strategies. Accessed January 28, 2014, at http://ec.europa.eu/health/communicable_diseases/docs/assessment_vaccine_en.pdf.

European Medicines Agency. (2004). *Guideline on submission of marketing authorization applications for pandemic influenza vaccines through the centralized procedure.* London: EMEA.

Fidler, D. P. (2010). Negotiating equitable access to influenza vaccines: global health diplomacy and the controversies surrounding avian influenza H5N1 and pandemic influenza H1N1. *PLoS Medicine, 7*, e1000247.

Halabi, S. (2014). Multipolarity, intellectual property, and the internationalization of public health law. *Michigan Journal of International Law, 35*, 1.

Hancock, K., Veguilla, V., Lu, X. (2009). Cross-reactive antibody responses to the 2009 pandemic PH1N1 influenza virus. *The New England Journal of Medicine, 361*, 1945–1952.

Hanquet, G., Van, D. P., Brasseur, D., De, C., Gregor, S., Holmberg, M., Martin, R., Molnár, Z., Pompa, M. G., Snacken, R., van der Sande, M., Van Ranst, M., Wirtz, A., Neels, P. (2011). Lessons learnt from pandemic A(H1N1) 2009 influenza vaccination: highlights of a European workshop in Brussels. *Vaccine, 29*, 370–377.

International Federation of Pharmaceutical Manufacturers and Associations. (2006). Pandemic influenza vaccines and liability protection for manufacturers. Accessed January 28, 2014, at http://www.ifpma.org/fileadmin/content/Global%20Health/Influenza/Ref_56_IFPMA_IVS_Request_on_Liability_May_19_2006.pdf.

Luteijn, J., Dolk, H., Marnoch, G. (2011). Differences in pandemic influenza vaccination policies for pregnant women in Europe. *BMC Public Health, 11*, 819–28.

McConnell, J. (2010). Pandemic influenza: learning from the present. *Public Health, 124*(1), 3–4.

Osterhaus, A. B., Fouchier, R., Rimmelzwaan, G. (2011). Towards universal influenza vaccines. *Philosophical Transactions of the Royal Society of London, Series B, 366*, 2766–2773.

Standing Senate Committee on Social Affairs, Parliament of Canada. (2010). Proceedings. Accessed January 28, 2014, at http://www.parl.gc.ca/Content/SEN/Committee/403/soci/13eva-e.htm?Language=E&Parl=40&Ses=3&comm_id=47.

Swendiman, K., Jones, N. L. (2009). The 2009 influenza pandemic: selected legal issues. Congressional Research Service, 19. Accessed March 9, 2014, at http://www.fas.org/sgp/crs/misc/R40560.pdf.

World Health Organization. (2010). Main operational lessons learnt from the WHO pandemic influenza A(H1N1) vaccine deployment initiative. Accessed January 28, 2014, at http://www.who.int/influenza_vaccines_plan/resources/h1n1_vaccine_deployment_initiaitve_moll.pdf.

World Health Organization. (2011a). Implementation of the international health regulations. Accessed March 9, 2014, at http://www.who.int/ihr/en/.

World Health Organization. (2011b). Report of the review committee on the functioning of the international health regulations in relation to pandemic H1N1. Accessed March 9, 2014, at http://www.who.int/ihr/preview_report_review_committee_mar2011_en.pdf.

World Health Organization. (2012a). Observed rate of vaccination reactions influenza vaccine. Accessed January 28, 2014, at http://www.who.int/vaccine_safety/initiative/tools/Influenza_Vaccine_rates_information_sheet.pdf.

World Health Organization. (2012b). Report of the WHO pandemic influenza A(H1N1) vaccine deployment initiative. Accessed January 28, 2014, at http://www.who.int/influenza_vaccines_plan/resources/h1n1_deployment_report.pdf.

CHAPTER 13 | Implications for Policy and Practice

MICHAEL A. STOTO

Introduction

The 2009 H1N1 pandemic required a concerted response effort from—and tested—the entire public health emergency preparedness (PHEP) system in the United States and other countries. The pandemic was identified quickly and characterized by laboratories in the United States and Mexico, triggering pandemic influenza response plans around the globe. However, public health surveillance systems were arguably less effective in tracking the pandemic accurately over time and identifying groups that were at greater risk of its consequences. Some school systems moved quickly to close to protect children and to limit the spread of pH1N1 in the community, but the epidemiologic impact of this strategy might not have justified the costs. In less than a year, a new vaccine was developed and produced, and despite production delays in and widespread concerns about its safety, more than 80 million Americans were eventually immunized, including 34% of the population groups initially targeted (Institute of Medicine, 2010). Globally, 78 million doses of pandemic influenza vaccine were deployed to 77 countries, but numerous systemic difficulties impeded the timely distribution of donated vaccines (Fineberg, 2014). In the United States, approximately half of the 162 million doses of 2009 H1N1 vaccine produced went unused (Institute of Medicine, 2010).

Whether the outcome can be counted as a success, a failure, or, more appropriately, some combination of the two, the experience did provide an opportunity to learn about U.S. and global PHEP capabilities. The primary goal of this book was to capture these lessons—something the first U.S. National Health Security Strategy (Department of Health and Human Services, 2009) called for specifically. A second goal was to outline efforts for measuring and improving the level of preparedness in current public health systems centered on the 2009 H1N1 experience. Based on the preceding analyses, this final chapter presents crosscutting conclusions about the implications for policy and practice.

The authors of each chapter took a systems perspective when analyzing the public health response to 2009 H1N1. "Public health systems" are understood to include not only government health agencies—federal, state, and local—but also hospitals and healthcare providers, fire departments, schools, community organizations such as schools and the media, and many others. Consistent with the "quality improvement spirit" called for in the U. S. National Health Security Strategy (U.S. Department of Health and Human Services, 2010a) the intent is neither to praise nor blame, but to identify opportunities to improve PHEP systems. Hence, the focus was not on what went well or poorly per se, but rather on whether the underlying root causes of problems that occurred that, if addressed, have the potential to improve future PHEP system performance.

Drawing on the PHEP logic model (Figure 13-1), we also sought to distinguish between the PHEP system's response capabilities, which we believe are the basic dimensions of preparedness, and the system's preparedness capacities.

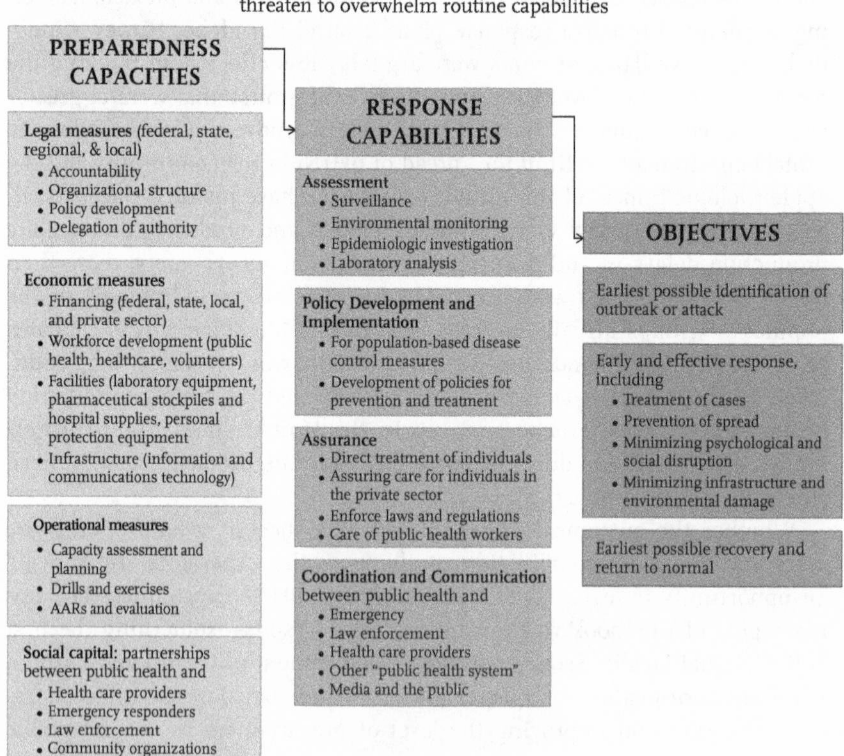

FIGURE 13-1

Capacities represent the resources—infrastructure, response mechanisms, knowledgeable and trained personnel—on which a public health system has to draw. These capacities include legal, economic, and operational dimensions (Potter et al., 2013), and "social capital"—the intangible partnership and informal relationships among individuals and organizations that research shows are critical to effective emergency operations and community resilience. Capacities are, in general, easy to measure, but we often have no credible evidence that the capacities—individually or in combination—in fact ensure the desired outcome.

Capabilities, on the other hand, describe the actions a public health system is capable of taking effectively to identify, characterize, and respond to emergencies: surveillance, epidemiologic investigations, disease prevention and mitigation, surge capacity for healthcare services, risk communication to the public, and coordination of system responses through an effective incident management system. Capabilities are latent characteristics of the PHEP system that are best measured and assessed when the PHEP system responds to an emergency, as it did in 2009.

We begin with the three major PHEP capabilities that were most tested during the 2009 H1N1 pandemic: biosurveillance, medical countermeasure dispensing, and public communication. We then discuss a series of more general issues that must be addressed to ensure an effective response to future public health emergencies. We conclude this chapter with a discussion of the implications of our analyses for ongoing efforts to measure and improve PHEP. This analysis draws primarily on the chapters in this book, supplemented with other reviews of different aspects of the U.S. and global response.

Basic PHEP Capabilities

Biosurveillance: Public Health Surveillance and Epidemiologic Analysis

In one major respect, the public health system response to 2009 H1N1 was a major success; only 10 days passed between Mexican health authorities' recognition of a possible new epidemic and their announcement of it—a sharp contrast to the many months in 2003 between the outbreak of severe acute respiratory syndrome in China and its public declaration (Wenzel, 2010). In Chapter 2, Zhang and Stoto demonstrate that investments in global surveillance and notification systems made an important difference in the 2009 H1N1 pandemic. In particular, enhanced laboratory capacity in the United States and Canada—including enhanced capacity at the federal, state, and local levels in the United States, and a trilateral agreement enabling collaboration among the United States, Canada, and Mexico—led to earlier detection and characterization of 2009 H1N1. In addition, and perhaps more important, improved global notification systems such as the Global Public Health Intelligence Network, ProMED Mail, and HealthMap that enabled Mexican officials to "connect the dots" to realize outbreaks they were aware of throughout the country were all manifestations of the pandemic virus (pH1N1) that had just been isolated in two children in California. The expectations set up by the 2005 international health regulations (IHRs) (World Health Organization, 2008)—that countries would report a potential "public health emergency of international concern" (PHEIC)—were also important.

This same analysis showed that syndromic surveillance played an important role in detecting the pH1N1 outbreak, but a different one than is commonly used to justify these systems. Syndromic surveillance systems, which collect and analyze statistical data on health trends—such as symptoms reported by people seeking care in emergency departments (EDs) or other healthcare settings, or even sales of prescription or over-the-counter flu medicines or Web searches—are typically used to detect outbreaks before conventional surveillance systems to enable a rapid public health response (Stoto, 2007). Because pH1N1 emerged in the winter, there were too few cases to be detected against the background of the normal flu season. Rather, increases in influenza like illnesses (ILIs) led authorities to conduct active surveillance for severe pneumonia, and later provided positive confirmation that the virus had spread widely throughout Mexico.

Despite this generally good performance, there was a period of one to two weeks in April 2009 when Mexican authorities were aware of an unusual pattern of disease outbreaks in different parts of the country (events that were reported globally through the Global Public Health Intelligence Network, ProMED Mail, and HealthMap) but didn't understand the full implications of the evidence. In particular, the point at which it becomes clear that something is a PHEIC is often not very distinct. The IHRs require countries to report a PHEIC within 24 hours of assessment of the public health information by the national authority (World Health Organization, 2008). Judging that an event must be reported requires a number of complicated assessments, including the following:

1. Is the pathogen a new subtype of human influenza or another pathogen listed in IHR Annex 2?
2. Is the public health impact serious?
3. Is the event unusual or unexpected?
4. Is there a significant risk of international spread?

In 2009, the Center for Disease Control and Prevention's (CDC's) report of a new influenza strain in humans in the United States helped Mexico answer the first question in the affirmative, making the others redundant. Going forward, it is important to recognize that, even in the best of circumstances, some period of uncertainty of this sort is to be expected and planned for. The implications of such uncertainty, which is likely to characterize many future public health emergencies, are discussed in the following pages.

After a new pathogen is identified, it must be characterized to develop testing kits and surveillance procedures; to create and manufacture a vaccine, to set policies for its use; and to guide interventions such as infection control policies, social distancing, and quarantine. In 2009, the enhanced laboratory capacity just discussed led to the rapid characterization of the pH1N1 virus itself, development of a vaccine, polymerase chain reaction testing kits, and so on. On the other hand, the epidemiologic characteristics of pH1N1 were harder to identify, and included disease incidence and rates of change of incidence, severity of infection, and risks to specific population groups. Estimates of these quantities inform decisions about control measures, and resource procurement and allocation. They also affect public perceptions of illness severity and risk, which influence the willingness of people to comply with control measures (Lipsitch et al., 2009).

As is often the case, under ascertainment of infected individuals with less severe cases led to an initial overestimate of case fatality rate, and the mischaracterization of virus "severity" (Garske et al., 2009; Lipsitch et al., 2009; Wong et al., 2013). Early evidence from Mexico, based on an observational study of hospitalized patients, suggested that 6.5% were critically ill and 41% of these patients died (Domínguez-Cherit et al., 2009; Fineberg, 2014). And although epidemiologists understand this phenomenon, policymakers and the public understandably find such figures—especially "41% of these died," taken out of context to make the point—as quite alarming. It was not until around September 2009—five months into the pandemic—that epidemiologists began to confirm the accurate case fatality rate, which was roughly comparable with the case fatality rate for seasonal influenza (Butler, 2010).

Confusion about the case fatality rate was compounded by differences in whether "severity" referred to virulence or ability to spread globally—the basis for the World Health Organization's (WHO's) pandemic phase classification in force at that time. This led to public confusion about exactly what the WHO meant by a pandemic, and complicated decision making about response logistics that depend on both spread and severity (Fineberg, 2014).

With regard to public health assessment capabilities (especially surveillance and epidemiologic analysis), Stoto shows in Chapter 3 how most public health surveillance data are potentially biased because they depend on a series of decisions made by patients, healthcare providers, and public health professionals about seeking and providing health care, and about reporting cases or otherwise taking action that comes to the attention of health authorities. Outpatient, hospital-based, and ED surveillance systems, for instance, all rely on individuals presenting themselves to healthcare facilities, and these decisions are based in part on their interpretations of their symptoms. Similarly, virologic surveillance and systems based on laboratory confirmations depend on physicians deciding to send specimens for testing. Even the number of Google searches and self-reports of ILI can be influenced by individuals' interpretation of the seriousness of their symptoms. Every element of this decision-making process is potentially influenced by the informational and policy environment (e.g., media coverage, current case definitions and practice recommendations, implementation of active surveillance), processing and reacting to the information on an individual level (e.g., healthcare seekers' self-assessment of risk, incentives for seeking medical attention, and self-isolation; healthcare provider's ordering of laboratory tests), and technical barriers (e.g., communication infrastructure for data exchange, laboratory capacity). And all these decisions are potentially influenced by what these people know and think, both of which change during the course of an outbreak. Recognizing the possibility of these biases but not knowing their extent of full impact adds to the uncertainty that characterizes public health emergencies.

Stoto (Chapter 3) concludes by calling for seroprevalence surveys, which are crucial to making informed policy decisions. For instance, case fatality rate is a key measurement of the severity of a pandemic, but getting a handle on it requires precise estimates of how many people have been infected. It was not until around September 2009—five months into the pandemic—that epidemiologists began to get such data (Butler, 2010).

Writing after the first wave of the pandemic, Hanfling and Hick (2009) addressed surveillance capabilities from the perspective of the healthcare delivery sector. To know what impact the pH1N1 outbreak had on ED, laboratory, and other hospital resources, they prepared an ongoing tally of ED patient visits, screening tests for influenza, and inpatient admissions of cases with febrile respiratory illness. This information was often facilitated by electronic medical record (EMR) systems—where available—and the ability to build screening questions flexibly (e.g., travel history and symptoms) into the ED triage process and adjust them to the evolving situation. Exposure tracking was also important; "internal" surveillance efforts had to include a clinical reporting mechanism for identifying staff exposures to potential influenza patients. Regular reporting of such data contributed to the ongoing efforts to provide situational awareness to the healthcare system or hospital leadership.

Medical Countermeasure Dispensing—Antivirals

The first wave of the 2009 H1N1 influenza pandemic presented an unusual opportunity to learn about the role of local public health in the management of antiviral response activities during a real public health emergency, and to provide practitioners, policymakers, and academicians with an understanding of the challenges they faced and a practice-based assessment of these events. As Hunter and colleagues describe in Chapter 6, although most communities dispensed a modest number of publicly purchased antivirals, local health departments (LHDs) nevertheless drew on their previous work and engaged in a number of antiviral activities, including acquiring, allocating, distributing, dispensing, tracking, developing guidance, and communicating to the public and clinical community. LHDs also identified specific antiviral challenges presented by the H1N1 pandemic, including reconciling multiple sources and versions of antiviral guidance, determining appropriate uses and recipients of publicly purchased antivirals, and coping with staffing shortages.

Hunter and colleagues (Chapter 6) identified two potential contributors to confusion at the local level that were also seen in a national analysis of LHDs conducted by National Association of County and City Health Officials (NACCHO) (2010). First, federal antiviral guidance during the H1N1 response focused primarily on clinical recommendations for antiviral use and did not address directly how public stockpiles should be used. Second, clinical antiviral guidance changed during the course of the pandemic, focusing originally on post exposure prophylaxis, and later on early treatment.

Hunter and colleagues (Chapter 6) also demonstrated that the recommended uses and recipients of publicly purchased antivirals during the H1N1 response differed from what LHDs had anticipated in their prepandemic plans, and that this resulted in additional difficulties. During the 2009 H1N1 pandemic, antivirals were generally available through normal wholesale and retail markets; as a result, the California state health department recommended that LHDs use publicly purchased drugs for the treatment of uninsured or underinsured persons and for communities experiencing shortages. For many health departments, this represented a significant shift in their prepandemic antiviral implementation strategy. Previous policy had focused on the use of publicly purchased antivirals for treatment of ill persons after retail supplies had been depleted, and emphasized the role of antivirals in protecting healthcare workers and other first responders. As a consequence, LHDs revised their plans to support these new strategies, although implementing and communicating these strategies caused a strain on some LHDs and community partners.

Hunter and colleagues (Chapter 6) found that agencies cited staffing issues as a challenge during their antiviral response. As noted by one participant, current public health resources were insufficient for local health agencies to deliver antiviral services confidently in a "secure, accountable, consistent, and equitable manner" during a pandemic with a larger scope or greater severity. These concerns should be taken into account in the future development of antiviral and medical countermeasure plans and policies.

Hunter and colleagues (Chapter 6) also found greater than expected variability in the approaches used by LHDs to manage publicly purchased antiviral drugs. Some of this variability is attributable to differences in the circumstances faced by LHDs (e.g., influenza illness incidence, community demographics, availability of antivirals in the retail market), whereas other variation is a result of differences in disease control and prevention strategies.

Hanfling and Hick (2009) also addressed the question of antivirals during the first wave of the pandemic. Neither hospital nor community pharmacies, they wrote, had significant stocks of antiviral medications on hand, in part because of a history of ambivalent support for their use in treating seasonal influenza, and the decreased sensitivity of circulating seasonal H1N1 strains to olseltamivir. The release of 25% of the strategic national stockpile to those states with confirmed cases was not particularly helpful in some areas because, in the absence of CDC guidance for preferred methods of distribution and use, state and local plans for distribution of the strategic national stockpile were inconsistent, and often not appropriate for limited distribution of pharmaceuticals. In addition, there was confusion related to shifting guidelines for antiviral administration. This was in part a function of the apparently "exploding" communicability of pH1N1 disease across the United States.

Medical Countermeasure Dispensing—Vaccine

The fall wave of 2009 H1N1 challenged the public health system to expand vaccine production and distribution capabilities sharply. The pandemic offered a stark reminder that current techniques for making a flu vaccine take too long—around six months from the identification of the new virus to production of any sizeable vaccine quantities (Butler, 2010). Many observers have called for investments in technologies that will ensure a more timely availability of the needed quantities of vaccine (Rambhia et al., 2010).

In Chapter 12, Halibi wrote that, although vaccines are the first line of defense to prevent infection and to control spread of pandemic influenza, the capability to develop and manufacture them is almost entirely under the control of private for-profit business entities. This situation created obstacles to vaccination donation and distribution by the major global pharmaceutical companies, the WHO, and donor and recipient governments in 2009. First, if a seasonal vaccine is inadequate against a new strain (which happened with pH1N1), manufacturers must modify the new virus to create a vaccine seed stock, coordinate with reference laboratories and regulatory agencies, conduct human trials, and decide whether (and how far) to switch seasonal vaccine production to pandemic vaccine production. Vaccines must then be tested in human trials to assess safety and effectiveness. Each of these steps generated contracting obstacles when the WHO and individual governments approached firms with requests for vaccine donation or purchase. Manufacturers face differing regulatory and approval processes, uncertain protection from legal liabilities, constraints imposed by advance purchase agreements in place with wealthier countries, and equally uncertain and undeveloped systems for distribution, even if they could manufacture a limitless number of doses. This experience, therefore, shows how the global public health response to pandemic influenza is dependent on private-sector actors who require both legal assurances and relief from legal requirements to participate fully in that response. An effective global strategy for the next influenza pandemic will hinge on the identification of these contracting and donation obstacles, and the creation of ex ante agreements to facilitate vaccine development and distribution.

Because vaccines are produced and distributed in a global pharmaceutical market, it is important to explore the influence of national policies. According to a review by Hanquet and colleagues (2010), pandemic vaccination policies differed across European Union countries and throughout the pandemic. All countries, however, faced similar challenges: how to interpret, collate, and analyze

TABLE 13-1 Reported Local Strategies to Vaccinate through the Healthcare System during 2009 H_1N_1.

STRATEGY	NOTES
Increased communication with healthcare providers	Local health departments built ties to health providers, especially those most likely to come in contact with individuals in the priority groups, including obstetricians, pediatricians, and other health providers. Including obstetricians, pediatricians, and other health providers.
Use of a tiered approach for vaccine distribution to health providers	Pediatricians, obstetricians, community health clinics, and providers serving larger numbers of priority group individuals were the first to receive vaccine. Other providers, including pharmacies, were given vaccine as supplies from manufacturers increased.
Targeted communications	Federal, state, and local communications targeted obstetricians and women who were pregnant. As vaccine supplies increased, communications expanded to the general public.
Registries of providers	Local providers participated in an immunization registry, organized by local and state health departments, to order vaccine, communicate with health officials, and maintain immunization records.

Source: Rambhia, K. et al., 2010.

burden of disease data; how to prioritize target groups for vaccination; how to convince target groups to get vaccinated when they feel at low risk and lack confidence in the vaccine; how to communicate effectively on pandemic vaccine safety and efficacy; how to deliver vaccine more effectively; and how to generate timely data on vaccine uptake and safety. To improve preparedness for future influenza pandemics, Hanquet and colleagues (2010) call for national-level improvements in vaccine safety and efficacy communication plans, transparent decision processes on prioritization of target groups, and strategies to obtain timely estimates of vaccine uptake. International health agencies should increase the flexibility between pandemic vaccine licensure and pandemic phases, and address vaccine licensing and availability at the end of a pandemic.

Rambhia and colleagues (2010) have documented the variety of vaccination strategies used at the local level in the United States (Table 13-1). According to participants at an Institute of Medicine workshop, the diversity in approaches meant that neighboring jurisdictions often had different distribution systems, causing confusion and communications challenges (Institute of Medicine, 2010).

Whether programs were based in schools, in public health departments, or with healthcare providers, the most successful initiatives were built on preexisting relationships. Close relationships between health departments in neighboring jurisdictions helped to coordinate the response within a region.

In many cases, joint conference calls among providers, health departments, and government officials facilitated information sharing and vaccine sharing between jurisdictions. Among other suggestions, the authors recommend developing local public health capacity and relationships with healthcare providers, and enhancing federal support of state and local activities (Rambhia et al., 2010).

Perhaps the biggest problem encountered in 2009 was out of the control of the state and local public health systems: uncertainties and delays in the production and delivery of vaccine to those who could administer it. To some, the solution is simple; public health authorities should "underpromise and overdeliver" on vaccine supplies. Others recommended that federal authorities develop a stronger and more formal partnership with vaccine producers to ensure they have the most up-to-date information on production and inventory, and can generate more accurate supply projections, and integrate existing systems and technologies further, such as barcoding and electronic tracking to improve the ability to track vaccine throughout the distribution and administration system (Institute of Medicine, 2010).

Another challenge was that the Advisory Committee on Immunization Practices (ACIP) recommendations did not entirely match previous federal pandemic planning documents, which had been developed with H5N1 avian flu in mind. The latter called for priority immunization of first responders and critical infrastructure workers, but ACIP's guidance did not. Another challenge was the exclusion of elderly people from the ACIP recommendations (Institute of Medicine, 2010).

In Chapter 7, Chamberlain and colleagues reported that most state and local immunization program managers found their pandemic influenza plan was helpful during the 2009 response. In addition, from the perspective of immunization program managers, emergency preparedness staff members were more helpful when they had collaborated with the immunization program on actual or simulated mass vaccination events in the previous two years. Among the few respondents who perceived their pandemic influenza plan as unhelpful, the primary reasons cited were the inappropriateness of the plan for the specific characteristics of this pandemic and the plan being outdated or inadequate in scope. The top three challenges cited were cultural differences between the programs, resource allocation, and leadership conflict or ambiguity. Communication was the theme indicated most commonly as both a success and a challenge.

Chamberlain and colleagues' results (Chapter 7) also suggested that expanded use of immunization information systems (IISs) can enhance immunization program ability to manage a large-scale vaccination campaign successfully. Managers from jurisdictions that did mandate IIS data entry were more likely to rate their IIS as valuable for facilitating registration of nontraditional vaccine providers such as obstetricians and pharmacists (42% vs. 25%, $p < 0.05$), and for tracking recalled influenza vaccine (50% vs. 38%, $p < 0.05$).

Higdon and Stoto's case study of Massachusetts (Chapter 8) demonstrated how the most effective way to implement a given capability—mass administration of a medical countermeasure, specifically the pH1N1 vaccine—depends on the local context. For instance, because children made up a large proportion of the target population, most communities found school-based clinics to be an effective way to administer the vaccine. Boston, on the other hand, found that its network of community health centers with established trusting links to the populations they serve worked well. And a large group practice used its existing EMR system effectively to call and set up appointments on any given weekend for patients for whom the available vaccine was appropriate. On Martha's Vineyard and in other rural settings, small LHDs found it useful to collaborate and pool resources to conduct regional clinics. Flexibility and adaptively were more important than LHDs having capacities that met a statewide or national standard for points of distribution (PODS).

In their analysis of high-performing LHDs, Klaiman and colleagues (Chapter 10) found that one of the keys to success in public vaccination clinics was defining the priority groups clearly before implementing public clinics. Success in reaching priority groups required access to vulnerable populations, which depended on strong, previously established partnerships with community organizations. Community partners were also vital in lending support to LHDs in areas such as safety and line control, vaccine administration, space donation, and help in setting up and taking down the clinics. LHDs that had existing relationships with community partners had fewer challenges getting stakeholders to agree on priorities, and had more streamlined clinic planning processes. Flexibility in decision making, staffing, and clinic implementation early during the vaccination campaign helped LHDs to be successful. LHDs used situational awareness to build from existing plans, but altered them as needed. LHDs had to implement new-staff training, recruit new staff and volunteers, and establish new policies while they were responding to an emergency.

With respect to school clinics, Klaiman and colleagues (Chapter 10) reported that many successful LHDs had previously established relationships with the school districts in their jurisdiction, making the vaccination location decision clear. For example, they discovered that small, rural LHDs depended on informal relationships with school administrators and nurses, whereas larger, more urban LHDs used more formal relationships. This is a reflection of the local community in which the school nurse may be the neighbor or fellow community group member of the local emergency planner. Personal relationships allow for less formality in partnerships, whereas formal relationships may solidify partnerships that would not exist otherwise. In rural communities, a neighbor may also be the local police chief who has a child in the same school. Such personal relationships allow for less formality in working with partners. Large, urban LHDs may require formal memoranda of understanding because organizational staff do not know each other.

According to Klaiman and colleagues (Chapter 10), global buy-in of the school system, intensive planning, constant communication, and trusting relationships between health department staff and the school districts were vital to the success of the school vaccination campaign. Some LHDs previously held mass vaccination drills or seasonal flu clinics in local schools, so clinic setup and implementation had already been practiced. Most successful LHDs had worked with school officials in the emergency preparedness planning process. School nurses served a vital role in the relationship between LHDs and local schools. The school nurses helped with planning and organizing the clinics, and acted as liaisons between LHDs and the schools.

Klaiman and colleagues (Chapter 10) reported that schools used a variety of mechanisms for distributing forms and communicating with parents about vaccinations. Schools that reached out directly to parents through a preexisting listserv or automated phone system received more feedback than those who sent slips home with children without following up with another form of communication. School nurses were typically responsible for data collection and management, and were also responsible for ensuring that each child who received a vaccine had a permission slip. School nurses reviewed each form to make sure the information was correct before the child received the vaccine, and in some instances had to call a parent or guardian to verify information on the form. Some LHDs used electronic databases to manage and store this information. However, entering the data manually was very time intensive, and many LHDs had to hire extra staff to complete this process. Because it took so long for most LHDs to enter the information about those vaccinated, they resorted to counting the forms to determine how many children were vaccinated at each clinic, thus undermining the value of the system for providing real-time tracking information.

Public Communication

An effective national immunization campaign required intensive efforts to communicate with the public about the need for the pH1N1 vaccine, when and where it was available, priority groups, and vaccine risks. It also bears noting that vaccines are not the only defense against a flu virus. Other, simpler strategies—such as hand washing, sanitation, and distancing measures such as keeping sick people at home—can stem the spread of a virus quickly, but these practices, too, must be communicated for the public to adopt them. Indeed, according to Steel-Fisher and colleagues (2010), surveys taken during the 2009 H1N1 pandemic suggest that public health communication efforts related to other personal influenza prevention behaviors were effective in reaching a large swath of the public.

In the United States, communication with the public involved the efforts of the CDC, state and local health departments, healthcare providers, and the media. Savoia and colleagues reported in Chapter 11 that there was a wide array of outlets to which people were exposed to messages about pH1N1. Local television news was reported as the primary source of information, followed by local newspapers. Most participants did not rate television as a highly trusted source. The most trusted source for pH1N1 information was healthcare professionals, including doctors and nurses. As a result of these efforts, a good portion of the U.S. population had very good knowledge about pH1N1, yet there were substantial inequalities. Socioeconomic position in general, and level of education in particular, were associated strongly with knowledge about pH1N1. Knowledge about pH1N1 was also related to home ownership—an indicator of social cohesion as well as economic status. Owning a home may signal better integration into the community and greater trust in local authorities, which in turn may affect willingness to heed the message and consequent ability to learn from the information received.

Savoia and colleagues reported in Chapter 11 that pH1N1 vaccine uptake was associated with socioeconomic position and demographic factors, pH1N1-related beliefs, and seasonal vaccination uptake. Fewer than half the people surveyed with a high school degree perceived the vaccine as safe, whereas two-thirds of those with a bachelor's degree or higher did. Blacks were the ethnic/racial group least likely to report believing the pH1N1 vaccine was safe, and blacks with less than a bachelor's degree were the least likely to have received the vaccine. Blacks were also more likely to have tried and failed to find vaccine.

In Italy, on the other hand, Savoia and colleagues noted in Chapter 9 that inconsistency of messages regarding vaccine priority groups, together with regional and local public health officials being asked to execute decrees with which they disagreed, created logistical and communications challenges in vaccine administration. Rumors surrounding vaccine safety, generated in part by the media, undermined public trust in government that may have generated additional barriers in communication.

Focusing on Mexico, on the other hand, Stern and Markel (2009) wrote that, vested with authority to act for the president during the crisis, Mexico's Health Secretary served as the only governmental spokesman at the height of the outbreak, delivering consistent information in accordance with regularly updated epidemiologic and clinical data. He invited stakeholders from key arenas of health, government, media, and education literally to share the stage with him at daily, sometimes hourly, press briefings. As a result, information sources and messages were strictly aligned to avoid public confusion.

In addition, Mexico's health promotion department disseminated a wide array of public health pamphlets and posters throughout the country. Reflecting Mexico's heterogeneous population and uneven literacy rates, these materials relied heavily on visual representations and appear to have influenced social behavior positively. In addition, the national media, including television, radio, and print, collaborated well with the health promotion department to educate citizens on personal hygiene techniques. The general consensus is that Mexicans implemented non-pharmaceutical interventions willingly and with little pushback. There are strong indications this may have been related to Mexico's multisector approach to health crises, which seeks to involve citizens based on various social, occupational, and geographic characteristics (Stern and Markel, 2009).

Hanfling and Hick (2009) have also written about how public education and risk communication messages are vital from the healthcare system's point of view as well. The 2009 H1N1 experience also reinforced the importance of effective public messaging and risk communication to lessen the possibility of overwhelming medical community resources, especially with large numbers of patients with signs and symptoms of the flu, but who did not absolutely have to be seen. This requires a cohesive communications strategy. Focusing on internal, hospital-based communications and working with the media and community partners on an external communications plan played a huge role in the initial response to the H1N1 outbreak. In 2009, coordinating access to identified hospital experts as part of a media relations plan was also important and often the only way to provide credible recommendations to the viewing and listening public regarding what to do, how to act, and when it is or is not appropriate to present for evaluation at hospital EDs.

Steel-Fisher and colleagues (2010) reported that surveys taken during the 2009 H1N1 pandemic suggest that, in the event of a future influenza pandemic, a substantial proportion of the public may not take a newly developed vaccine because they may believe the illness does not pose a serious health threat, because they (especially parents) may be concerned about the safety of the available vaccine, or both. And WHO influenza chief Keiji Fukuda noted that the Internet had a disruptive impact on the handling of the flu pandemic by fanning speculation and rumors in blogs, social networking and websites: "Anti-vaccine messaging was very active," he said, and "made it very difficult for public health services in many countries" (Agence France-Presse, 2010). Similarly, in the United States, local responses to H1N1 were dictated in part by what writer Marc Fisher called "the germ of fear"; a fearful public crammed hospital EDs and overloaded LHD phone lines (Fisher, 2009). Behavioral researchers attributed part of a general overreaction to the advent of social media, especially Twitter, which quickly magnify rumors. Public concerns complicated decisions about school closures and other control measures. Public reactions included some resistance to vaccination, especially among pregnant women. Indeed, the greatest challenge revealed by the media accounts involves public overreaction to events, unrealistic public expectations for testing and treatment, and spotty public adherence to public health recommendations. Clearly, LHDs must develop and implement effective communications strategies to meet H1N1 exigencies (National Association of County and City Health Officials, 2009).

According to *Time Magazine*'s one-year review (Walsh, 2010), it all boils down to communication and trust. The perception that officials overhyped and overreacted to the H1N1 pandemic may make the public less inclined to react appropriately the next time around. The only way to defuse public skepticism is for health officials to communicate better about what they know about an outbreak and—even more important—what they don't know about it. There wasn't enough explanation of what a "pandemic" really meant—that it referred only to the transmissibility of the new virus, not its virulence (Walsh, 2010).

Speaking at the 2010 Public Health Preparedness Summit, Steven Redd (2010), Director, CDC Influenza Coordination Unit, Incident Commander for H1N1, also stressed the need for maintaining the public's trust. Redd noted that, although the national response was based in science, many decisions had to be made without all the information one would like, which required an attitude of humility and being willing to monitor and change if necessary. He also stressed the importance of effective risk communication. Although there was a lot of uncertainty at the start of the pandemic about the epidemiology and who would be affected, maintaining the public's trust required openness. Specifically, it required telling people what was known and what was not, and what was being done to fill in the gaps. In this regard, Redd (2010) noted that what matters is what people hear, not what public health officials say.

Public health officials and professionals rely on the media to distribute, explain, and support public health messages. To journalists, a defining test of a policymaker's credibility is his or her openness, just as a test of the wisdom of a policy is its transparency. Consequently, LHDs should recognize the consequences of refusing to disclose information about the gender, age range, occupational category, or risk factors of confirmed cases and fatalities (National Association of County and City Health Officials, 2009).

More General Lessons about PHEP

The U.S. and Global Public Health System

Beyond the specific PHEP capabilities discussed earlier, the 2009 experience and the pandemic–flu response in general point to the many problems with the nation's patchwork of a public health system. There are more than 2,500 state and local health departments in the nation, and they are plagued by huge disparities in funding and competence (Milbank, 2009). Similarly, NACCHO (2010, p. 26) concluded, "The swine flu outbreak fell short of a full-blown international crisis, but revealed the precarious state of local U.S. health departments, the community bulwarks against disease and health emergencies in the United States." The implications of this diverse and fragmented system can be seen in all the capabilities discussed earlier. The Public Health Agency of Canada's (2010) review raised similar concerns in the context of collaboration between the federal government and the provinces and territories.

Stern and Markel (2009, p. 1222) wrote, "Perhaps the most immediately valuable lesson learned from spring 2009 is that Mexico's transparency and rapid response not only helped other countries react properly but also set a high bar for how the 21st-century global community must cooperate to share information about impending epidemics." Mexico's success in communicating with its public was discussed earlier. On the other hand, with a federal system such as the United States, epidemiologic surveillance and case reporting were inconsistent and incomplete across the country. Although some states have computerized systems that gather critical morbidity and mortality data on a standardized basis and transmit it to federal agencies, a few states still use pen and paper, and several did not generate any case data. These lacunae as well as other technological barriers led to an early gross overestimation of case fatality rates.

At the global level, Fineberg (2014) wrote that the WHO proved to be an indispensable global resource for leading and coordinating the response to a pandemic. The organization provided guidance to inform national influenza preparedness plans, which were in place in 74 countries at the time of the outbreak, and helped countries monitor their development of IHR core capacities. The WHO Global Influenza Surveillance Network detected, identified, and characterized the virus in a timely manner, and monitored the course of the pandemic. Within 48 hours after the activation of provisions in the 2005 IHRs, the WHO convened the first meeting of the emergency committee of experts who would advise the WHO on the status of the pandemic. Within 32 days after the WHO had declared a PHEIC, the first candidate vaccine viruses were developed, and vaccine seed strains and control reagents were made available within a few weeks. The strategic advisory group of experts on immunization at the WHO provided early recommendations on vaccine target groups and dose. The WHO provided prompt and valuable field assistance to affected countries, and efficiently distributed more than three million courses of antiviral drugs to 72 countries.

"Against this background of accomplishments," Fineberg (2014, p. 1339) wrote, "the WHO confronted systemic difficulties and made a number of missteps in the course of coping with the unfolding pandemic." These included being concomitantly the moral voice for health in the world and the servant of its member states, having a budget incommensurate with the scope of its responsibilities, and relying on a structure designed to respond to short-term emergencies rather than a sustained response. This last point is discussed in more detail later in "Emergency Operations."

Focusing on the 2005 IHRs, Wilson (2010) concluded that the IHRs provided a more robust framework for responding to PHEICs by requiring reporting of serious disease events, strengthening how countries and the WHO communicate concerning health threats, empowering the WHO director-general to declare the existence of PHEICs and to issue temporary recommendations for responding to them, and requiring countries not to implement measures that restrict trade and travel unnecessarily or that infringe on human rights. The 2009 H1N1 pandemic also revealed limitations to the effectiveness of the IHRs, including continuing inadequacies in surveillance and response capacities in some countries, violations of IHR rules, and a potentially narrowing scope of application to influenza like pandemic events only.

In his review, Gostin (2009) was less sanguine. Regarding monitoring and enforcement, for instance, he wrote that the new IHRs afford the WHO little authority to monitor and enforce rules. Although most countries reported pH1N1 cases conscientiously, the WHO has no authority to penalize countries that fail to notify. More important, the IHRs impose binding limits on travel and trade restrictions, but many countries flagrantly violated this norm with impunity. The WHO director-general has the power to make recommendations, but the IHRs state explicitly that those recommendations are nonbinding.

A more comprehensive review of the WHO's response to the pandemic also serves as the first analysis of how the IHRs have so far fulfilled their purpose to provide the world adequate health security with the least possible disruption to economies, specifically to travel, transport of goods, and human rights. The international review committee found that the IHRs did help make the world better prepared to cope with public health emergencies. The core national and local capacities called for in the IHRs, however, are neither fully operational nor on a path to timely implementation worldwide. And despite the positive features of the IHRs, many countries lack the core capacities to detect, assess, and report potential health threats. The most important structural shortcoming of the IHRs is the lack of enforceable sanctions (World Health Organization, 2011).

In particular, the international review committee identified a number of systemic difficulties that confronted the WHO in 2009, including the following two:

1. The absence of a consistent, measurable, and understandable depiction of the severity of the pandemic. What is needed is a proper assessment of severity at national and subnational levels.
2. Inadequately dispelling of confusion about the definition of a pandemic. "One online WHO document described pandemics as causing 'enormous numbers of deaths and illness,' whereas the official definition of a pandemic is based only on the degree of spread" (World Health Organization, 2011, p. 15).

To address these issues in the future, the committee recommended that the WHO develop and apply measures that can be used to assess the severity of every influenza epidemic, as discussed further in the following pages (World Health Organization, 2011).

Managing under Uncertainty

Chapters 2 and 3, by Stoto and Zhang, clearly illustrate the challenges of early detection and characterization in public health emergencies. As with most novel pathogens, the emergence of the pandemic H1N1 virus was characterized by uncertainty that took weeks to months to resolve. Many emergency preparedness professionals, however, still think in terms of single cases triggering a response in hours or at most days, and this thinking is reflected in such key public health preparedness documents. More broadly, this recognition means it is important to expect and plan for uncertainty in preparing for the emergence of a new pathogen. Because some future public health emergencies may be more like 2009 H1N1 than the acute events on which many planning assumptions are based, plans should be developed for situations that emerge over extended periods of time and are characterized by uncertainty. Rather than outbreak detection per se, the challenges are to determine whether the outbreak is a PHEIC and to determine its epidemiologic characteristics. In this context, the first evidence of an outbreak should trigger efforts to learn more, rather than disproportionate control measures based on worst-case scenarios (Fineberg and Wilson, 2009). The risk management approach in the WHO's new interim pandemic influenza guidance (World Health Organization, 2013) is one example.

In Chapter 8, Stoto and Higdon demonstrated the challenges of managing a public health crisis under uncertain conditions. For instance, Martha's Vineyard officials, as in many other state and local public health systems, had been preparing for years for mass dispensing of vaccine or other counter measures in public health emergencies. Consistent with such planning, and based on federal and state assurances in the summer and early fall that vaccine would be produced and delivered in large amounts starting in early October, the Massachusetts Department of Public Health (MDPH) adopted a mass dispensing approach to the 2009 H1N1 vaccination effort by increasing sharply the number of registered vaccination sites and trained vaccinators. Initially, the Vineyard planned to use one island wide mass dispensing site, as called for in public health emergency plans. The reality, of course, is that vaccine did not arrive nearly as quickly or in as large numbers as had been promised, and demand waned after the perception developed that the crisis has passed. By pooling vaccine among the six towns on the island, sharing resources such as vaccination teams that would go from one school to another in a region, and other means, the case study presented in Chapter 8 demonstrated the importance of strong communitywide partnerships to address public health problems. The case also demonstrated the need to balance precise policies with flexible implementation, the importance of local involvement in decision making, and the need to increase the transparency of communications.

In Chapter 9, Savoia and colleagues documented the challenge of managing a crisis under conditions of uncertainty in another setting. In Italy, the early estimates of the severity of the pandemic (as measured by the case fatality rate) ranged between the mildest possible pandemic envisaged in preparedness planning to a level of severity requiring highly stringent interventions. Another form of uncertainty was whether the severity, drug sensitivity, or other characteristics of the infection might change as the pandemic progressed across countries. With such uncertainty and the historical precedent of a mild infection turning virulent in a matter of months, public officials in both Italy and the United States ended up making an investment in vaccine procurement and other prevention activities regardless of the estimated severity of the disease.

Describing the severity of a pandemic was a major focus of the WHO review. Severity is especially difficult to estimate during the early phase of an outbreak, typically varies by place and over time, and has multiple dimensions (deaths, hospitalizations, and illness, with each varying by age and other attributes, such as preexisting health conditions and access to care; burden on a health system; and social and economic factors). Despite these challenges, the WHO review committee urged that descriptive terms used to characterize severity, such as mild, moderate, and severe, be defined quantitatively in future WHO guidelines so they may be used consistently by different observers and in different settings. The committee also urged that consideration be given to adaptive measures that would move as rapidly as possible from early counts of cases, hospitalizations, and deaths to population-based rates. Severity should be assessed as early as possible during a pandemic and should be reassessed as the pandemic evolves and new information becomes available. Severity might be assessed using a "basket of indicators" in a pre-agreed minimum data set such as hospitalization rates, mortality data, identification of vulnerable populations, and an assessment of the impact on health systems (World Health Organization, 2011).

To address these issues, Wenzel (2010) recommended that public health authorities become clearer about the lexicon of uncertainty—what they know and don't know about a pandemic. Authorities also need to be transparent about how they devise their recommendations, which often have to balance infection control and the daily activities of offices and schools. And, Wenzel added that we need to identify which social distancing techniques truly help control pandemics. For example, does the closing of schools and malls minimize the spread of viruses from infected children to adults?

Speakers at the 2010 Public Health Preparedness Summit agreed that the 2009 H1N1 pandemic also showed the need to plan with flexibility. Pandemic influenza plans had been developed with the expectation that a pandemic virus would emerge outside the United States and that its transmissibility and severity would be reasonably well characterized before it arrived in the United States. However, the pandemic essentially began at stage 4 of the federal plan, and officials did not realize how unclear the epidemiologic facts would be at the outset. Given these circumstances, agility and focus were important characteristics of the response that enabled a 180-degree change from a plan based on a 1918-like virus (which stressed closing the borders to keep it from entering the United States) to a response that focused on vaccinating the population. Bruce Dart, Director, Lincoln–Lancaster County Health Department in Nebraska, and President of NACCHO, stressed the need for flexibility at the local level to implement federal recommendations and for an appreciation that the CDC would change its recommendations if they didn't work at the local level. According to Carter Mecher, Director, Medical Preparedness Policy for the White House Homeland Security Council, the challenge was to determine what was really important. Similarly, Nicole Lurie, Assistant Secretary for Preparedness and Response, U.S. Department of Health and Human Services, stressed the importance of not only the federal pandemic plan, but also the capabilities behind it and the ability to mix and match them as needed while the pandemic unfolded.

Similar points were made in the U.K.'s influenza pandemic preparedness strategy report (U.K. Pandemic Influenza Preparedness Team, 2011), which identified the following three (among other) major challenges to be addressed when developing response plans to pandemic influenza: uncertainty about when an influenza pandemic could occur, unpredictability about how severe a future influenza pandemic could be, and the speed with which the pandemic can develop. The team also noted the problem of local hotspots—that is, that the demands of the pandemic are unlikely to be uniform, but different areas will be under pressure at different times (and some not at all), requiring flexibility of approach, and planning for easy access to antiviral medicines.

Authority Conflicts

In a complex, evolving response as was seen during the 2009 H1N1 pandemic, no single agency was equipped to do everything. No entity had the assets, the authority, or the information to craft and execute comprehensive actions. The best public health outcome would depend on collaborative and coordinated activity among multiple agencies at the federal, state, and local levels; on private and nonprofit organizations; and, not the least, the general public.

Significant conflict can arise over authority, priorities, the variety of potential risks, and the narrative to describe what is occurring. Information flow between organizational units can be difficult, particularly in times of stress. Hierarchies may be in competition and priorities in conflict. Conflict can arise as various authorities apply different criteria, priorities, and objectives in their decision making. Authority and accountability structures become more reciprocal and relational because many of these actors are not ordered within the same hierarchical structures or legal frameworks. In this context, creating unity of effort across this extended enterprise was perhaps the greatest leadership challenge. Amid the complex web of jurisdictions and authorities involved, influence was as important, and conceivably more so, than formal authority. This, in turn, required that vertical linkages—both up and down—be complemented by horizontal connections between organizations.

At the global level, the regional WHO offices are autonomous, with member states of the region responsible for their own budget and program. And although this system allows for regional variation to suit local conditions, it also limits the ability of the WHO to direct a globally coherent and coordinated response during a global health emergency (Fineberg, 2014).

In both Mexico and the United States, many schools were closed in an attempt to limit the spread of pH1N1 in the community. Klaiman and colleagues' analysis of U.S. school closings (Chapter 4) documented significant variation in the stated goal of closure decision, including limiting community spread of the virus, protecting particularly vulnerable students, and responding to staff shortages or student absenteeism. Because the goal of closure is relevant to its timing, nature, and duration, unclear rationales for closure can challenge its effectiveness. There was also significant variation in the decision-making authority to close schools in different jurisdictions, which, in some instances, was reflected in open disagreement between school and public health officials. Last, decision makers did not appear to expect the level of scientific uncertainty encountered early during the pandemic, and they often expressed significant frustration over changing CDC guidance. Klaiman and colleagues concluded that the use of school closure as a public health response to epidemic disease can be improved by ensuring that officials clarify the goals of closure and tailor closure decisions to those goals. In addition, authority to close schools should be clarified in advance, and decision makers should expect to encounter uncertainty as disease emergencies unfold and plan accordingly.

Emergency Operations

For many health departments in the United States, the 2009 H1N1 pandemic provided a major test of the incident command system (ICS), a standardized, on-scene, all-hazards incident management approach developed by the Federal Emergency Management Agency. According to NACCHO (2010), many agencies found that the use of ICS improved the flow of information, particularly when multiple agencies were involved. Communication along lines of authority proved to be critical in ascertaining situational awareness; confusion arose when the chain of command was broken. On the other hand, some jurisdictions experienced difficulties in adapting the ICS to their response operation. The feeling among these agencies is that the ICS should be modified to fit public health incidents. Many jurisdictions felt that the ICS worked for a short duration only and did not translate to the long-term response.

Speaking at an event organized by the National Health Policy Forum, Karen Remley, Health Commissioner, Commonwealth of Virginia, noted that the ICS was critical early on because it instilled a sense of urgency, but that Virginia went to a modified version after first few months of the response (Remley, 2011). Nicole Lurie, Assistant Secretary for Preparedness and Response, added that the ICS was needed and worked well for execution, but did not help to solve the difficult policy problems that came up every day, especially early during the outbreak. Solving these problems required getting the right people from a variety of agencies to work together, and the ICS structure did not facilitate this (Lurie, 2011).

Furthermore, according to NACCHO (2010), many public health agencies realized the importance of an emergency operations center (EOC) in the response effort. Even during a small incident, EOC activation was found to be paramount in organizing the response, streamlining efforts, and coordinating logistics. When agencies operated without a single point for information sharing and resource ordering, operations became more difficult and efforts were duplicated. Depending on the type of activation, health departments may have varying levels of EOC staffing, and it is important these levels—and roles and responsibilities, be determined well in advance of an actual activation.

The survey of immunization program directors conducted by Chamberlain and colleagues (Chapter 7) suggests that ICS and EOC structures, pandemic influenza plans, and collaborations with emergency preparedness partners during nonemergencies can enhance an immunization program's ability to manage a large-scale vaccination campaign successfully. The extent to which ICS/EOC structures were used for this vaccination campaign was substantial, given that these management structures were largely foreign to public health agencies before the 2003 adoption of the national incident management system, which uses the ICS for emergency response. Because the hierarchical nature of the ICS is not typically used to manage state and local health departments, implementation of the relatively unfamiliar ICS was met initially with some reticence by public health agencies. Results from the survey suggest that although some immunization program managers indicated resistance and frustration with the culture of the ICS, more felt that using the ICS helped them to work effectively and efficiently with collaborators, especially their emergency preparedness partners.

In Chapter 5, Lewis and colleagues showed how the 2009 H1N1 pandemic illustrates the challenges of mounting simultaneously a long-term, large-scale response while also maintaining most routine functions. The general challenges encountered related to division of labor, channels of input in decision making, workload, and the timeliness and execution of decisions. These challenges stem from the need to work concomitantly within two organizational structures—the "routine" structure used for daily department operations, and the "emergency" structure prescribed by the ICS used by all first responder organizations from fire to police and to (more recently) governmental public health agencies. Although focused on the Los Angeles County Department of Public Health's 2009 H1N1 response, these challenges likely apply to most LHDs, particularly those in large, complex metropolitan areas. Recommendations for addressing these challenges include the following:

- Identify escalating continuity of operation plans, with clear triggers for balancing emergency and routine operations.
- Provide coaching on the ICS and crisis decision making.
- Create a rapid process improvement cell.
- Create regular opportunities to practice crisis decision making.

Fineberg (2014) made a similar point about the WHO's emergency operations. He wrote that the WHO is better designed to respond to focal, short-term emergencies, such as investigating an outbreak of hemorrhagic fever or managing a multiyear, steady-state disease control program, than mounting and sustaining the kind of intensive, global response required to deal with a rapidly unfolding pandemic.

Social Capital for PHEP

The 2009 H1N1 pandemic reminds us of the challenges of getting the many components of complex PHEP systems to work together efficiently. The pandemic required the coordinated efforts of federal, state, regional, local, and tribal health departments. Private-sector hospitals, community health centers, individual healthcare providers, schools, and many other entities were also essential. The CDC public health preparedness capabilities (Centers for Disease Control and Prevention, 2011) get at this mostly through capabilities 3 (emergency operations coordination) and 6 (information sharing). Emergency operations coordination focuses on establishing a "standardized, scalable system of oversight, organization, and supervision consistent with jurisdictional standards and practices and with the National Incident Management System" (Centers for Disease Control and Prevention, 2011, p. 10). Information sharing addresses the ability of the entities in the PHEP system to exchange of health-related information and situational awareness data focusing on rules and data elements, and technology for information sharing. But, although these capabilities are clearly important, the 2009 H1N1 experience reminds us that preparedness also requires the creation and maintenance of social capital, "a collective dimension of society external to the individual . . . [that] consists of features of social organization—such as networks of interpersonal trust and norms of mutual aid and reciprocity—which act as resources for individuals and facilitate collective action" (Lochner et al., 1999, p. 260).

One aspect of social capital is the need for more community involvement in decision making and program management. This can be seen in the Massachusetts case study (Chapter 8). To maximize pH1N1 vaccine delivery capacity, the MDPH rapidly expanded the number of sites registered to receive vaccine in summer 2009. They achieved this by building on an existing system used to allocate state-purchased childhood vaccines under the federal Vaccines for Children program, which was used to distribute vaccine to more than 1,000 registered sites shortly after it arrived in the state. The downside of this approach, however, is that the registration system did not include complete information on the population served by each registered site, nor did it provide any information on the number and types of vaccine delivered to substate areas, such as the island of Martha's Vineyard. As a result, no one either at the MDPH or on the Vineyard had the information needed to coordinate local efforts to share vaccine or to ensure the available vaccine was going where it was most needed.

The 2009 H1N1 pandemic also demonstrates the need to balance clear and precise policies with flexible implementation, taking into account the local situation. The Massachusetts case study (Chapter 8) shows that when the H1N1 vaccine was in short supply, clear definitions of priority groups were essential to ensure the available supply went to those most in need. The case illustrates how Vineyard officials were grateful that the MDPH established tiers within the CDC's vaccine priority groups. On the other hand, lack of clarity about the definition of "healthcare worker" and the intended uses of vaccine allocated to hospitals caused problems. Should opened batches of vaccine left over at the end of a school clinic be used for the emergency medical services workers who helped with the clinic, even if they are not in the MDPH's first tier? The entire PHEP system—from the federal and state levels down to the local level—needs a shared understanding of the situation and situational awareness.

Savoia and colleagues made a similar case in Chapter 9, where they noted that Italy and the United States prioritized vaccinations in very different ways. Limited vaccine supplies created a tradeoff between vaccinating those at greatest risk (to provide direct protection) and those most likely to transmit the infection (herd immunity). U.S. guidance on priority groups was more flexible, and local agencies embraced the herd immunity strategy because it was more convenient logistically. Italian health officials, however, decided to embrace the direct protection strategy. They could do that thanks to the existence of a health information system and a network of primary care physicians that allowed them to have access to the exact number of individuals who were affected by chronic conditions served by each healthcare provider, and therefore who were at greater risk of severe complications or death if infected.

Maintaining social capital also requires efforts to increase both the transparency and clarity of communications. The Los Angeles case (Chapter 5) illustrates the challenges of addressing potentially valuable improvement suggestions that come from thought leaders who do not hold positions in the ICS chain of command. The Massachusetts case (Chapter 8) illustrates the importance of not assuming that informal communication channels are either accurate or complete. For instance, Martha's Vineyard hospital believed the town health departments were still planning a single island wide pH1N1 vaccine clinic even after the focus had switched to a school-based plan. In addition, parents were confused about whether their children should be immunized at school, at the hospital's preschool clinic, or by Vineyard Pediatrics, and whether it mattered which doctor's patient they were.

In Chapter 9, Savoia and colleagues showed how clear and consistent communication across agencies is important to sustain population trust in governmental institutions. The use of vaccine adjuvant in Italy (unlike the United States) was the source of the greatest concern in the population, reminding us that countries are not silos, and that differences in policies and communication messages are noticed by the public. Such differences, especially when highlighted by the media, can generate a safety or equity argument.

The Massachusetts case (Chapter 8) provides many examples of how trusting relationships can enhance—and their absence impede—an effective public health emergency response. Trusting relationships are also central to the effectiveness of regional activities, as described earlier in the discussion of local involvement in decision making and program management. For instance, the Martha's Vineyard experience illustrated the importance of encouraging and enhancing relationships among all the organizations connected with health, including school nurses, hospitals, and emergency medical services. The Vineyard's approach to pooling resources in the form of vaccine and creating "shooter" teams that moved from the small to the larger schools as vaccine came available would not have been possible without everyone involved trusting that this was the most appropriate way to ensure that the most populations were best protected.

Similarly, in Chapter 9 Savoia and colleagues demonstrated the importance of generating trusting relationships between individuals and public agencies. Trust contributes to transparency. The absence of preexisting relationships or a clear definition of roles and responsibilities may undermine the execution of simple public health policies. Community involvement is needed to build trust in decision making and program management so that when a crisis hits, such relationships generate a solid foundation for a more centralized response compared with daily routine activities. Especially in Italy, where regulations are strict and applied by decree, the preexistence of trusting relationships is extremely important to generate the possibility of the feedback necessary from local to regional and national levels to improve the response while the emergency is still evolving.

The importance of social capital, often expressed as "trusting relationships," emerged in a number of retrospective analyses. Speaking at the 2010 Public Health Preparedness Summit, Nicole Lurie, Assistant Secretary for Preparedness and Response, noted the "incredible collaboration" across the entire federal government during the 2009 H1N1 pandemic (Lurie, 2010). Steven Redd, U.S. Incident Commander, said that a team approach characterized the national response, and that this required respect and trust (Redd, 2010). Representing the White House Homeland Security Council, Carter Mecher added that the pandemic planning process had created networks of people who knew one another creating cohesion—or social capital—that led to a convergence of effort both vertically and horizontally within the federal government, and with state and local health departments (Mecher, 2010).

More specifically, Fineberg (2014) argued that the WHO's policy of keeping confidential the identities of the members of the emergency committee convened under the IHR, together with a lack of systematic and open procedures for disclosing, recognizing, and managing conflicts of interests, stoked suspicions about the potential links between individual members of the emergency committee and industry. Confidentiality practices designed to shield experts from commercial or political influences during a one-day emergency meeting were ill-suited to an advisory function that extended over a period of months.

The Institute of Medicine (2011) also noted that both existing and new partnerships played a crucial role in the vaccination campaigns. Important partners included healthcare providers, pharmacies and pharmacists, health plans, large companies with occupational health programs, community organizations, emergency medical services, school systems, colleges and universities, contract nurses, Medical Reserve Corps, and federal agencies and programs providing clinical services, including the Department of Defense, the Department of Veterans Affairs, and the Indian Health Service. Healthcare providers played an integral role in the distribution and administration plans of this emergency vaccination campaign. For instance, large, integrated healthcare systems may already have systems set up specifically for vaccinating their members. Health plans already have systems for communicating with healthcare providers, employers, and members, including call centers and targeted communications and reminders based on electronic records.

Some observers, however, noted that communication between public health and physicians was problematic. In many instances, physicians didn't receive faxed health alerts; in other instances, e-mail systems weren't in place to deliver them. Medical associations that had existing relationships with physician groups helped fill some of the void during the pandemic. Private practice providers and commercial vaccinators also faced significant challenges resulting from uncompensated costs associated with participation in the 2009 H1N1 vaccination campaign, such as the costs associated with the additional staff needed to handle the large volume of telephone calls and the logistical requirements of receiving and administering vaccine (Institute of Medicine, 2010).

Pharmacies and pharmacists were also integrated into the response much more deeply than ever before. Some observers noted, however, that some healthcare providers objected to pharmacies receiving vaccine when healthcare providers did not have adequate supplies (Institute of Medicine, 2010).

Similarly, in the higher education sector, the response to H1N1 required strong internal and external collaborations that were built well before the pandemic and were nurtured longterm. Prepandemic planning efforts were invaluable to establish relationships and determine roles and resources. Written plans, particularly specific response actions based on external triggers, often did not match this pandemic. The use of multidisciplinary response teams was reported as an overwhelming success (Center for Infectious Disease Research and Policy, 2010).

Implications for PHEP measurement

Implementing systematic quality improvement efforts to improve health security, as called for in the National Health Security Strategy, requires valid and reliable measures of PHEP system preparedness (Stoto et al., 2012). Indeed, during the last decade there has been much progress in this area. This includes the development of specific, validated measurement systems such as strategic national stockpile program technical assistance reports (Nelson et al., 2010), and valid and reliable methods for measuring performance during exercises (Savoia et al., 2009). In addition, the performance measures required by the CDC's PHEP cooperative agreements have evolved from inventories and capacity assessments to a capability-based framework (Centers for Disease Control and Prevention, 2011). Current measures of these capabilities, however, are largely capacity based or not yet developed, and only 2 of the 10 measures in the most recent report from the Trust for America's Health *Ready or Not?* report reflect capabilities: the whooping cough vaccination coverage rate for children and the state's ability to notify and assemble public health staff rapidly (Trust for America's Health, 2012).

One of the important implications of the analyses in this book is that capacity measures do not adequately represent how well a complex PHEP system will perform during an actual public health emergency. Current biosurveillance measures, for instance, focus on ensuring that state and local public health laboratories can respond rapidly, identify or rule out specific biological agents that the systems were designed to find, or have the workforce and surge capacity to process large numbers of samples during an emergency. These capacities do not reflect what was needed in 2009. Rather, as Zhang and Stoto show in Chapter 2, the surveillance system capabilities that were most essential were the availability of laboratory networks capable of identifying a novel pathogen, notification systems that made health officials aware of the epidemiologic facts emerging from numerous locations in at least two countries, and the intelligence necessary to "connect the dots" and understand their implications.

Similarly, Stoto (Chapter 3) demonstrated how public health surveillance data are potentially biased because they depend on a series of decisions made by patients, healthcare providers, and public health professionals about seeking and providing health care and about reporting cases or otherwise taking action that comes to the attention of health authorities. Outpatient, hospital-based, and ED surveillance systems, for instance, all rely on individuals deciding to present themselves to obtain health care, and these decisions are based in part on their interpretations of their symptoms. Similarly, virologic surveillance and systems based on laboratory confirmations depend on physicians deciding to send specimens for testing. Even the number of Google searches and self-reports of ILI in the Behavioral Risk Factor Surveillance System survey can be influenced by individuals' interpretation of the seriousness of their symptoms. Every element of this decision making is potentially influenced by what these people know and think, both of which change during the course of an outbreak. As a result, the ability of these systems to provide reliable information for situational awareness is compromised.

Similarly, at the global level, biosurveillance capabilities needed to detect and characterize emerging biological threats rapidly are a central part of the Global Health Security Agenda, announced in February 2014. The Agenda seeks to build capacity by developing and strengthening diagnostic and laboratory systems; developing, strengthening, and linking global networks for sharing biosurveillance information; and training and deploying a workforce to ensure the effective functioning of these systems (Department of Health and Human Services, 2014). However, the 2009 H1N1 experience reminds us that it is not just detection, but epidemiologic characterization, that is necessary. Similarly real-time biosurveillance systems are important, but as the 2009 H1N1 experience shows, they may contain inaccurate information about epidemiologic risks. Rather, it was the ability of scientists in Mexico, the United States, and other countries to make sense of the information emerging laboratory and epidemiologic information—an example of global social capital—that was critical for an effective global response. Thus, to ensure that it is meeting its goals, the Global Health Security Agenda must track not only capacities (laboratory, reporting networks), but also capabilities, such as the ability to consolidate and make sense of rapidly emerging information to characterize epidemiologic risks (Stoto, 2014).

The public health system's capabilities to develop and implement policies, especially population-based disease control measures, were also tested during the 2009 H1N1 pandemic. With regard to school closings, for instance, as Klaiman and colleagues documented in Chapter 4, significant variation existed in the stated goal of closure decisions, including limiting community spread of the virus, protecting particularly vulnerable students, and responding to staff shortages or student absenteeism. Because the goal of closure is relevant to its timing, nature, and duration, unclear rationales for closure can challenge its effectiveness. There was also significant variation in the decision-making authority to close schools in different jurisdictions, which in some instances was reflected in open disagreement between school and public health officials. Last, decision makers did not appear to expect the level of scientific uncertainty encountered early during the pandemic, and they often expressed significant frustration over changing CDC guidance. The challenge is not whether jurisdictions have emergency authorities, but rather whether a public health system, operating under uncertainty, can clarify the goals of school closure, tailor closure decisions to those goals, and implement these decisions seamlessly and effectively.

The primary public health assurance capability tested during the 2009 H1N1 pandemic was the national vaccination campaign and, as described previously, this was a success in many respects. However, the slow and unpredictable distribution of pandemic vaccine to LHDs created challenges. Stoto and Higdon's analysis of the Massachusetts public health response to 2009 H1N1 in Chapter 8 illustrated the challenges of managing the distribution of vaccine under these circumstances and identified a number of lessons about community resilience. The ad hoc approach health officials adopted—pooling vaccine among the six towns on Martha's Vineyard; sharing resources, such as vaccination teams that went from one school to another in a region—was easy to explain and well accepted by the public, and thus was an efficient, fair, and flexible response to uncertainty about when vaccine would arrive. The case also demonstrates the importance of strong communitywide partnerships to address public health problems and the need to balance precise policies with flexible implementation, and the importance of local involvement in decision making and increasing the transparency of communications. None of these capabilities, however, are well reflected by typical measures, such as whether health departments had a mass dispensing plan or had experience with the ICS.

The Massachusetts experience also demonstrates how the most effective way to implement a given capability—mass administration of a medical countermeasure, specifically the pH1N1 vaccine—depends on the local context. For instance, because children made up a large proportion of the target population, most communities found school-based clinics to be an effective way to administer the vaccine. Boston, on the other hand, found that its network of community health centers, with established trusting links to the populations they serve, worked well. And a large group practice used its existing EMR system effectively to call and set up appointments on any given weekend for patients for whom the available vaccine was appropriate. On Martha's Vineyard and in other rural settings, small LHDs found it useful to collaborate and pool resources to conduct regional clinics. Flexibility and adaptively were more important than LHDs having capacities that met a statewide or national standard for PODs.

What this means is that current capacity-based structured measurement approaches are not sufficient to predict how the PHEP system actually performs in an emergency. It is not whether we have laboratory capacity and surveillance systems, but how well they perform when called on to detect and characterize a new pathogen and to provide accurate situational awareness. It is not whether we have emergency authorities, but whether a public health system, operating under uncertainty, can use them effectively to clarify the goals of and implement school closures. And it is not whether health departments have a mass dispensing plan, but whether they can collaborate with all the public and private organizations in their community to dispense vaccine.

Thus, a new approach is needed that combines the structure of Homeland Security Exercise and Evaluation Program (HSEEP) formatting to ensure that critical capabilities are covered with a system for assessing PHEP system capabilities realistically in actual situations—and how that system is likely to perform in the future. This is not to say that capacities are not important; indeed, without them, the PHEP systems would not have the needed capabilities, so the new capability-based measures should supplement rather than replace current approaches to measuring a nation's PHEP.

One such approach would be a PHEP critical incident registry that fosters in-depth analyses of individual incidents and provides incentives to share results with others working in similar contexts and for cross-incident analysis. For comparative purposes, critical incident registry reports could address specific PHEP capabilities, and could be a platform for a structured set of performance measures. When the focus is on quality improvement and on complex PHEP systems, rather than their components or individuals, qualitative assessment of the system capabilities of PHEP systems can be more useful than quantitative metrics. Ensuring that such assessments are rigorous can be challenging, but a well-established body of social science methods provides a useful approach (Piltch-Loeb et al., 2014).

To enable organizational learning, the capabilities must be defined at a high enough level so that lessons learned in one example can be transferred to similar situations and in future emergencies. Defining capabilities in a more generic way can also make measures of these capabilities more comparable. The Massachusetts case study shows, for instance, that what matters is how well a PHEP system can administer a countermeasure to the target population, not whether LHDs meet national capacity standards for, say, PODs. The 2009 experience also shows that the local public health system in Massachusetts had this capability, including the flexibility to adapt to local context. Although future emergencies will likely require other countermeasures and will target different populations, the positive experience in 2009 is probably a better measure of the state's ability to respond effectively to future emergencies than capacity-based measures focusing on PODs standards and similar capacities.

Acknowledgments and Disclosures

This research was conducted with funding support awarded to the Harvard School of Public Health under cooperative agreements with the U.S. CDC (grant no. 5P01TP000307-01). The author is grateful for comments from John Brownstein, Melissa Higdon, Tamar Klaiman, John Kraemer, Larissa May, Christopher Nelson, Hilary Placzek, Ellen Whitney, Ying Zhang, the staff of the CDC Public Health Surveillance Program Office, and others who commented on presentations.

References

Agence France-Presse. (2010). Flu probe focuses on role of the media. Accessed April 14, 2010, at http://www.iol.co.za/scitech/technology/flu-probe-focuses-on-role-of-the-media-1.480501#.UyotpqidVZQ.

Butler, D. (2010). Portrait of a year-old pandemic. *Nature, 464*, 1112–1113.

Center for Infectious Disease Research and Policy. (2010). H1N1 and higher education: lessons learned. Accessed March 3, 2013, at http://www.cidrap.umn.edu/sites/default/files/public/downloads/big102webfinal_0.pdf.

Centers for Disease Control and Prevention (CDC). (2011). Public health preparedness capabilities: national standards for state and local planning. Accessed March 3, 2013, at http://www.cdc.gov/phpr/capabilities.

Department of Health and Human Services. (2009). National health security strategy. Accessed March 3, 2013, at http://www.phe.gov/Preparedness/planning/authority/nhss/Pages/default.aspx.

Department of Health and Human Services. (2014). Global health security agenda: toward a world safe and secure from infectious disease threats. Accessed March 3, 2013, at http://www.globalhealth.gov/global-health-topics/global-health-security/GHS%20Agenda.pdf.

Domínguez-Cherit, G., Lapinsky, S. E., Macias, A. E. (2009). Critically ill patients with 2009 influenza A (H1N1) in Mexico. *Journal of the American Medical Association, 302*, 1880–1887.
Fineberg, H. V. (2014). Pandemic preparedness and response: lessons from the H1N1 influenza of 2009. *The New England Journal of Medicine, 370*, 1335–1342.
Fineberg, H. V., Wilson, M. E. (2009). Epidemic science in real time. *Science, 324*, 987.
Fisher, M. (2009). Flu not as contagious as fear. *The Washington Post*. Accessed November 22, 2011, at http://www.washingtonpost.com/wp-dyn/content/article/2009/05/02/AR2009050202136.html.
Garske, T., Legrand, J., Donnelly, C. A. (2009). Assessing the severity of the novel influenza A/H1N1 pandemic. *British Medical Journal, 339*, b2840.
Gostin, L. O. (2009). Influenza A (H1N1) and pandemic preparedness under the rule of international law. *Journal of the American Medical Association, 301*, 2376–2378.
Hanfling, D., Hick, J. L. (2009). Hospitals and the novel H1N1 outbreak: the mouse that roared? *Disaster Medicine and Public Health Preparedness, 3*, S100–S106.
Hanquet, G., Van Damme, P., Brasseur, D. (2010). Lessons learnt from pandemic A(H1N1) 2009 influenza vaccination: highlights of a European workshop in Brussels. *Vaccine, 29*, 370–377.
Institute of Medicine. (2010). The 2009 H1N1 influenza vaccination campaign: summary of a workshop series. Accessed March 3, 2013, at http://iom.edu/Reports/2010/The-2009-H1N1-Influenza-Vaccination-Campaign.aspx.
Lipsitch, M., Riley, S., Cauchemez, S. (2009). Managing and reducing uncertainty in an emerging influenza pandemic. *The New England Journal of Medicine, 361*, 112–115.
Lochner, K., Kawachi, I., Kennedy, B. P. (1999). Social capital: a guide to its measurement. *Health and Place, 5*, 259–270.
Lurie, N. (2010). Remarks in panel discussion on "The crash of the pandemic wave: the public health response to the H1N1 influenza virus," Public Health Preparedness Summit, February 16, 2010, Atlanta, Georgia.
Lurie, N. (2011). Remarks in panel discussion on "Lessons learned from the 2009 H1N1 flu pandemic," the National Health Policy Forum, November 11, 2011, Washington, DC.
Mecher, C. (2010). Remarks in panel discussion on "The crash of the pandemic wave: the public health response to the H1N1 influenza virus," Public Health Preparedness Summit, February 16, 2010, Atlanta, Georgia.
Milbank, D. (2009). Pandemic tests a patchwork health system. *The Washington Post*, October 11. Accessed September 28, 2014, at http://www.washingtonpost.com/wp-dyn/content/article/2009/10/09/AR2009100903139.html
National Association of County and City Health Officials. (2009). Local decisions, local action: local health departments' H1N1 activities, as reported by news media, April–August 2009. Accessed March 3, 2013, at http://www.naccho.org/topics/H1N1/upload/NACCHO_LHD_ACTIVITIES_REPORTED-BY_MEDIA_H1N1report.pdf.
National Association of County and City Health Officials. (2010). NACCHO H1N1 policy workshop report. Accessed March 3, 2013, at http://www.naccho.org/topics/H1N1/upload/NACCHO-WORKSHOP-REPORT-IN-TEMPLATE-with-chart.pdf.

Nelson, C., Chan, E., Chandra, A. (2010). Developing national standards for public health emergency preparedness with a limited evidence base. *Disaster Medicine and Public Health Preparedness, 4*, 285–290.

Piltch-Loeb, R., Kraemer, J. D., Nelson, C. D., Stoto M. A. (2014). A public health emergency preparedness critical incident registry. *Biosecurity and Bioterrorism, 12*, 132–143.

Potter, M. A., Houck, O. C., Miner, K., Shoaf, K. (2013). Data for preparedness metrics: legal, economic, and operational. *Journal of Public Health Management and Practice, 19*, S22–S27.

Public Health Agency of Canada. (2010). Lessons learned review: public health agency of Canada and Health Canada response to the 2009 H1N1 pandemic. Accessed March 3, 2013, at http://www.phac-aspc.gc.ca/about_apropos/evaluation/reports-rapports/2010-2011/h1n1/index-eng.php.

Rambhia, K. J., Watson, M., Sell, T. K. (2010). Mass vaccination for the 2009 H1N1 pandemic: approaches, challenges, and recommendations. *Disaster Medicine and Public Health Preparedness, 8*, 321–330.

Redd, S. (2010). Remarks in panel discussion on "The crash of the pandemic wave: the public health response to the H1N1 influenza virus," Public Health Preparedness Summit, February 16, 2010, Atlanta, Georgia.

Remley, K. (2011). Remarks in panel discussion on "Lessons learned from the 2009 H1N1 flu pandemic," the National Health Policy Forum, November 11, 2011, Washington, DC.

Savoia, E., Testa, M., Biddinger, P., Cadigan, R., Koh, H., Campbell, P., Stoto, M. (2009). Assessing public health capabilities during emergency preparedness tabletop exercises: reliability and validity of a measurement tool. *Public Health Reports, 124*, 138–148.

Steel-Fisher, G. K., Blendon, R. J., Bekheit, M. M., Lubell, K. (2010). The public's response to the 2009 H1N1 influenza pandemic. *The New England Journal of Medicine, 362*, e65.

Stern, A. M., Markel, H. (2009). What Mexico taught the world about pandemic influenza preparedness and community mitigation strategies. *Journal of the American Medical Association, 302*, 1221–1222.

Stoto, M. A. (2007). Syndromic surveillance in public health practice. In: Institute of Medicine, editor. *Infectious disease surveillance and detection (workshop report)* (pp. 63–72). Washington: National Academy Press.

Stoto, M. A. (2014). Biosurveillance capability requirements for the global health security agenda: lessons from the 2009 H1N1 pandemic. *Biosecurity and Bioterrorism, 12*, 225–230.

Stoto, M., Nelson, C., LAMPS Investigators. (2012). Measuring and assessing public health emergency preparedness: a methodological primer. Accessed March 3, 2013, at http://lamps.sph.harvard.edu/images/stories/MeasurementWhitePaper.pdf.

Trust for America's Health. (2012). Ready or not? Protecting the public's health from diseases, disasters, and bioterrorism. Accessed March 3, 2013, at http://www.healthyamericans.org/assets/files/TFAH2012ReadyorNot08.pdf.

U.K. Department of Health Pandemic Influenza Preparedness Team. (2011). UK influenza pandemic preparedness strategy 2011. Accessed March 3, 2011, at https://www.gov.uk/government/uploads/system/uploads/attachment_data/file/213717/dh_131040.pdf.

Walsh, B. (2010). One year later: five lessons from the H1N1 pandemic. *Time Magazine*, April 27. Accessed September 28, 2014, at http://content.time.com/time/health/article/0,8599,1985009,00.html

Wenzel, R. P. (2010). What we learned from H1N1's first year. *New York Times*, April 13, p. A25. Accessed September 28, 2014, at http://www.nytimes.com/2010/04/13/opinion/13wenzel.html?emc=eta1

Wilson, K. (2010). Strengthening the international health regulations: lessons from the H1N1 pandemic. *Health Policy and Planning*, 25, 505–509.

Wong, J. Y., Kelly, H., Ip, D. K. (2013). Case fatality risk of influenza A (H1N1pdm09): a systematic review. *Epidemiology*, 24, 830.

World Health Organization. (2008). *International health regulations*, 2nd ed. Geneva: World Health Organization.

World Health Organization. (2011). Report of the review committee on the functioning of the international health regulations (2005) in relation to pandemic (H1N1) 2009. Accessed March 3, 2013, at http://apps.who.int/gb/ebwha/pdf_files/WHA64/A64_10-en.pdf.

World Health Organization. (2013). *Pandemic influenza risk management WHO interim guidance*. Geneva: World Health Organization.

INDEX

Page numbers for major discussions are in **boldface**. Boxes are indicated by b, figures by f, and tables by t following the page number.